# Asthma—
# An Emerging Epidemic

# Asthma—
# An Emerging Epidemic

## A Manual for

Patients with Asthma
Parents of Children with Asthma
Asthma Educators
Health-care Providers
School Nurses and Coaches

by
## Paul J. Hannaway, M.D.

Author of the American Medical Writers
Association Book Award Winner
*The Asthma Self-Help Book*

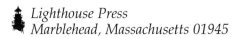 *Lighthouse Press*
*Marblehead, Massachusetts 01945*

Note to Readers:

The information in this book should not be substituted for, nor used to alter, medical therapy without your doctor's advice. For a specific health problem related to the contents of this book, consult your physician or health-care provider for guidance.

Illustrations by Bunny Hannaway
Book Design by Wilkscraft Printing, Inc., Beverly, Massachusetts
Editing and Production by Lighthouse Press

**Library of Congress Cataloging in Publication Data.**

ISBN 0-9621799-1-4

Address all inquiries to:
Lighthouse Press
P.O. Box 602
Marblehead, MA 01945
Tel: 1-800-225-9886 or 978-740-0648
Fax: 978-745-6208 or 781-631-2225
E-mail: Lhtpress@aol.com
Web sites: www.asthmaepidemic.com
www.lighthousepress.org

# Early Praise for
# Asthma—An Emerging Epidemic

"Doctor Hannaway has once again found a way to make asthma education not only informative but interesting and captivating as well. This book is comprehensive and up-to-date, and a great resource for anyone looking to better understand asthma and be better able to control it."

**Rachel Butler, Editor of *Asthma Magazine***

"If you have asthma, there are a million reasons why you need to read this book. So, take your inhaler and run to the bookstore to get your copy. Believe me, you'll breathe a sigh of relief knowing you've got this great information resource at your side."

**Dr. Bill Berger, President-Elect of the American College of Allergy, Asthma & Immunology, and author of *Allergies and Asthma for Dummies***

"Dr. Hannaway, widely recognized as a physician's physician and patient advocate, has provided another exceptional information source for those that live with asthma, their families, health-care providers, school and health educators. *Asthma—An Emerging Epidemic* provides a broad array of information, all pertinent to state-of-the-art asthma prevention and care. I will own this manual, my nursing staff will use it, and it will be recommended to all my patients living with asthma and to their families."

**Phillip E. Korenblat, M.D., Professor Clinical Medicine, Washington University School of Medicine, St. Louis, Missouri**

"Education of the laity as well as the medical profession is central to successful asthma therapy. *Asthma—An Emerging Epidemic* clearly facilitates communication of essential asthma-care information to the patient."

**Albert L. Sheffer, M.D., Clinical Professor of Medicine, Harvard Medical School**

"Once again, Doctor Hannaway has given readers an in-depth look at asthma. I found the book enlightening and enjoyed reading it."

**Nancy Sander, President AANMA— Allergy and Asthma Network Mothers of Asthmatics**

"The unique aspect of this text is its wonderful first four chapters. These chapters alone justify the price of the book. Anyone suffering from this disease or caring for a patient with asthma will be fascinated by the content of these chapters. The remainder of the text, written in clear, concise and communicative, excellent style, presents the broad array of management techniques used by physicians specializing in asthma care.

"Doctor Hannaway gives the reader a comprehensive source of resources and a wonderful exposition regarding asthma therapy guidelines. I would definitely suggest this text for all my patients and enthusiastically recommend it. This book is clearly written in keeping with the latest scientific knowledge, in a style that not only communicates, but also captivates. It is a must for the asthmatic."

**Phil Lieberman, M.D., Clinical Professor of Medicine and Pediatrics, University of Tennessee, Memphis, Past President of the American Academy of Allergy, Asthma & Immunology**

"Paul Hannaway's book is a 'must read' for everyone who wants to understand why asthma has grown into an epidemic—and where the hope lies for the future. Exploring all aspects from genes to indoor and outdoor air pollution to changes in our immune system and the role for medications, Hannaway is not afraid to state how his own views have changed. This book is rooted in science, but told in a bold and fast-paced style for everyone who wants to learn how to control asthma."

**Patricia G. Goldman, Executive Director, Asthma and Allergy Foundation—New England Chapter**

**Mary Worstell, National Executive Director Asthma and Allergy Foundation of America**

"The title page of *Asthma—An Emerging Epidemic* by Dr. Paul J. Hannaway states that this is a manual for patients with asthma, parents of asthmatic children, health-care providers, school nurses, teachers and coaches involved with asthma, and asthma educators. How can one book appeal to such a diverse audience? The answer is that anyone involved with asthma will be interested in the opinions and practice the philosophy of a master clinician like Dr. Hannaway. The book is written in a reader-friendly style that allows the author to address individual topics in a concise manner that defines the issues, lays out the supporting research background, gives Dr. Hannaway's assessment of the situation and leads to concrete, useful recommendations for asthma management.

"This single author textbook, a rarity these days, is remarkable in its breadth of topics, including virtually every area that I, as a practicing allergist, would consider important in clinical asthma management. Throughout the book, Dr. Hannaway pays deference to the history of asthma and, thereby, confers a perspective on the modern state of knowledge that is usually lacking in some of our current sources of information like the esoteric review article, 12-week clinical drug study or multiple author textbook. In addition, by referring to specific research, he reveals the studies and researchers he respects and the thought processes that have formulated his present management philosophy.

"Sections of this book that I found especially valuable include environmental control, medication choices, immunotherapy for asthma, controversial asthma treatments, fatal asthma, and consumer advice regarding publications, devices and support organizations. Besides new factual information, the language and concepts that Dr. Hannaway employs in patient education in these areas adds to the 'take home message.' A commitment to scientific proof for treatment recommendations is an underlying theme in this book. This is, however, coupled with an open-mindedness and desire to help asthma patients that is truly inspirational.

"This book often reads like a novel as Dr. Hannaway recounts his long experience in treating asthma. I, for one, am grateful that he found the immense time and energy it took to include us on this journey. If you are a person with asthma or care for or about a person with asthma, you need to read this book."

**Michael Mellon, M.D.**
**Associate Clinical Professor Pediatrics**
**UCSD School of Medicine, La Jolla, California**

**Chairman Pediatric Asthma Task Force**
**Kaiser Permanente, San Diego, California**

*"Asthma—An Emerging Epidemic* is a unique contribution to asthma awareness. Dr. Hannaway, in one book, summarizes his lifetime experience in caring for thousands of asthma patients as well as the rapid advances in scientific knowledge. His insight is thoughtful, timely and honest. All patients and parents of children with asthma should read this book. It will answer the many questions that cannot possibly be addressed in the current time allowed for an office visit. This book will serve as an excellent medium for continuing communication between patients and their physicians."

**Stanley J. Szefler, M.D.**
**National Jewish Medical and Research Center**

"Doctor Hannaway has provided a current, comprehensive well written treatise on asthma for patients and those who care for them. A worthy up-to-date successor to his award winning book *The Asthma Self-help Book."*

**Elliot F. Ellis, M.D., Past President**
**American Academy of Allergy, Asthma & Immunology**

"A much needed comprehensive update on the treatment of asthma, its causes and management written for patients and those who care for them—both physicians and asthma educators."

**Kathleen Conboy-Ellis, R.N., Ph.D., MHA, CPNP**
**Asthma Educator and Consultant, Past President**
**of the Association of Asthma Educators**

"Dr. Hannaway is well known for his creative energy and wonderful sense of humor. He has applied these talents to his new book. I found the book easy to read, very enjoyable with personal and historical references, and full of very practical information. His work has made information on this subject of asthma easily available to a broad range of individuals."

**Robert C. Strunk, M.D., Donald Strominger Professor of Pediatrics,**
**Washington University School of Medicine, Division of**
**Allergy and Pulmonary Medicine, St. Louis**
**Children's Hospital, St. Louis, Missouri**

To my patients and families afflicted with asthma.

# Acknowledgements

I would like to thank the following individuals for their contributions to this manuscript: Rachael Butler, Carlene Roundy and Marilyn Nagle (editing); Nancy Sarles (book promotion); Jean Conwell and Carol Sikora (office staff); Fred Wesemann and Anne Drueding (book design); Speros A. Zakas (proofreading); Camilla Ayers (indexing); Doctor Albert Sheffer (foreword) and my wife Bunny for her thoughtful input and wonderful illustrations.

"I have no magic cure to report; all I have in mind is a rational conduct of life."

—Moses Maimonides
*Treatise on Asthma*, A.D. 1190

# Table of Contents

## CHAPTER 9. **Food Allergy and Asthma**/131

## CHAPTER 10. **Infections and Asthma**/151

## CHAPTER 11. **Drug Therapy and Asthma**/159

## CHAPTER 12. **The Controlling Drugs**/173

## CHAPTER 13. **The Side Effects of the Cortisone Drugs**/185

# Foreword

Doctor Paul Hannaway has devoted his medical career to the care of allergic patients, particularly those suffering from asthma. His special interest has been the delivery of quality medical care to those afflicted with asthma. This has required educating patients, family members and health-care providers regarding the diagnosis and management of asthma. *Asthma—An Emerging Epidemic* is the successor to his two previous editions of *The Asthma Self-Help Book.* Education of the laity as well as the medical profession is central to successful asthma therapy. *Asthma—An Emerging Epidemic* clearly meets these requirements.

In spite of the advances in the appreciation of asthma causes and treatment, this disease remains a significant worldwide health problem. During the past decade, the prevalence of asthma in the United States has nearly tripled, while the annual fatality rate has remained unchanged at about 5000 deaths. Asthma continues to be under-diagnosed and under-treated in spite of national and global guidelines for the diagnosis and management of asthma. Publications such as this book clearly facilitate the appreciation of asthma and its successful treatment.

Nobody should die from asthma since present-day drug therapy should reverse life-threatening asthma exacerbations. The major impediment to successful asthma management is the lack of effective education of asthma sufferers, their families and particularly their health-care providers in the recognition of asthma severity and its appropriate treatment. Few other diseases as serious as asthma require such patient self-management. The increments in the prevalence and the persistence of asthma severity have occasioned innumerable publications germane to asthma. *Asthma— An Emerging Epidemic* and Dr. Hannaway's two previous books devoted to the appreciation and management of asthma have contributed considerably to patient education in this regard.

The National Heart, Lung, and Blood Institute (NHLBI) and the Global Initiative of Asthma (GINA) have developed the guidelines for the diagnosis and management of asthma. Such programs have enlightened physicians and the public regarding asthma. *Asthma—An*

*Emerging Epidemic* further translates scientific descriptions of asthma causes and management into simple, easily understood vernacular. For example, these new guidelines have clearly defined successful asthma therapy in four major categories: environmental control, objective measures of pulmonary function, pharmacotherapy of both maintenance and acute exacerbations of asthma, and patient education. This monograph clearly exemplifies this latter category as it interprets and applies information from the three former categories.

Successful asthma treatment requires health-care practitioners specifically trained in asthma care to continually educate asthma patients and their families. *Asthma—An Emerging Epidemic* facilitates the translation of the principles of asthma management from the professional to the patient. It is this partnership between the patient and the health-care provider that enhances asthma care. This monograph clearly enhances such communication of essential asthma-care information to the patient. In accomplishing this goal, the asthma patient becomes able to identify and control asthma symptoms early, thus preventing an attack. With this information, lung functions as well as symptoms, can be monitored closely until normal breathing capacity is restored. Such well-controlled asthma will permit patients to resume normal activity, including strenuous exercise. Hopefully, the inflammation, now recognized as being central to asthma, can now be treated. With newer controller anti-inflammatory medications, the progressive remodeling or scarring of the asthma airways can be prevented and irreversible airflow obstruction blunted and asthma fatalities reduced, if not, prevented. Thus, *Asthma—An Emerging Epidemic* provides insight and instruction to patients suffering from asthma to meet the defined goals of therapy. In properly managed cases asthma can be well controlled, patients can be free of asthma relapses and no one should succumb to asthma.

ALBERT L. SHEFFER, M.D.
CLINICAL PROFESSOR OF MEDICINE
HARVARD MEDICAL SCHOOL

# Introduction

## What's New Since '92?

**A**fter I wrote *The Asthma Self-Help Book* in 1989, rapid advances in asthma research and therapy made it necessary to revise this American Medical Writers Association Book Award Winner in 1992. I have now written an entirely new book on asthma, entitled *Asthma—An Emerging Epidemic.* You might ask: Why write another book on asthma? What's new since 1992? The answer is—plenty. Spectacular breakthroughs in the causes of asthma, new asthma drugs, questions, controversies, concepts, asthma treatment guidelines and futuristic therapy are just some of the new topics that I will cover in *Asthma—An Emerging Epidemic.*

Our understanding of the basic science and the clinical aspects of asthma has expanded enormously in the past decade. Several fascinating questions are now under investigation. Is asthma one disease with one cause, or is it like hypertension or high blood pressure—a syndrome with many different causes? Does inflammation in the nose and sinus cavities lead to lower airway inflammation and asthma, or is it all just part of one disease process? Does the lack of naturally acquired infections push our immune system in the direction of an allergic or asthmatic response?

Despite exciting progress in our understanding of asthma; the availability of safer, more potent and very effective asthma medications and implementation of innovative educational programs, the number of new cases of asthma has reached epidemic levels. This asthma epidemic is occurring at a time when most other chronic diseases of mankind are decreasing in frequency and severity, making it the world's biggest medical mystery.

This asthma epidemic is not confined to the United States. The asthma outbreak is worldwide. Epidemiologists or experts on health care statistics would label it a pandemic! The most striking increase in asthma has been reported in Australia, where approximately one in every four children has been diagnosed with asthma. In the United States the number of asthma cases has nearly tripled, from 6.7 million in 1980 to an estimated twenty-six million cases in the year 2000. Six million American children now have asthma. This rise in asthma cases has been observed in all levels of society, from affluent white suburbanites to inner-city black and Hispanic families.

The asthma epidemic has been much more devastating in poorer inner-city neighborhoods. Alarming increases in asthma hospitalizations and mortality in inner-city populations have prompted the United States government and the National Institutes of Health to appropriate millions of tax dollars to evaluate methods of improving asthma care for American inner-city children.

## New Asthma Theories

Perhaps the most exciting development in asthma research in the past decade has been the discovery that if your body (or your mother's body) receives the wrong signals or environmental exposures during infancy or pregnancy, your immune system may be programmed to follow an asthma-allergy pathway for several years or the rest of your life. Epidemiologic studies suggest that the ongoing asthma and allergy epidemic may be due to changes in modern 20th-century lifestyle, including exposure or non-exposure to viruses, bacteria, antibiotics, air pollutants and childhood vaccines.

We may be raising our infants and young children in too clean an environment. Why did the citizens of heavily polluted East Germany have far less asthma and allergic disorders than did Germans living in the cleaner and more hygienic West Germany? Such observations have resulted in an emerging and popular theory called the "hygiene hypothesis." Once you read about this hygiene hypothesis you may want your child to eat a little dirt or enroll in a virally infected day care center at an early age.

## New Asthma Therapy

Pharmaceutical companies have developed nearly a dozen new drugs for the treatment of asthma in the past decade. Such drugs range from knock-offs of old asthma drugs like nedocromil or Tilade, to an entirely new class of asthma drugs called leukotriene (pronounced lu-ko-try-een) modifiers. The leukotriene drugs (Zyflo, Accolate and Singulair) are designed to block asthma-inducing chemicals called leukotriene mediators. They are the first new class of asthma drugs to be developed in 25 years. Other new asthma drugs introduced in the past decade include long-acting bronchodilators, salmeterol (Serevent), formoterol (Foradil) and the potent inhaled-cortisone preparations fluticasone (Flovent) and budesonide (Pulmicort). These new inhaled cortisone drugs are available in various dosing strengths and delivery systems, including metered dose and dry-powder inhalers.

In September 2000, a solution form of inhaled budesonide (Pulmicort Respules) was approved by the FDA. This is the first inhaled cortisone drug that can be delivered via nebulizer to younger children who cannot use metered dose inhalers (MDIs) and spacing devices. In 2001, the FDA approved another unique asthma drug, Advair, which is a combination of the inhaled cortisone drug fluticasone (Flovent) and the long-acting beta-agonist salmeterol (Serevent). This new medication will replace the need to use two different inhalers in patients requiring both these asthma drugs. Other new drugs in the asthma pipeline include mometasone (Asmanex) and Symbicort, a combination of budesonide and formoterol, a short- and long-acting bronchodilator.

## New Asthma Controversies

Controversial issues which center on the potential side effects of inhaled cortisone drugs continue to be debated. The potential for cortisone drugs to cause growth retardation in children, and osteoporosis, glaucoma and cataracts in adults, will be addressed. The role of immunotherapy or allergy injections in asthma similarly

---

Throughout the book, drug names will usually be written as generic names followed by their brand names in parentheses: i.e., fluticasone (Flovent).—ED.

remains the subject of argument. The world-renowned asthma research center at Johns Hopkins University has published data suggesting that allergy injections are not effective in asthma, while scores of publications from other asthma centers throughout the world imply that when patients are carefully selected, immunotherapy may be very beneficial. New approaches in immunotherapy may be the ultimate road to the cure for allergic diseases and asthma. European allergy centers are now advocating the use of immunotherapy in very young children. Some European researchers believe starting allergy injections at an early age can prevent the development of future allergies and even asthma. If this concept proves to be correct, American allergy specialists will radically change their approach to immunotherapy.

Alternative therapy, including homeopathic and herbal medicines, has entered the asthma arena. The potential value of "non-traditional" therapy in asthma will be discussed. New concepts in environmental controls will be reviewed in detail, including the expanding risks of house dust mites, molds and animal allergens in asthma. I will review unique features of asthma, including new concepts in exercise-induced asthma, childhood asthma, asthma in women and during pregnancy and asthma in adulthood.

## New Asthma Guidelines

In 1992, the National Heart, Lung, and Blood Institute (NHLBI), a division of the National Institutes of Health, published the first set of national guidelines for the treatment of asthma. Medication protocols were based on a detailed classification of the severity of each particular asthma case. In 1997, these NHLBI guidelines were extensively rewritten and revised by a national task force of asthma experts. New parameters on asthma diagnosis and treatment based on these 1997 guidelines, as well as the new pediatric asthma guidelines published in the year 2000, will be reviewed.

## Futuristic Therapy

Right now the only sure way one could avoid getting asthma would be to pick the right parents or grandparents and be born into a pet-hating family in the Alps where there are no dust mites, animals or mold exposure. Contrast this "ideal" childhood environment to the child born in an inner city into a family with a history of asthma, and being raised in a home with high levels of exposure to dust mites, cockroaches, animal dander and a mother who smokes.

Today's asthma drugs act at the local tissue level. In other words, the horse is already out of the barn—present-day therapy is not designed to be curative. It only relieves or controls coughing and wheezing—the end result of the release of potent asthma-inducing chemicals into the lung. Bronchodilating drugs, like beta-agonists and theophylline, relieve the bronchospasm of the smooth muscle lining the respiratory tract. Inhaled or oral cortisone drugs reduce the inflammation in the asthmatic bronchial tubes. These old-fashioned treatment concepts are rapidly changing. Exciting clinical and laboratory discoveries have opened up new horizons in asthma and allergy treatment.

One research team at the National Institutes of Health, led by Doctors Henry Metzger and Jean-Pierre Kinet, has isolated gene receptors on the cell surfaces of the asthma mediators. Such a discovery, the result of years of painstaking research, may make it possible to block the asthma-allergy reaction right at the site of the receptor, and completely prevent the release of asthma-allergy inducing chemicals. In 2001, biotech researchers announced the isolation of an asthma gene. Applications of this discovery and other genetic research findings may not be far away. We now know that genetic traits determine how we respond to different drugs. Some patients either do not respond to an asthma drug, or they have serious reactions to certain drugs.

Genetic coding will allow doctors to pick out these patients and prescribe the right drug for the right patient. Getting a genetic profile will be as simple as a routine blood count. High-powered biotech-driven research may eventually lead to the ultimate cure and prevention of asthma and other allergic disorders. Doctor Frank Austen, a leading research scientist from Harvard University, feels we are on the threshold of exciting new treatments in the field of asthma and allergy. Rapid developments in the field of molecular biology now allow researchers to find answers to important questions in just a year or so, whereas older research tools required a decade or more to solve difficult problems. What is the present status of research efforts to find a cure for asthma? I used to think that while this concept was attractive, any potential cure for asthma was decades away. I now believe that genetic and biotechnical laboratory techniques will produce a magic asthma bullet (or bullets) much sooner than ever thought possible. Is there one magic bullet? I doubt it. There are so many steps in the asthma-allergy immune response that the final cure is more likely to come from a shotgun than a pistol.

Environmental controls may somehow fit into the final answer. Identification of the changes in our modern Western lifestyle that have led to this allergy-asthma epidemic may force alterations in maternal and infant dietary habits, including the way we administer childhood vaccines and antibiotics to infants and young children.

When I began practice nearly 30 years ago, the therapy of asthma was simple and primitive. It was essentially a no-brainer. The only effective asthma drugs were combinations of oral ephedrine, theophylline and isoproterenol, an inhaled bronchodilator. More difficult cases of asthma required oral cortisone drugs like prednisone, or the administration of intravenous cortisone and aminophylline in a hospital setting. All of these older asthma drugs had frequent and sometimes severe side effects. In those days we knew very little about the value of environmental controls. The extracts we used for allergy injections or immunotherapy were crude and poorly standardized. There were no asthma education programs in that era, as we had very little educational information to impart to our patients or families afflicted with asthma.

Asthma therapy has come a long way in the past 20 years. We now have more and better drugs, and more efficient environmental control methods. Allergy extracts are purified and highly standardized. As a result of these advances, asthma therapy, while more effective, is much more complicated. It is difficult for even asthma specialists to stay current. The patient or family of an asthmatic must learn to identify asthma triggers, anticipate asthma relapses and know when to increase or decrease asthma medications. Asthma self-help and education programs that have expanded dramatically at the local, regional and national level must establish partnerships between families, patients, asthma specialists and primary care providers.

## *Asthma in America*

Despite the incredible advances in asthma care, as well as the growth in asthma education programs and detailed asthma treatment guidelines, I believe many people with asthma are still receiving poor care. The American Asthma Survey proved this point. This survey, sponsored by GlaxoSmithKline, interviewed 2,509 asthma sufferers, 512 doctors, 101 nurses, 113 pharmacists and 1,000 members of the general public, and came to the conclusion that America is coming up short in asthma care.

Figure 1

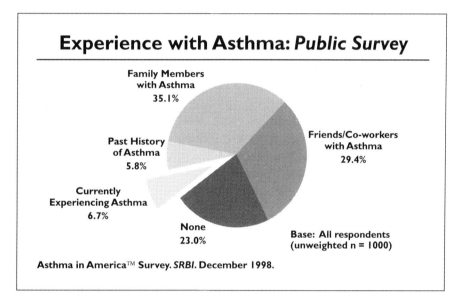

This survey found that 49 percent of children with asthma and 25 percent of adults with asthma missed school or work because of their asthma in the past year. Almost one in three asthma patients were awakened at least once a week with asthma symptoms. Thirty-two percent of children with asthma went to the emergency room, and 41 percent of all people sought urgent care for asthma in the past year. Nearly 50 percent were limited in their sports or recreational activity. Amazingly, only one in every three asthmatics had a lung function test in the past year, and only 28 percent were using peak flow meters. Nearly half of the American public had experienced asthma in their own home or in their immediate family (Figure 1). Three out of ten knew friends or co-workers with asthma. Thus, 80 percent of surveyed Americans were directly or indirectly affected by asthma. Nine out of every 10 doctors agreed that anti-inflammatory drugs were essential in the long-term management of persistent asthma, yet only 18 percent of asthma patients had used an anti-inflammatory drug in the past week. There was widespread misunderstanding of their underlying condition and confusion about asthma treatment. Half of the asthma patients thought that it was only possible to treat asthma symptoms, and not the underlying cause of asthma. Only nine percent knew that chronic inflammation was the cause of their asthma. In an incredible understatement, three-quarters of the responders believed that there was a definite need for more patient education.

A recent survey of 5,181 adult asthma patients reported that 30 percent were dissatisfied with their asthma treatment. Dissatisfaction was related to poor patient-provider communication, poor asthma control and a lack of belief in asthma medications. Another survey of 438 asthmatic children found that 40 percent had frequent nocturnal awakenings from asthma. The frequency of their nighttime wheezing was directly related to missed school days, parent's work attendance and poor performance in school.

This book, by no means a quick fix, is my personal effort to further advance asthma education and improve asthma care. My target audience is not merely people with asthma and their families. Health-care providers and caregivers such as nurse practitioners, physician assistants, school nurses, coaches, teachers, babysitters and grandparents need to learn more about asthma if they are to assume responsibility for treating, supervising and caring for children and adults with persistent asthma. I have tried to provide the thoughtful reader with an in-depth look at asthma and allergy from all angles. I firmly believe that those who read this book will come away more informed about this complex, yet very treatable, disease.

PAUL J. HANNAWAY, M.D.
ASSOCIATE CLINICAL PROFESSOR
TUFTS UNIVERSITY SCHOOL OF MEDICINE

# The
# Emerging
# **Epidemic**

## 1

## *United States Experience*

**M**ost, if not all, of the developed countries in the world have experienced a dramatic increase in the incidence of asthma. My own experience with asthma supports the idea that the industrialized world is in the midst of an emerging asthma epidemic. As a child and young adult, I was the only kid on the block who suffered from asthma. I don't recall any other friend, schoolmate or teammate in grade school, high school or even college who was rushed to the local emergency room or the school health center for acute asthma treatment or needed to puff on an asthma inhaler before or after athletic activities.

This picture has changed dramatically over the past 20 years. Two of my five children and scores of their friends have asthma. If you attend any type of athletic or youth sporting event you will observe that an incredible number of participants running on a soccer field or skating in a hockey rink are puffing on some sort of asthma inhaler. While the true incidence of asthma in the United States during the 1950s and early 1960s is not well documented, trends indicate that the number of asthma suffers has probably increased tenfold since the 1950s. I cannot think of any other chronic disease with such alarming numbers.

Most epidemiologists agree that the number of asthma cases in the United States has tripled in the past 20 years (Figure 1.1). In 1980, it was estimated that 6.8 million Americans had asthma. According to the National Center for Health Statistics, the number of asthmatics increased to nearly 18 million cases in the United States between 1980 and 1996. The number of asthma deaths has also increased

**Figure**
**1.1**

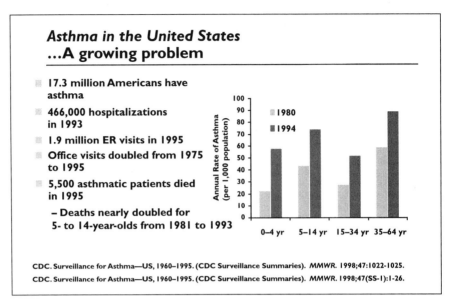

Asthma in the United States
...A growing problem

- 17.3 million Americans have asthma
- 466,000 hospitalizations in 1993
- 1.9 million ER visits in 1995
- Office visits doubled from 1975 to 1995
- 5,500 asthmatic patients died in 1995
  - Deaths nearly doubled for 5- to 14-year-olds from 1981 to 1993

CDC. Surveillance for Asthma—US, 1960–1995. (CDC Surveillance Summaries). MMWR. 1998;47:1022-1025.
CDC. Surveillance for Asthma—US, 1960–1995. (CDC Surveillance Summaries). MMWR. 1998;47(SS-1):1-26.

threefold, from 1,674 deaths in 1977 to 5,500 fatalities in 1995. An alarming study by the Johns Hopkins School of Public Health estimates that the number of people afflicted with asthma and the number of asthma deaths will double in the next decade. If these Johns Hopkins figures are correct, 29 million Americans will have asthma, and 10,000 will die from their disease in the year 2010. The increase in asthma is most dramatic in children under age five, where the number of cases has tripled since 1980.

The rate of asthma in children has increased five percent each year. This means there are a half-million new cases of childhood asthma in the United States every year. Six million youngsters under the age of 18 now have asthma. California, New York and Texas, the most populated states, have the most cases of asthma. Deaths from asthma in the five- to fourteen-year-old age group have doubled in the past 15 years.

This increase in asthma coincides with an across-the-board rise in all types of allergic diseases, including allergic rhinitis or hay fever, atopic dermatitis or eczema and food allergies. A survey from the American College of Allergy, Asthma & Immunology (ACAAI), a national organization of asthma and allergy specialists, found that allergies were twice as prevalent as previously believed. According to this ACAAI study, 38 percent of all Americans now suffer from some sort of allergic condition. Fifty-six percent of all homes surveyed reported that at least one member in each household had an allergic condition.

## *The Inner-city Epidemic*

The asthma epidemic has hit American inner cities the hardest. Inner-city dwellers, especially minority children and young adults, have experienced an explosive, unprecedented and unexplained increase in asthma cases. There is twice as much asthma in the heavily industrialized Northeast than the less densely populated rural West. In 1988, there were 9,275 hospital admissions for childhood asthma in New York City, compared to 15,000 admissions 10 years later. The poorer sections of New York City have been hit the hardest. The rate of hospitalization for asthma in the Bronx and Harlem is 20 times higher than asthma admissions in the more affluent neighborhoods of New York City.

Inner-city blacks and Hispanics have a disproportionally high rate of asthma-related emergency room visits and hospitalizations. These unfortunate minorities are four times more likely to die from asthma. Potential reasons for this tragic inner-city epidemic may include ethnic patterns, combined with high exposure to outdoor air pollutants, indoor allergens (dust mites, cockroaches) and animal allergens, especially cats and rodents.

Poverty, dire psychosocial problems and poor medical care undoubtedly play a major role in the frequency and severity of asthma, and are important predictors for an asthma death. Some asthma experts believe inner-city children spend too much time indoors. An Inner-City Asthma Study funded by the National Institutes of Health found that only 40 percent of inner-city children played outside after school hours, because of the potential threat of neighborhood violence.

The asthma epidemic is not localized to inner cities. A substantial, although less dramatic, increase in asthma cases has been observed in suburban populations. The important question in this whole picture is why are we experiencing an asthma epidemic and an increase in the rate of asthma hospitalizations and asthma deaths, when we have many more effective drugs to treat asthma than we did 20 years ago?

## *Impact of the Asthma Epidemic*

This emerging asthma epidemic has had a tremendous impact on health-care costs and the quality of life for asthma sufferers. Asthma is the leading chronic disease among children. Childhood asthma accounts for ten-million lost school days, and is the third leading cause of hospitalization for children under age 15. Next to upper respiratory infections, asthma is the leading cause of school absenteeism. The number of office visits for asthma has gone from 4.6 million per year in 1980 to over 10 million per year in the late 1990s.

Work by Doctor Kevin Weiss of Rush Medical College in Chicago estimated the economic burden of asthma in the United States at $6 billion in 1990. In the year 2000, the price of asthma has nearly tripled. When you add the cost of office visits, emergency room care and hospitalizations to the increasing prices of asthma drugs, the economic burden of asthma care in the United States approaches $20 billion per year. Asthma-care costs now exceed the combined total costs of AIDS and tuberculosis.

Twenty percent of all asthmatics, undoubtedly the sickest, account for nearly 80 percent of all money spent on asthma care. There are nearly 600,000 emergency room visits per year for childhood asthma. Hospitalizations account for more than half of all expenses. In children under age four, hospitalizations eat up more than three-fourths of all childhood asthma costs. Thus, considerable savings would occur if hospitalizations were reduced, especially in patients with more severe asthma.

What about the effect of asthma on one's quality of life? A Philadelphia survey found 27 percent of asthmatics were awakened with asthma at least once a week. One in every three asthmatics missed school or work, and nearly half agreed that asthma interfered with exercise or daily activities. One in every three asthma sufferers made an unscheduled visit to their doctor or clinic in the past year because of their asthma. Forty-two percent required a hospitalization or an emergency room visit in the past year. Parents and caregivers lose time from work and day-to-day activities. Disturbed sleep from nocturnal asthma leads to decreased productivity from the working parent(s) and poor academic performance by the student with asthma. How many of these patients were seeing an asthma specialist on a regular basis? The survey found that only 50 percent of patients with mild asthma had ever seen an asthma specialist, and one-third of patients with severe asthma had never seen a specialist. The final conclusions of this Philadelphia study were that most asthmatics had an impaired quality of life and were not receiving proper asthma care.

## The Worldwide Epidemic

The increase in the frequency and severity of asthma is not confined to the United States. Ireland, England, Scotland, New Zealand and Australia have all reported an increase in the frequency and severity of asthma. The World Health Organization estimates that there are 150 million asthmatics in the world, and 180,000 will die each year from this disease. This represents a 50-percent increase in asthma deaths in the past decade. In South and Central American countries like Brazil and Costa Rica, the prevalence of asthma is between 20 and 30 percent of the general population. The incidence of asthma in the Western Pacific Region varies from 50 percent in the Caroline Islands to virtually zero asthma cases in New Guinea.

A survey of 3,400 school children in Scotland found that Scottish school children were becoming more allergic. The incidence of asthma in Scottish children rose from 4.1 percent in 1964 to 10.2 percent in 1998. Likewise, allergic rhinitis or hay fever increased from 3.2 percent to 12 percent. Atopic dermatitis or eczema more than doubled, from 5.2 to 12 percent. Thus, children and adults throughout the world, especially in developed countries, are developing more asthma and allergic diseases. Contrast this with less developed, rural countries such as Indonesia, Albania, rural Africa, New Guinea and rural China, where the incidence of asthma is less than two percent of the total population. Statistical trends clearly show that the emerging asthma-allergy epidemic is taking place in the more developed countries influenced most by Western civilization.

In the next chapter, I will address ongoing studies of the cultures and lifestyles of those areas of the world that have not experienced the asthma and allergy epidemic. Such research may help solve this baffling asthma mystery and determine why asthma is one of the few chronic diseases of modern times that is headed in the wrong direction. The final answer undoubtedly lies within the interaction of our genetic background, our immune system and our environment. Before we discuss how these factors may predispose infants and young children to years or a lifetime of asthma and other allergic diseases, the basic features and functions of the normal and the asthmatic lung and our immune system should be reviewed.

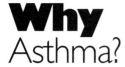

# Why
## Asthma?

## 2

## The Normal Lung

The main function of our lungs is to inhale oxygen-rich air and to remove or exhale the body's waste gas—carbon dioxide. This all-important exchange of oxygen and carbon dioxide takes place deep in our lungs, in tiny air sacs called alveoli (Figure 2.1). Before air reaches these air sacs, it must pass through the trachea, or windpipe, that divides into the right and left bronchial tubes that in turn connect to the right and left lung. These main bronchial tubes then further subdivide into smaller tubes called bronchioles on the way to the air sacs.

Your lungs can be pictured as two big pouches of air containing millions of smaller sacs connected to tubes. Another way to look at the lung is to picture it as an upside-down tree, in which the tree trunk is the trachea or windpipe, the largest branches are the main bronchial tubes, the smaller branches are the bronchioles and the leaves are the air sacs or alveoli. Once air enters the alveoli, inhaled oxygen crosses the walls of the alveoli into the blood stream. It is then transported to the heart, which pumps blood rich in life-sustaining oxygen to all parts of the body. A separate network of blood vessels brings the body's waste gas, carbon dioxide, back to the alveoli. The carbon dioxide is removed from the body when you exhale or breathe out.

## The Lung in Asthma

What goes wrong in the asthmatic lung? First, let us look at the walls of the bronchial tube. These walls are made up of various cells, muscle

15

tissue and mucus-secreting glands. In the normal lung, air moves in and out of the alveoli and bronchial tubes, and your lungs maintain a perfect balance of oxygen and carbon dioxide throughout your entire body. In asthma, the bronchial tubes are abnormal (Figure 2.1). They are constantly inflamed or swollen, and air movement is blocked. The bronchial tubes are lined by tens of thousands of cells, including white blood cells and specialized cells called mast cells, which are loaded with toxic chemicals called mediators. When these mast cells release their chemicals, the walls of the bronchial tubes swell up, go into spasm and become inflamed. The end result of a swollen and obstructed bronchial tube that blocks the passage of air is shortness of breath, coughing and wheezing—the cardinal symptoms of asthma.

A good analogy is to think of your bronchial tubes as a garden hose. When the hose is open, water flow is unimpeded, but if you pinch or bend the hose, the flow of water is obstructed, and the obstructed hose produces a hissing or wheezing sound. In asthma, this bronchial obstruction can often be reversed, and the bronchial

Figure 2.1

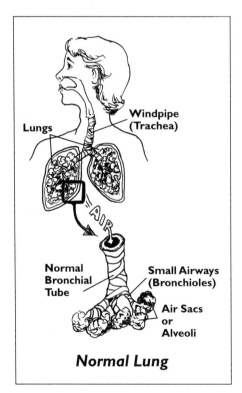

**Normal Lung**

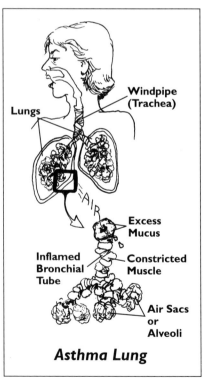

**Asthma Lung**

tubes can return to a normal state. Thus, the best medical definition of asthma is "reversible obstructive airways disease," often abbreviated as ROAD. Two other more catchy names for asthma are "twitchy lung syndrome" and "wheezy bronchitis." It is now recognized that tissue inflammation in the bronchial tubes is the major cause of chronic asthma.

## The Inflammation Theory

In the 1980s the rediscovery of an old concept led to an important breakthrough that dramatically altered the way asthma specialists treat asthma. In 1873, Sir Charles Blackley demonstrated that hay fever and asthma sufferers challenged with an allergen did not begin to sneeze or wheeze until several hours after inhaling the allergen, and sometimes their sneezing and wheezing lasted several days after the allergen was removed. In 1952, Karl Herxheimer expanded these observations when he reported that there were two very distinct components to the response to an inhaled allergen. He called these components the early phase or immediate asthma response and the late phase asthma response. Additional studies have shown that asthmatics react in two ways to inhalation challenges, both in real life and in the laboratory (Figure 2.2).

■

Figure
2.2

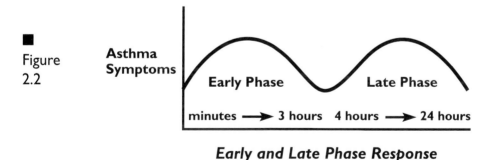

**Early and Late Phase Response**

The coughing and wheezing that develops within minutes, peaks in 30 minutes and resolves in one to three hours is called the early phase asthma response. The wheezing that starts three to four hours after an inhalation challenge, peaks in four to eight hours and lasts 24 to 72 hours is called the late phase asthma response. Most asthma authorities now believe that this late phase response that leads to chronic inflammation of the bronchial tubes is the single most important feature of chronic asthma. This important finding has produced dramatic changes in asthma therapy, as it has been shown that asthma drugs have different actions in the early and late asthma responses.

The asthma relieving or bronchodilating drugs like the beta agonist drugs, theophylline and the anticholinergic drugs open up or dilate the bronchial tubes. For this reason, they are called *relievers* or bronchodilators. These drugs prevent or relieve the symptoms of the early response, but have little or no effect on the late phase inflammatory response. On the other hand, anti-inflammatory medications such as the cromolyn-like drugs, the cortisone drugs and the new leukotriene modifiers will not relieve asthma symptoms once they occur, but they prevent or control the late phase or inflammatory response. Such drugs are called *controllers* or anti-inflammatory drugs. How should these findings be applied to the real world of asthma therapy? The clinical implication is obvious. As we shall see, all patients with persistent asthma will require both a relieving and a controlling asthma drug.

## What Causes Inflammation?

There is no simple answer to this question. No one group of cells or chemical mediators fully explains asthma. It is best to think of asthma as a symphonic orchestra where the end point of inflammation is the result of many sections of instruments—the cells and chemical mediators. Once this immune orchestra starts playing, the bronchial tube becomes swollen and inflamed. In the next chapter, I will detail how the body's immune system handles invading allergens or an asthma trigger.

In *The Asthma Self-Help Book* I wrote that asthma was a reversible obstructive airways disease, or ROAD. This older asthma definition meant that lung functions could be reversed or improved with treatment. This was wrong. Lung function may never return to the normal range in some patients with severe asthma, even with ideal treatment. The newer definition of asthma depicts it as a chronic disorder of the airways in which many inflammatory cells play a role. In susceptible individuals this inflammation causes recurrent wheezing, chest tightness and coughing, especially at night or in the early morning. Symptoms are usually associated with an airflow limitation that usually reverses with treatment. The inflammation also causes an increase in airway response to a variety of stimuli that asthma researchers call bronchial hyperreactivity.

## Remodeling—A New Concept

Studies have shown that many nonsmoking asthmatics have low lung function levels seen in patients with chronic lung disease, such as bronchitis or emphysema. In some cases, this loss of lung function is permanent. This discovery has led to a new asthma term called "remodeling." What do asthma researchers mean when they talk about airway remodeling? Remodeling is the buzzword used to describe permanent structural damage to the airway in asthma. I like to think of airway remodeling as a scarring reaction to chronic inflammation and the loss of the ability to repair or reverse lung inflammation. When the bronchial tubes remain chronically inflamed, they overreact or become hyperreactive to all types of irritants or inhaled particles and aeroallergens. When airway inflammation persists, the lungs may become permanently scarred. Fortunately remodeling or scarring is not a common occurrence, but it does explain why many asthmatics that have never smoked have poor lung functions.

Asthma specialists know the greatest loss in lung function in asthma occurs within three years after the onset of asthma symptoms. This loss in lung function may occur as early as six or seven years of age in asthmatic children. The concept of airway remodeling has promoted several important questions. Would early and aggressive use of the inhaled cortisone drugs, especially in young children, prevent remodeling? Preliminary studies have found that young children with persistent asthma who were treated with inhaled cortisone drugs for three years had better lung function than those children treated with only bronchodilating drugs. Children who delayed starting inhaled cortisone for two to three years after the onset of their asthma had poorer lung functions than children started on inhaled cortisone right after their asthma was first diagnosed.

The concept of preventing remodeling is especially important in young children, many of whom are not diagnosed as having asthma until several years after the onset of coughing and wheezing. In my experience health-care providers for young children, especially pediatricians, continue to be hesitant to make the diagnosis of asthma, preferring to use terms like bronchitis, bronchiolitis or reactive air-ways syndrome. This is an unfortunate scenario for those persistent wheezers who go on to develop full-blown asthma. In my opinion early and aggressive anti-inflammatory therapy in this age group may prevent chronic asthma in adulthood, whereas a delay in diagnosis and lack of proper therapy may lead to lung remodeling and severe debilitating asthma later on in life.

Now that we have reviewed what goes wrong in the asthmatic lung, the diligent reader should now ask: why asthma? While there is no correct answer to this compelling question, the bottom line is that you can place some of the blame on your parents or grandparents. Your ancestors are guilty of passing on an asthma gene or genes, and your parents may have kept too clean a home or not allowed you to you play in the dirt during infancy or early childhood. As we shall discuss in detail, asthma is a result of a complex interaction between your genetic background, your immune system and environmental exposures.

## The Elusive Asthma Genes

What are genes? Every living organism, including all plants and animal life, contains a substance called deoxyribonucleic acid, more commonly known as DNA. Human DNA is composed of nearly 40,000 genes that act like computer chips that program your body to develop individual characteristics such as baldness, brown hair or blue eyes. DNA that is passed down from one generation to another determines what diseases you may or may not develop during your lifetime. Asthma is labeled as a complex genetic disease. That means that there are several genes that predispose one to develop asthma, and they interact in a complex manner. In genetic language this means that asthma is due to several family traits or genes which, when combined with the right (or wrong) environmental exposures, lead to clinical disease. The inheritable component of asthma and other allergic diseases has long been recognized, due to clusters of asthma and allergic diseases in families and identical twins.

In 1916, Cooke and Vanderveer studied the family histories of 504 asthmatics and concluded that inheritance was a definite factor in asthma and allergy. Not all individuals who inherit an asthma or allergy gene will develop asthma or an allergic disease. This is called non-penetrance. Penetrance refers to those individuals with a certain gene who do develop the disease state. In a complex genetic disease, like asthma, penetrance is never complete. This explains why asthma may skip generations. No one single asthma gene has been isolated. Undoubtedly several genes are involved. Other diseases that have a similar genetic makeup include diabetes, cancer and heart disease. This contrasts to cystic fibrosis, a disease that is transmitted by a single dominant gene. Either you have cystic fibrosis or you don't, and environmental exposures play no role.

The results of the United States Human Genome Project, started in 1990, are now unfolding. This project will identify the 40,000 to 50,000 human genes and determine the three billion DNA building blocks that underlie all human biology. The full sequencing of human DNA will result in the identification of the two to three hundred thousand proteins that are used to make up a human being. This new era in genetic research will lead to new ways to diagnose and treat allergies and asthma, and have a profound impact on all complex diseases. Geneticists at the University of Washington who have studied the DNA of asthmatics and compared it to non-asthmatics have discovered a mutated gene that controls the inflammation that leads to asthma. Persons with this mutated gene are 10 times more likely to have asthma or allergic diseases.

Additional research has found an abnormal gene in patients experiencing near-fatal or fatal asthma attacks. Genes not only determine if and when you get asthma; they also program the severity level of your asthma. Once a specific asthma gene (or genes) is found, the proteins produced by the gene can be identified. Some of these gene proteins are "good proteins" that prevent one from developing asthma. Other proteins are "bad proteins" that trigger a genetic disease like asthma. Genetic researchers will someday develop chemicals to block the bad proteins and prevent the development of the inherited disease.

## The Immune System

In the early part of the twentieth century, asthma was thought to be a purely psychosomatic disorder. One famous victim of this erroneous concept was President Theodore Roosevelt. Leading psychiatrists of Roosevelt's day theorized that his childhood asthma was the result of an unstable home and a domineering father. Such speculations were proven wrong after young Roosevelt's asthma improved dramatically when he left his eastern home to live in Wyoming. This recovery was undoubtedly due to a combination of growth, vigorous exercise and breathing the clean Wyoming outdoor air. Eventually such erroneous psychiatric concepts would give way to a more plausible explanation of asthma that focuses on man's most important body system—the immune system.

Humans are equipped with a powerful biological defense, or immune system, made up of a complicated network of organs, cells and glands that defend and protect or confer immunity against all kinds of foreign invaders (Figure 2.3). The four major components of our immune system are the bone marrow, thymus gland and spleen, and lymph nodes or glands.

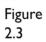

Figure
2.3

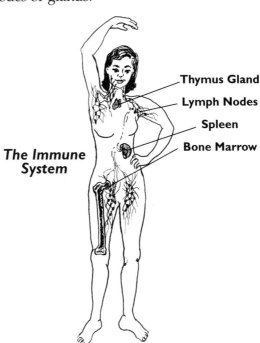

**The Immune
System**

Thymus Gland

Lymph Nodes

Spleen

Bone Marrow

These organs produce a variety of blood cells, chemicals and protective proteins called antibodies, whose main purpose is to defend against or ward off outside invaders. Such invaders include viruses, bacteria, parasites, allergens and a host of other stimuli, including cancer-inducing substances. When our immune system fails to work properly, we get sick. The failure of our immune system to protect us from an outside invader ranges from a simple virus that triggers the common cold to the deadly Acquired Immune Deficiency Syndrome or AIDS virus. AIDS is the most blatant example of what happens to man when his immune system fails to defend itself against an invading virus. There are two basic components of the immune system—the humoral system and the cell-mediated immune system (Figure 2.4).

## The Humoral Immune System

Before discussing humoral immunity, we must define the difference between an antigen and an antibody. A foreign substance, such as a virus or allergen, that enters the body is called an antigen. When the body's immune system encounters an antigen, certain white blood cells called B-cells make a protective protein against the antigen. This protein is called an antibody. The next time your body encounters this antigen, the protective antibody will neutralize the antigen. When the immune system is functioning normally, you develop immunity to invading antigens that lasts for years or even a lifetime. This is the basis of all vaccinations or immunizations. The immune system can be programmed to induce permanent immunity or protection by injection or vaccination with foreign proteins (antigens) derived from viruses and bacteria.

An ideal example of humoral immunity centers on childhood vaccines. In infancy and early childhood, vaccines are administered to children to protect them against common childhood diseases like polio, measles, mumps, diphtheria and chicken pox. After vaccination, the immune system manufactures protective antibodies against these vaccines. Later on, when you are exposed to the natural virus or bacteria, the immune system will kill or neutralize the virus or bacteria. The end result is that you do not get these once-common childhood diseases.

Our humoral immune system produces antibodies against naturally acquired infections. During our lifetime we produce tens of thousands of antibodies that protect us from all types of infections, parasites and diseases, thereby allowing us to lead a normal, healthy life. However, sometimes the immune system overacts to an antigen, and we may develop an autoimmune disease like lupus or rheumatoid arthritis. In some individuals the B-cells overreact to harmless allergens in our environment, and start making too much allergic antibody. As we shall see, asthma and other allergic diseases are the direct result of an overreaction of our immune system to normally harmless outside invaders or antigens.

## Cell-mediated Immunity

The second component of our immune response is called cell-mediated immunity (Figure 2.4). In cell-mediated immunity, antigens or invaders are processed by a series of cells in the immune system called T-cells. They are called T-cells because they are derived from the thymus gland. These T-cells are present in your lymph nodes or glands. Once an antigen reaches the lymph gland, several types of T-cells come into play. Some T-cells kill the antigen (killer T-cells), some suppress it (suppressor T-cells), and some actually help the antigen (helper T-cells). The T-cells are even more important to our discussion than the antibody-producing B-cells, as it is the T-cells that determine whether or not you will develop asthma and/or other allergic diseases.

■

Figure
2.4

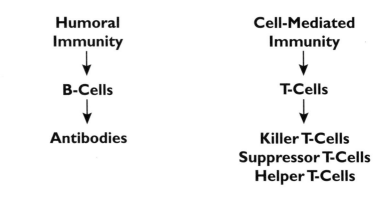

**Humoral and Cell-Mediated Immunity**

## The Allergic Reaction

Throughout our lifetime, the humoral component of the immune system manufactures thousands of antibodies or immunoglobulins each time we are exposed to viruses, bacteria, parasites or allergens. These immunoglobulins (abbreviated Ig) are divided into five groups: IgA, IgD, IgG, IgM and IgE. The immunoglobulin most involved in protecting us against common viruses and bacteria is the IgG antibody, commonly known as gammaglobulin antibody. The immunoglobulin that plays the major role in asthma and allergic diseases is called immunoglobulin E, or IgE antibody. Approximately one in every five individuals inherits an asthma-allergy gene (or genes) that primes their immune system to overproduce this allergic or IgE antibody. The fascinating aspect about allergic or IgE antibody is that it once protected people against common tropical and parasitic diseases. Through the process of evolution and diminished exposure to worms and parasites, this once-friendly IgE antibody has turned on mankind. It is now a "bad antibody" that overreacts to common environmental allergens such as dust mites, molds, animal parts, foods, drugs, insect stings and innocuous pollen grains. The forty-million unfortunate Americans who have inherited the tendency to make a lot of IgE antibodies have a greater risk of developing allergic conditions like asthma, hay fever, eczema or food and drug allergy.

## The Mast Cell and IgE Antibody

What makes the IgE antibody so influential in asthma and other allergic conditions? Unfortunately, IgE antibody has a special affinity for one of the more important cells in the human body, called the mast cell. Millions of mast cells line your skin, nose, intestines and bronchial tubes. Each mast cell contains more than a thousand tiny granules that are loaded with dozens of potent chemicals or mediators. These mediators range from the oldest and most widely known chemical, called histamine, to the newly discovered group of mediators—the leukotrienes. In essence the IgE antibody attaches itself to the mast cell, which is a chemically laden bomb just waiting to explode. When you inherit the capacity to become allergic and make IgE antibodies, the first time or season you are exposed to a potential allergen like ragweed pollen, you do not get hay fever.

However, after repeated seasonal exposures your immune system's B-cells start to produce IgE antibodies to the ragweed pollen (Figure 2.5). These IgE antibodies then attach themselves to the surface of the mast cell. The next time you inhale ragweed pollen, it binds to the IgE antibody sitting on the surface of the mast cell. This combination of antigen (ragweed pollen) and IgE antibody

## *The Sneeze-Wheeze-Itch Reaction*

■

Figure
2.5

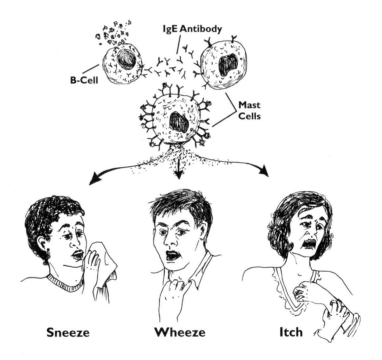

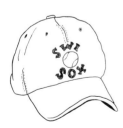

triggers a chemical reaction in the mast cell that releases its powerful mediators, like histamine, into the surrounding tissues. The surrounding tissues then get very inflamed and swollen. When the mast cell erupts in your nose, you sneeze; when the lungs are targeted, you wheeze; and if the skin is the site of the reaction, you itch. The end result of this mast cell eruption is the classical SWI, or sneeze, wheeze and itch reaction, that typifies allergies. You may be interested to know that as a former baseball-softball player, I sponsor a softball team in my local town called the SWISOX. Just like my beloved Boston Red Sox, I am still waiting for them to win it all.

Common aeroallergens that trigger this SWI reaction include dust mites, molds, animals, pollen, stinging insects, foods and drugs. When doctors first discovered that allergens could induce attacks of hay fever, asthma or hives, they set out to develop ways to determine if a person was allergic or sensitive to these substances. Thus, the specialty of allergy was born, and the allergist became the doctor who could isolate and identify the specific allergens that caused people to sneeze, wheeze or itch. Over the past three decades, advances in immunology have produced a greater under-standing of our immune system. Such discoveries are beginning to explain the potential reasons for the asthma-allergy epidemic, and define why allergen exposures during pregnancy and early infancy may alter the way our immune system handles allergens for the rest of our lives. Therefore, we now must take an even closer look at how our immune system, especially the cell-mediated side, handles foreign invaders or antigens.

Foreign invaders or antigens enter our bodies through various portals, including our skin, nose, lungs and gastrointestinal tract. Since we are mainly concerned with asthma, let us explore what happens when we inhale a foreign antigen like a virus, bacteria or allergen into our lungs. After an antigen or allergen is inhaled, it settles on the lining of the lung, a region called the mucosal surface. The body's first attempt to defend itself against the inhaled antigen is the production of mucus by glands known as mucous glands. We all know that when we get a cold or breathe in any kind of foreign substance like an air pollutant, the lining of our respiratory tree produces excess mucus, or phlegm, called mucin. Mucus does not kill or inactivate a virus, bacteria or allergen, but simply wraps it up in a coating of gel. This mucus is then coughed up, spit out or swallowed and degraded in the intestinal tract where the inhaled antigen is destroyed. When this system is operating normally, we protect ourselves from inhaled viruses, bacteria, air pollutants or allergens.

However, if the invader evades this mucus trap, it crosses the surface of the mucosa, where it is met by a class of cells called DC or dendritic cells—biology students will remember them as the macrophages. This cell then absorbs and digests the invading antigen and breaks it up into smaller particles called peptides. The DC cell then acts like a taxicab that transports the peptides to nearby lymph nodes or glands where the critical phase of the immune response takes place (Figure 2.6).

## *The Lymph Gland Reaction*

One of the major components of our immune system is the network of lymph nodes or glands located throughout our body. These glands essentially act as filters against invading agents, by mounting an immune response to neutralize the invading antigen while at the same time avoiding local tissue injury. This response explains why you get swollen glands in your neck when you experience a viral or bacterial infection in your throat. This lymph node reaction involves the interaction of dozens of various cells and chemicals. As we discussed earlier, the two most important cells involved in the immune response are the B-cells and the T-cells. The B-cells make antibodies like allergic or IgE antibody, and gammaglobulin or IgG antibody.

■

Figure
2.6

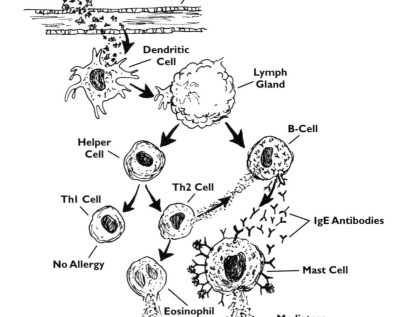

*Tissue Inflammation*

The T-cells are more complicated. T-cells that kill the invader are called killer T-cells. Other T-cells that suppress an invader are labeled suppressor T-cells. Lastly, the helper T-cells program various other pathways in the immune system. The helper T-cells send out signals that bring other cells into the area to combat the invader. These helper T-cells are labeled Th (h is for helper) cells, and are the most influential of all the T-cells, as they determine the path the immune system travels after being exposed to an outside invader or antigen. Immunology research has found that the helper or Th cells can be divided into two major cell types labeled the Th1 and Th2 cells. These Th1 and Th2 immune cells determine if you do or do not develop asthma or other allergic diseases.

When the Th1 cells are activated, they release chemicals called cytokines that drive the immune system away from an allergic response to an invading allergen. Too much Th1 cell activity may lead to autoimmune diseases. On the other hand, the Th2 cells are pro-allergic cells. They produce cytokines that signal the B-cells to manufacture allergic-IgE antibody. The Th2 cells also send out signals to attract allergy blood cells like the eosinophils, basophils and mast cells from other parts of the body. The cells that heed the call of the Th2 cells migrate into the local area of antigen invasion and secrete mediators like histamine and leukotrienes into the surrounding tissues. Once these chemicals hit the local tissues, they cause swelling and inflammation.

Again, the site of the reaction determines if you will sneeze, wheeze or itch. Thus, the allergic reaction is the end result of those all-important Th2 cells driving the immune response in the direction of an inflammatory or pro-allergic response. Doctors can indirectly measure Th2 cell activity by measuring the level of eosinophils and IgE antibody in your serum. Individuals with allergic or atopic conditions like asthma, hay fever and eczema have high levels of eosinophils and IgE antibody.

## Th1 versus Th2

What drives our immune system in either of these two directions? Genes or hereditary factors play a big role, as asthma-allergy genetic codes passed from one generation to the next send the immune system down the Th2 allergy highway. People who do not carry an allergy-asthma gene are more likely to mount a Th1 or non-allergic response to an invading allergen. The second factor that determines what road your immune system takes is your environmental exposure. The reason some individuals who carry an asthma-allergy gene never develop asthma or other allergic diseases is that they had little or no exposure to allergy-triggering antigens such as foods, animal allergens, dust mite, molds and pollens at key periods of their lives. On the other hand, those who have inherited the asthma-allergy gene may have no chance if they are exposed to an offending allergen at the right (or wrong) time of their lives.

What is the right or wrong time? Immunologists now believe that allergen exposures during pregnancy, early infancy and childhood are the key factors. The most fascinating aspect of the recent discoveries in this immune scenario is that a pro-allergy or Th2 response may be determined by what your mother eats or inhales during pregnancy, or by what you are exposed to or injected within infancy or early childhood. As we shall discuss later, whether or not your immune system travels down the Th2 allergy highway may even be determined by the size of your family, your month of birth, attendance at a day care center or early life on a farm.

The developing fetus usually has markedly different blood and tissue types from the mother. All unborn babies are essentially a mass of foreign protein living in their mother's womb. Transplant immunology has taught us that when you try to graft or unite different types of organs or blood types, the host or recipient will promptly reject the graft or organ transplant. This is called the graft-versus-host reaction. One of the miracles of the animal kingdom is that a fetus or unborn infant is rarely rejected by the mother's immune system. The reason for the mother's acceptance of this foreign organism is that the unborn baby mounts a strong Th2 immune response that prevents rejection by the host mother.

Thus, all healthy infants are born with a pro-allergic Th2 immune system. Why don't all newborns then follow the allergy-prone Th2 highway? Here's where Mother Nature takes over. In newborns destined to be non-allergic, the immune system shifts over to the non-allergic Th1 pathway shortly after birth. Just the opposite occurs in infants born with an asthma or allergy genetic makeup. When the fetus or newborn carrying the asthma-allergy gene is exposed to a variety of antigens or allergens early in life, or possibly even in utero, the end result is that the pro-allergy or Th2 system remains in control. Let's take this one step further. What has happened in the last 20 years that favors the Th2 pathway and the onset of the asthma-allergy epidemic?

■
Figure
2.7

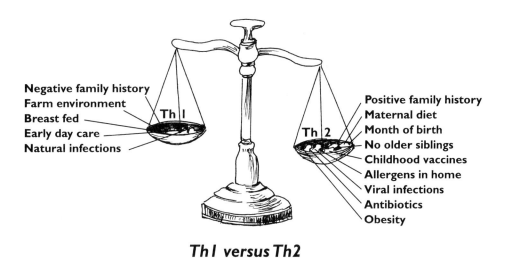

**Negative family history**
**Farm environment**
**Breast fed**
**Early day care**
**Natural infections**

Th 1

Th 2

**Positive family history**
**Maternal diet**
**Month of birth**
**No older siblings**
**Childhood vaccines**
**Allergens in home**
**Viral infections**
**Antibiotics**
**Obesity**

*Th1 versus Th2*

The asthma-allergy epidemic has taken place in less than a generation—too short a time to be blamed on genetic or evolutionary factors. The answer to the epidemic may lie in changes in our environment and lifestyle (Figure 2.7). Alterations in maternal and infant eating habits, environmental exposures (or lack thereof) and the expanded use of childhood vaccines and antibiotics may be keeping the Th2 system operating. A pro-allergic Th2 response then sends the infant or young child down the allergy highway and increases the likelihood of developing one or all of the "big four" allergic conditions—asthma, allergic rhinitis or hay fever, eczema and food allergy.

# Eat
# a Pound of **Dirt**
# Before You Die

**3**

n the 1800s hay fever was virtually unknown in Europe and North America. In just 200 years, hay fever and asthma have become the most common chronic diseases of developed Western societies. One-third of all adolescents and young adults in the United Kingdom and the United States now have hay fever. Obviously something different is happening in infancy and childhood that has led to the increasing prevalence of asthma and allergic diseases in the past 20 years.

If we are to uncover what has brought about this asthma-allergy epidemic, we must look at the features unique to the environment or lifestyle of modern Western civilization that may be diverting our immune system down the Th2 or asthma-allergy pathway. Undoubtedly, there are many pieces to this puzzle. Potential reasons for the asthma-allergy epidemic include changes in ethnic patterns, exposures to indoor and outdoor allergens, air pollutants, alterations in childhood bacterial and viral infections, childhood obesity, modifications in the lifestyles of infants and children, and the expanded use of childhood vaccines and antibiotics in infancy and early childhood.

## Potential Reasons for the Asthma-Allergy Epidemic
▲ Genetic and Ethnic Patterns
▲ Aeroallergen Exposure
▲ Air Pollution
▲ Month of Birth

▲ Western Lifestyle Changes
▲ Obesity
▲ Maternal-Infant Diet
▲ Lack of Natural Infections
▲ Childhood Vaccines
▲ Excess Use of Antibiotics

## Genetic and Ethnic Patterns

There is no doubt that the tendency to develop asthma and other allergic conditions is inherited. However, the asthma-allergy epidemic has taken place much too quickly (in less than a generation) for it to be due to evolutionary changes or genetic mutations. What about ethnic patterns? Ethnicity may be related to the rise of asthma cases, especially in the inner cities. Hospital admissions rates and asthma deaths are statistically higher for American inner-city blacks and Hispanics, and among the Maori in New Zealand. Poverty and socioeconomic status are important determinants of access to appropriate medical care in the inner cities. While inner-city lifestyles and environmental exposures can determine the risk of asthma, some ethnic groups are more likely to develop asthma and other allergic diseases regardless of their socioeconomic status.

One study found an extremely high rate of asthma in children born to Puerto Rican and African-American mothers, where the rate of asthma was 18.4 percent in Puerto Rican children and 11.3 percent in blacks, versus 7.4 percent in white children. Review of potential asthma risk factors in all three of these ethnic groups showed no differences in allergen exposures or socioeconomic status. Thus, regardless of poverty level, African-American and Puerto Rican families may be more prone to asthma strictly from an ethnic standpoint.

This ethnic concept was given additional support by a survey from the Henry Ford Health System in Detroit that found that African-American children had higher levels of allergic IgE antibodies than Caucasian children, regardless of poverty level. Prior studies have shown that African-American children have smaller lung capacities than European-American children, regardless of socioeconomic status. In my experience, ethnic factors do play a role in asthma and allergic disorders.

Over the past 30 years I have treated a large number of first- and second-generation Portuguese families with severe allergies and asthma. These patients of Portuguese descent have high allergy blood counts (eosinophil and IgE levels), strongly positive allergy skin tests and are often the sickest patients seen in my office during heavy pollen seasons. Childhood allergies and asthma in this ethnic group often persist into adulthood. While no one has ever closely studied this ethnic group, I feel that Portuguese families have a higher prevalence of asthma and allergic diseases than other ethnic populations, at least in my practice.

## The House Dust Mite Theory

Doctor Morrison Smith fired the first warning shot on the increase in the number of asthma cases when he reported that the incidence of asthma in English schoolchildren dramatically increased during the 1960s. Doctor Smith's early studies and those of other researchers eventually established a strong link between exposure to house dust mites and asthma. In 1978, Doctors Thomas Platts-Mills and Martin Chapman investigated the role of the house dust mite in asthma. They proposed that changes in airtight home construction methods, combined with the use of wall-to-wall carpeting, allowed dwellings to become more humid and dust mite friendly. A warm, humid indoor climate favored the proliferation of dust mites in homes where children and adults were spending more time than ever indoors—an average of 23 hours per day.

Worldwide reports from Holland, Great Britain, Australia and New Zealand strongly supported this dust mite theory. It was firmly established that the level of dust mite exposure within a home was directly proportional to the risk of asthma, and reducing house dust mite levels improved asthma symptoms. Asthma researchers thought they had found one answer for the asthma epidemic. They postulated that increased exposure to the dust mite, secondary to changes in housing construction and lifestyle of the occupants, was a major cause for the increasing prevalence of asthma. The dust mite theory did not explain everything. Changes in home construction leading to the increase in house dust mite exposure were basically complete by the mid-1970s, but the incidence of asthma continued to rise throughout the 1980s and 1990s. Likewise, the asthma epidemic was evolving in areas of the world like Scandinavia and the mountainous regions of North America, where low humidity levels were not conducive to dust mite growth. In some cities, like Chicago, Illinois, that experienced an asthma epidemic, house dust mite levels were actually quite low. The Chicago asthma epidemic was blamed on high exposure to cockroaches in inner-city dwellings.

The asthma epidemic in Scandinavia has been linked to household pets. Other studies have shown that indoor and outdoor molds may be the most important asthma triggers in some locals. In my opinion the explosion in the world's cat population is another factor in the asthma epidemic. Thus, it appears that increased exposure to not just one but multiple allergens is playing a role in the ongoing asthma epidemic.

Changes in public housing design could be another factor in the rise in asthma cases. In Boston, Massachusetts, poor people suffer six times more asthma than the rest of the population. In one South Boston housing project, 26 percent of adults have asthma. In another Boston housing project in a different neighborhood, 50 percent of resident children have asthma. Asthma experts have attributed this high rate of asthma in housing projects to poverty, poor housekeeping, smoking, lack of access to medical care and exposure to dust mites or cockroaches. Yet in the 1990s (when compared to the 1960s and 1970s), Boston's poor have cleaner housing, smoke less and have access to some of the best hospitals in the world.

*Boston Herald* columnist Tom Keane reported the interesting possibility that the rise in asthma might be the fault of programs initiated by the U.S. Department of Urban and Housing Development, or HUD, 30 years ago. In the 1970s the oil embargo and energy crisis prompted President Jimmy Carter and HUD to appropriate millions of dollars to curb heating costs. Energy-efficient windows, roofs and walls were installed in HUD public housing projects throughout the United States. This HUD program was very successful, and energy costs sharply declined. This leads to the speculation that energy-efficient public housing has increased exposure to dust mites, molds, cockroaches and animals. The Boston Housing Authority, which oversees 27,000 residents, has teamed up with Boston's three schools of public health—Harvard, Boston University and Tufts—in an $8 million project that will track residents for five years. Hopefully this important study will uncover the causes of the high rate of asthma and asthma mortality in Boston's public housing.

## Outdoor Air Pollutants

Is the asthma epidemic due to outdoor air pollution? Studies have shown that exposure to air pollutants like ozone, sulfur dioxide, nitrous dioxide and diesel exhaust particles can stimulate the pro-allergic Th2 cells and promote the development of allergic or IgE-mediated diseases like asthma. While there is no doubt that outdoor air pollutants trigger preexisting asthma, new asthma cases and the need for hospital care have continued to increase in cities and countries where air pollution levels have significantly decreased. Thus, it appears unlikely that a change in exposure to air pollutants is a major reason for the asthma epidemic. One intriguing study that compared the incidence of asthma in heavily polluted East Germany to the more hygienic West Germany found a much lower rate of allergy and asthma in East German citizens.

## Month of Birth

Your date of birth may be another reason why you travel down the allergy-asthma highway. The first clue that exposure to aeroallergens in very early infancy might play a role in the development of allergy or asthma came from Scandinavia. Clinical studies in this northern climate found that infants born in late winter—just before the onset of the Scandinavian birch tree pollen season—had more birch pollen allergy later in life compared to children born in the summer, after the birch pollen season had subsided. The inference here is early exposure to birch pollen in the first few weeks of life may trigger birch pollen allergy later on in childhood.

Researchers at the Henry Ford Hospital in Detroit compared allergic IgE antibody levels in children born in the fall months to children born in the summer. They found that children born in the fall had higher IgE levels than those born in the summer months. Canadian children born in the winter were more likely to be allergic to dust mites and cats. The presumption is that children born in the fall and winter spend the better part of their early existence in a closed and heated indoor environment and are more likely to become allergic to indoor allergens and develop asthma, eczema or allergic rhinitis. Early exposure to high levels of indoor and outdoor allergens in the first few months of life may prevent the infant's Th2-driven immune system from switching over to the non-allergic Th1 response.

## The Couch Potato Theory

Asthma remains a rare disease in undeveloped countries such as New Guinea, China and most parts of rural Africa, where there is no television, electricity or motorized transport. Children in these countries play outdoors a great deal, and walk or run 10 to 20 miles a day to and from school. No wonder the Kenyans dominate the Boston Marathon! Prior to 1960, most American children played outdoors after school for several hours a day, or from dawn till dusk in the summer months.

I remember my own school days when, depending on the season, my friends and I would gather after school or during the summer for unsupervised sporting activities including pickup baseball, football, basketball or hockey. In that bygone era, we had no coaches, umpires, referees or uniforms, and even more importantly, no parental influence over our athletic activities. We organized our own games that went on for hours. As many families of that era only had one automobile, we walked or cycled several miles a day to and from schools and ball fields. Nowadays, SUV-driven children rarely walk or cycle to and from their schools or playing fields, even if they are a relatively short distance from home. You never see children participating in an athletic event without uniforms, coaches or referees. It is highly unlikely that today's children would be capable of organizing any type of pickup game.

Is this pattern of childhood activity playing a role in the asthma-allergy epidemic? Dr. Thomas Platts-Mills has proposed an intriguing theory that could be labeled the "couch potato theory."

Platts-Mills feels that the sedentary after-school habits of modern children (no outdoor play, lying on carpets or rugs and watching television or computer screens) have allowed children to spend more time indoors in poorly ventilated homes or apartments. Such environments may be infested with indoor allergens like dust mites, molds, household pets and cockroaches, which in turn lead to increased allergy sensitization and asthma. This lifestyle has concomitantly led to a new generation of obese children.

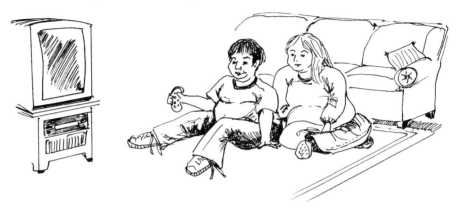

This theory is supported by several studies on asthma and obesity. Obesity has been found to be a definite risk for both children and adults with asthma. One study that followed the health of over 100,000 female nurses found that overweight nurses were three times more likely to develop asthma than their thinner colleagues. A British study of 8,000 people found that heavier adults were more likely to have asthma than thinner people. No one can explain why overweight people have more asthma.

Doctor Carlos Carmagos from Boston's Brigham and Women's Hospital studied 16,862 children between nine and fourteen years of age and found that asthma was more prevalent in overweight children. He suggested being overweight compresses the airways and make obese people more reactive to common asthma triggers. Over the past 25 years the number of overweight children and adults who have asthma has impressed me. I assumed that obesity was related to inactivity or lack of regular exercise due to asthma. One group of obese children especially prone to asthma are overweight adolescent females, who can develop a severe form of non-allergic asthma, called late-onset childhood asthma.

A study of enrollees in a military-managed, health-care program in the northwestern United States found that a higher body mass index, especially in younger females, was a strong predictor for asthma. Additional studies need to be done to determine if weight reduction in obese asthmatics will reduce asthma symptoms.

## Maternal and Infant Diet

Can unborn infants be sensitized to food or inhalant allergens during pregnancy? Blood from an infant's umbilical cord can contain allergic antibodies to egg, milk, dust mites, cats and birch pollen. One interesting study found that umbilical cord blood of infants born before their mothers were exposed to grass pollen had no antibodies to grass pollen, while infants born to mothers exposed to grass pollen during pregnancy had grass pollen antibodies in their umbilical cord blood. The mother's placenta apparently allows antigens from her body to cross over to the fetus and trigger an allergic immune response in the fetus. Such a response may start as early as the 24th week of pregnancy, when the fetus adopts a Th2 posture to prevent rejection by the mother. These findings imply that environmental control measures should be implemented in early pregnancy.

The possible role of diet in the asthma-allergy epidemic has been evaluated. Alterations in the dietary habits of civilized nations that could trigger asthma include the increased exposure to food additives, colorings and preservatives, combined with decreased consumption of fish and a shift to a high-potassium, low-sodium diet. While these theories are attractive, it is unlikely that diet plays a major role in asthma, as the ongoing asthma epidemic has occurred throughout the developed world in many countries where dietary habits are extremely varied.

## The Hygiene Hypothesis

During my childhood when I came home in a dirty and disheveled state from play, my mother was fond of quoting the old Irish proverb, *"If you want to live a long and healthy life, you should eat a pound of dirt before you die."* Mother may have been right on the money, as there is mounting evidence that a lower incidence of bacterial infections, combined with the increased use of antibiotics and vaccines in infancy and being raised in too clean an environment, may favor the pro-allergic Th2 pathway.

We can thank the fall of the Berlin Wall in 1989 for yielding the first clues that a hygienic or overly clean environment may be the reason for the asthma-allergy epidemic. The seeds of the *"hygiene hypothesis"* arose out of a preliminary study in Germany where investigators looked at the incidence of allergy and asthma in East and West German citizens—two identical ethnic populations with similar genetic backgrounds who had been living under vastly different living conditions for nearly 50 years. At the outset of the study the investigators proposed that the residents of the less hygienic, more industrialized and heavily polluted East Germany would have more allergy and asthma. Much to their surprise, they found just the opposite. West Germans had three times more asthma and allergic disorders than the East Germans.

This study suggested that infants and young children raised in the more hygienic environment of West Germany with clean air and sophisticated childhood immunization programs experienced fewer respiratory infections in early life. Proponents of the hygiene hypothesis believe that a lack of exposure to naturally acquired infections and air pollutants produce a lazy or lightly challenged immune system that is more likely to follow the pro-allergic Th2 pathway.

## Down on the Farm

Additional support for this attractive concept came from an unlikely source—the farm. Studies in Austria, Canada, Germany and Finland have found that farm-raised children have less asthma and allergic diseases. The Austrian study arose out of a local doctor's observation that children in his practice who lived on a farm had less asthma and allergy problems than children who were brought up in the local village. Indeed, when epidemiologists investigated this shrewd observation, they found that children raised on the farms had fewer allergy-asthma problems than their classmates who lived in the local villages. As neither group was exposed to any outdoor air pollutants, the thought was that farm-raised children were exposed to a variety of soil organisms and farm animals that somehow protected them from developing allergic disorders and asthma.

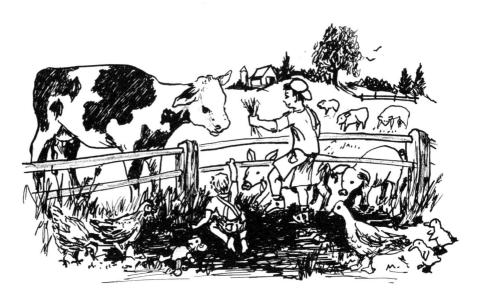

A study of school children in rural Canada confirmed these findings. Canadian investigators studied 1,199 children in 14 elementary schools in rural Quebec. They divided these children and their families into two groups—subjects raised on farms in rural Quebec and those who lived in local towns with no farm exposure. The children in both groups underwent allergy skin tests, breathing tests, and inhalation challenges. They found less asthma and allergy in the children who lived on a farm.

Children raised on farms are exposed to a wide variety of sources of potential toxins and allergens, including dairy barns, pigsties and chickens, which provide a constant source of airborne bacteria, endotoxin, molds, animal dander and irritant chemicals. The major farm exposure that may be protective is contact with animal dung that harbors a form of bacteria called gram-negative bacteria. The cell walls of these bacteria produce a potent chemical called endotoxin, that may drive the immune system down the non-allergic Th1 pathway.

Additional observations lend credence to the hygiene hypothesis. Second and subsequent children have a lower incidence of asthma than first-born children. The reasoning here is that younger siblings experience more respiratory infections at an early age than older siblings, as infections are brought home by older siblings attending virally infested day care centers or schools. Investigators in Tucson, Arizona, have tracked the respiratory status of 1,035 children from birth to age 13. Children with more than one older sibling at home, or those who attended day care at an early age, had more wheezing in early childhood than those children with no older siblings or less exposure to day care. However, by age six the younger siblings and children who attended day care at an early age had less wheezing. This study implied exposure to common viral respiratory infections at an early age, either in or out of the home, protected against wheezing and asthma later on in childhood.

German children enrolled in a day care center at an early age had less asthma and wheezing than children kept at home. Working mothers take notice. These findings should relieve some of your fear or guilt when you drop off your child at a day care center infested with all sorts of respiratory infections. You may actually be preventing your child from developing asthma or hay fever later on in life.

Less-than-ideal housekeeping may also prevent asthma. A little dust or dirt in the home may produce endotoxin, the chemical that is present in the cell walls of common bacteria. Most homes contain small amounts of endotoxin. When researchers looked at the homes of a group of wheezy-allergic infants, they found that their homes had less endotoxin than the homes of a control group who did not have allergies or asthma. Early exposure to endotoxin in house dust may protect against allergy and asthma by provoking the allergy Th1 cell response in early infancy.

Naturally acquired infections or vaccines may also protect against asthma. Military recruits in Italy who had evidence of prior infection with the hepatitis A virus had less asthma than those with no evidence of hepatitis. Japanese subjects injected with BCG, an anti-Tb vaccine, had less asthma than those who did not receive BCG vaccine. A multinational study centered in Munich, Germany, that has followed nearly 250,000 children in 85 centers in Europe,

North America, Australia and New Zealand discovered an inverse association between tuberculosis and asthma. Those children who had evidence of exposure to tuberculosis had a lower incidence of asthma. It is theorized that BCG vaccine or tuberculosis bacteria may favor the non-allergic Th1 cell response and shut down the pro-allergic Th2 system. Clinical trials in asthma with this BCG vaccine are now underway.

## *Vaccines and Antibiotics*

Modern medicine has developed scores of childhood vaccines in order to ensure that children in developed countries no longer suffer from measles, mumps, chicken pox, polio or a host of other childhood diseases. Many childhood vaccines contain alum, a substance that boosts or enhances the immune or protective response of the vaccine. Unfortunately, alum is a potent stimulator of the pro-allergic Th2 pathway. The implication here is that it may be possible to develop alum-free Th1-stimulating vaccines that would favor the Th1 pathway for infants and young children. Overuse of antibiotics in infancy and childhood and eradication of both friendly and unfriendly bacteria may be another reason for the allergy-asthma epidemic. A New Zealand survey found that children who received an antibiotic in infancy had a four-fold risk of having asthma in their teens.

The key bacteria in this immune scenario may be bacterial organisms in our intestinal tract. The intestine or gut is the largest organ in the body that interacts with the environment. The lymph glands in the gut constantly process bacterial microorganisms and food antigens. The concept is that strains of friendly bacteria in the intestinal tract might program the immune system to adopt the non-allergic Th1 response. One common harmless bacterial resident of the gut is *lactobacillus.*

Finnish investigators studied 159 pregnant women with a family history of eczema, hay fever or asthma and gave them *lactobacillus* or a placebo before and after their delivery. Those children whose mothers received *lactobacillus* had 50 percent less eczema in the first two years of life. If this exciting finding is confirmed by other studies, it may represent a unique advance in the treatment of allergic diseases.

In Estonia, where infants have a high level of intestinal *lactobacillus*, there is less allergy and asthma compared to Sweden, where the level of *lactobacillus* is lower and the incidence of allergy and asthma is higher. *E. coli*, another common intestinal bacteria, produces the endotoxin found in high concentrations in house dust, soil and air pollutants. This may explain why farm-raised children have less allergy and asthma, since they are constantly exposed to high levels of *E. coli* and endotoxin in the farm environment. It also explains why premature infants have less allergy and eczema. Premature infants who enter the world before their immune systems are fully primed for protection are more susceptible to infections, especially intestinal infection.

Hygienically raised children have no experience in fighting off any infectious diseases except naturally acquired viral infections. Some experts have postulated that the absence of bacterial diseases in early childhood makes children more prone to developing allergic diseases later on in life. Exposure to certain species of harmless bacteria in the soil and the intestinal tract favors the stimulation of the Th1 pathway. Should we turn the clock back and return to the less hygienic living conditions of the past? Certainly not—improvement in public health and childhood vaccines are two of the major reasons for the increase in our life span.

A more practical approach may be injecting high-risk infants and young children with bacterial vaccines to prevent allergic disease and asthma. One bacterial vaccine currently under study is *Mycobacterium vaccaea,* a harmless bacteria present in the soil. This bacteria evokes a strong Th1 or non-allergic response in mice. Early human clinical trials with this vaccine in subjects with allergic rhinitis and asthma appear promising.

Thus, my mother was probably right—eating a little dirt early on in life may not be all that bad. One hundred years ago human beings were constantly exposed to common infectious diseases, worms and parasites that repeatedly stimulated their immune system. These parasitic infections may have protected humans against allergy and asthma by promoting the production of a T-cell mediator called interleukin-10 or IL-10.

A recent study found that 520 Gabonese children with parasitic infections and high levels of IL-10 had less dust mite allergy. These findings have stimulated additional research in an attempt to harness the anti-inflammatory effects of IL-10 in asthma therapy. The low incidence of allergy and asthma in some third-world countries where parasitic infections are common suggests that our immune system may not be as tough or as well conditioned as it was decades ago. The improvements in public health and hygiene and the overuse of antibiotic drugs mean people are no longer exposed to potent immune stimulants. In essence, the tradeoff of living a longer, healthier life may be a higher incidence of allergic diseases and asthma. It is exciting to speculate that if a "lazy immune system" is responsible for the ongoing asthma and allergy epidemic, some type of vaccine strategy that stimulates a lethargic immune system in infancy or early childhood may prevent the onset of asthma and other allergic diseases.

I feel some concepts of the hygiene hypothesis clarify the asthma-allergy epidemic. It explains why some areas of the world like rural Africa and China have one-tenth the incidence of asthma when compared to more developed Westernized countries. It is highly likely that exposure to any type of allergen in infancy or early childhood triggers the pro-allergic Th2 reaction. Thus, exposure to cats or birch pollen in Scandinavia; dust mites in coastal regions such as Boston; molds in Tucson, Arizona; or cockroaches in Chicago is the major reason for the development of asthma and other allergic disorders in genetically predisposed children. Whereas, certain environments such as large families, farms, day care centers or poorly kept homes may be protective. One new and intriguing concept that will be discussed in the section on environmental control is that in-home exposure to a dog or cat at an early age may actually block the onset of asthma.

In summary, the hygiene hypothesis needs further confirmation. It does not explain the increasing prevalence of asthma in American inner cities and some rural areas of Africa, nor does it address the role of exposure to aeroallergens and pollutants in the rising tide of asthma. In all likelihood there are many reasons for the emerging asthma epidemic.

# Asthma—
# An
# **Ancient** Illness

# 4

## *Early Historians*

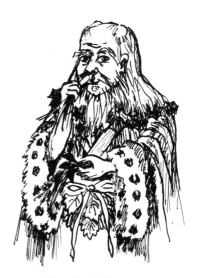

The Red Emperor

**U**nlike many modern chronic conditions, asthma is an ancient illness that has intrigued medical historians for centuries. The earliest recorded use of asthma medicines dates back to approximately 3000 B.C. in China. According to Chinese legend, Shen Nong (c. 2700 B.C.), also known as the Red Emperor, was considered to be the father of Chinese Herbal Medicine. Legend has it that Shen Nong was the first to taste ephedra, a horsetail plant with edible, raspberry-like berries. Ephedra, also called *Ma huang*, has been used to treat respiratory disorders, including asthma, for centuries and is still a common ingredient of many herbal medicines.

The first Western references to asthma are found in Egyptian writings. The Ebers Papyrus, which was unearthed in 1862, contains an extensive collection of prescriptions, medical and surgical remedies for asthma, plague, scurvy and cataracts. Egyptian healers

---

[Some of the material in this chapter is adapted from *Asthma:* Lippincott, Williams & Wilkins 1998, and *Ancestors of Allergy,* Global Medical Communications New York, NY USA 1994. Edited by F. Estelle Simons, MD FRCPC.]

who had a somewhat sophisticated approach to medicine were called *swnu*. They were both physicians and priests, and healed through divine intervention in a time when medicine was considered to be a sacred art controlled by primeval gods. The first physician to be deified as the God of Medicine was Imhotep (c. 2700 B.C.). Imhotep, who was also an astronomer and an architect, designed the first Step Pyramid.

Egyptians considered asthma to be a *whdu* (a disorder or foulness) of the *metu*, or ducts, that distributed air and water to the body's organs and lungs. Egyptian asthma remedies included compounds of sweet beer, bird dung, grapes, frankincense, goose grease and fresh bread taken by mouth or inhaled over hot stones. Fortunately, inhalation therapy has come a long way since Egyptian times.

## The Greco-Roman Era

Asthma, as first described by the ancient Greek, Egyptian and Hebrew healers, was initially considered to be a symptom and not a true disease. The term asthma comes from the Greek word *panos*, which means to pant or to breathe with an open mouth. The Greeks had a great deal of respect for panos, or asthma, as they believed it to be a sacred disease signifying a divine visitation from the Gods. Ancient Greek medicine was based on the philosophies of Aesculapius (c. 900–1200 B.C.) who was said to be a doctor of such talent that he could raise the dead. Greek healers used snakes and rituals, along with diet, rest, massage and hydrotherapy. Many physicians followed the cult of Aesculapius, and practiced in temples called Aesculapians, where snakes were kept. This explains why snakes are still strongly associated with medicine.

Hippocrates the Great, born in 460 B.C. and still regarded as the Father of Medicine, is the most renowned and influential physician in western history. He was the first Greek physician to move away from the supernatural force and divine intervention theories and toward a more scientific approach to medicine. Hippocratic medicine identified four humors: blood, phlegm, yellow bile and black bile. Health was believed to be the result of a proper balance between these four humors. Any illness was thought to be due to an excess level of one or more of these humors. Hippocrates believed that asthma was due to excess amounts of phlegm, the evil humor that flowed from the brain through the nose and sinus cavities into the lungs. The thought was that excess phlegm blocked the lungs and produced *catarrh*, which means flowing down. In his essay *Airs, Waters, and Places*, Hippocrates was the first to correlate asthma with climate and location.

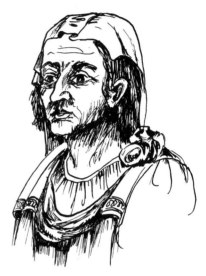

Hippocrates

*"Let us suppose we are dealing with a district which is sheltered from northerly wind but exposed to warm ones.... The inhabitants of such a place will thus have moist heads full of phlegm, and this, flowing down from the head, is likely to disturb their inner organs. The constitution will be flabby and they tolerate neither food nor drink well. It is a general rule that men with weak heads are not great drinkers as they are particularly liable to hangovers. Children are liable to convulsions and asthma which are considered as divine visitations and the disease itself as sacred."*

Hippocrates correctly noted that asthma was an inherited condition most commonly seen in children. He was 2,000 years ahead of his time when he reported that asthmatics were prone to obesity and wheezed after imbibing alcoholic beverages. One of the asthma remedies of the Hippocratic era included a cocktail of figs, grapes, sycamore fruit, frankincense, cumin, juniper, wine, goose grease and sweet beer. In addition, extracts of henbane or Hyoscyamus were placed on a heated brick and their vapors inhaled. Much less palatable treatments included the inhalation of heated camel and crocodile dung.

The first true medical historian and arguably the greatest of all the Latin medical writers, Aulus Celsus, (first century B.C.), compiled the oldest recorded medical document on asthma. Celsus, often called the "Hippocrates of the Romans," wrote the oldest known medical document—*De Medicinia*. This treatise, largely ignored by his contemporaries, was rediscovered by Pope Nicholas V in the 15th century. *De Medicinia* was among the first medical texts to be published in 1478 after the introduction of the printing press. Celsus' classic description of asthma and shortness of breath remained popular well into the Middle Ages.

> *"When the difficulty of breathing is moderate and not suffocating it is called dyspnoea, when it is more vehement so that the breathing is more sonorous and wheezing, it constitutes asthma; when the breathing can only take place in an upright position it is termed orthopnoea."*

In the first century A.D., Aretaeus, a Greek physician from Cappadocia, astutely recorded that women were more prone to asthma, men were more likely to die of it, and children had a better outlook for recovery. The teachings of Aretaeus, the first to classify asthma as a specific disease, went unnoticed for 1500 years, until his Greek manuscript was translated into Latin and printed in Venice in 1552. Aretaeus's description of an acute attack of asthma is easily the most vivid account of acute asthma in ancient and possibly modern times.

> *"If from running, gymnastic exercise, or any other form of work, the breathing becomes difficult, it is called asthma. The cheeks are ruddy, and the eyes protuberant as if from strangulation; a rale [noise in the chest] can be heard in the waking state, but the evil is much worse in sleep; the voice is liquid and without resonance. Patients eagerly go into the open air, since no house suffices for the respiration; they breathe as if desiring to draw in all they can possibly inhale. Pale in countenance except for the cheeks which are ruddy, they sweat about the forehead and clavicles, the cough is incessant and laborious, the expectoration small and thin. The neck swells, the pulse is small and compressed, and their legs are slender. If these symptoms increase, they can produce suffocation. When the crisis ends, the expectoration becomes copious, the urine increases, and the voice becomes louder."*

In the second century A.D., Galen of Pergamus, born in 129 in Asia Minor and considered to be the greatest clinician after Hippocrates, advanced a theory based on the Hippocratic misconception of anatomy and the doctrine of evil humors. After finishing his medical training at the medical center in Alexandria, Galen went to Rome and became the personal physician to the gladiators and Emperor Marcus Aurelius (A.D. 121–180). Many Greek physicians went to Rome in this era, as the Romans did not encourage their own citizens to study medicine. Proper knowledge of basic human anatomy was definitely a weak spot for these early medical researchers.

Galen believed that the brain communicated directly with the lung through the nose and sinus cavities, thereby permitting the removal of the excrements of the brain. He prescribed cleansing and detergent medicines, and forbade all things hot or cold, as well as astringents, as they might thicken these evil humors. Galen correctly noted, however, that opiates were harmful in asthma, as they cooled the body too much and thereby thickened the humors. Galen came close to the cause of asthma when he wrote that asthma was due to the accumulation of thick viscid humors in the lungs, resulting in *a lack of room in the cavities of the lungs.* Galen's works shaped the course of medicine for more than a thousand years.

Several Roman physicians and scholars, including Pliny the Elder (A.D. 23–79), criticized the practices of these Greek healers by attacking their honesty and integrity. Pliny's own work, however, was somewhat off the mark, as he delved into folklore and recommended drinking the blood of wild horses and eating insects soaked in Attic honey as an asthma remedy.

Early Hebrew medicine focused on the belief that diseases were the result of God's intervention and divine will. In the Talmud, the collective work of Jewish scholarship, diseases were divided into two categories—those due to natural causes and those caused by God. One Hebrew remedy for asthma was derived from a gum resin of oriental plants in the carrot family. Early medical texts from India interwove rational medical therapy with myths and magic. Indian therapies were exported to Greece and Egypt in the fourth and fifth centuries after the invasion of Alexander the Great.

Many Indian herbal remedies are derived from the medical text, *Ayurveda,* including stramonium, which was extracted from the thorn apple tree. In the seventh century the Muslim invasion of the Middle East and North Africa resulted in a merging of Arabic medicine concepts with the traditional teachings of the Greek and Roman Schools. Most Arabic physicians embraced the teachings of Hippocrates, Celsus, and Galen.

## The Middle Ages

The collapse of the Roman Empire created a deep void in medical research and thought. Medical care in the Middle Ages (A.D. 450 to 1300) focused on relieving suffering and not on basic causes or scientific theory of disease. One bright center of medical thinking in this period was Baghdad, where many Greek and Persian works were translated into Arabic. The most famous Arabic physician of this era was Rhazes (c. 855–923), a Persian scholar who wrote on a wide variety of topics, including astronomy, mathematics and medicine. Among Rhazes's 140 books on medicine is an incredible description of hay fever, called *A Dissertation on the Cause of the Coryza which occurs in the Spring when the Roses give forth their Scent.* Rhazes listed several asthma remedies, including two drachmas of dried and powdered fox lung and figs added to a drink.

Many Arabic physicians also treated asthma with the administration of arsenic by inhalation or pills. Another famous Persian in this era was Avicenna (980–1037), who was called the Prince of Physicians. His most famous work, *The Cannon of Medicine,* became required reading throughout the Islamic and Western World for 500 years. Both Rhazes and Avicenna believed that asthma and epilepsy were related conditions. This concept persisted well into the seventeenth century, when attacks of asthma were still referred to as "fits."

## A Remedy for All Ages

The next significant breakthrough in medicine and asthma did not come until the twelfth century. The most famous medical scholar of this period was Moses Maimonides (1135–1204), the great Jewish physician and philosopher who traveled to Morocco to escape Jewish persecution. Once his fame spread, Maimonides's medical skills were highly sought after, and he was asked to become the court physician to Saladin, the Great Sultan of Egypt, Syria and Palestine. As a result

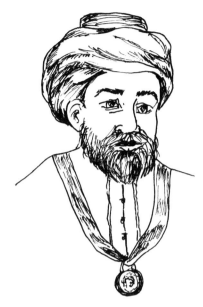

Maimonides

of his many victories in the Crusades, Saladin is considered to be the most famous Muslim hero of all time. Maimonides was asked to treat Saladin's son, who suffered from bronchial asthma and melancholia.

After Maimonides wisely moved Saladin's son from the more humid climate of Alexandria to the dry air of Cairo, he wrote *Treatise on Asthma* in A.D. 1190. This milestone paper stated that asthma should be treated according to the various causes that bring it about. It is humbly prefaced by a statement that still applies today. *"I have no magic cure to report; all I have in mind is a rational conduct of life."* Maimonides advised his patients on hygiene and recommended specific medicines and dietary therapy. One of Maimonides's dietary remedies has endured for centuries. In cases of acute asthma and other respiratory conditions, he recommended the *"spicy soup of the fat hen"* if the patient had no fever, and sweetened barley porridge if the patient had a fever. Maimonides correctly believed that chicken soup assisted in the expectoration of thickened mucus or phlegm. Recent research suggests that chicken soup may have some anti-inflammatory properties.

## A Famous Consultation

Prior to the twelfth century, most of the meaningful advances in medicine originated from the Middle East and Eastern Europe. Western European medicine was mired in the depths of Medieval monastery-based medicine that practiced the primitive cult and faith-healing practices common to the Middle or Dark Ages. In thirteenth-century England, John Gaddesden wrote a four-volume work on medicine that described a number of asthma remedies riddled with the mysticism, charms and superstitions typical of these times. The corner was about to be turned; however, the year A.D. 1552 marks what is perhaps the most famous consultation in the history of medicine.

Gerolamo Cardano (A.D. 1501–1576), a Professor of Medicine at the University of Pavia, was the most celebrated physician of his time in Western Europe. In 1552, Cardano was summoned to Edinburgh, Scotland, to treat John Hamilton, the Archbishop of St. Andrew's, whose asthmatic condition had been steadily deteriorating for 10 years. Cardano was strongly influenced by Maimonides's treatise on asthma. He believed that asthma, while incurable, could be relieved by adhering to proper diet and lifestyle. On his way to Edinburgh, Cardano attended a medical conference in Paris where a controversy arose as whether or not the wheezing Archbishop's brain was "too cold or too hot."

Many physicians of this era erroneously followed the Hippocratic theory, that teaches that harmful humors and fluids flow from the brain down to the lung. In asthma these fluids are said to be too thick, and their thickness causes irritation. Many Parisian doctors opted for the cold theory, and mandated that the Archbishop's brain and body needed warming. These "cold-docs" insisted that the Archbishop keep a burning peat or charcoal fire near him at all times, even when he was riding in his carriage. Thus, the Archbishop was denied fresh air and only allowed to ingest hot foods and mulled wines. No matter where he went, day or night, the Archbishop inhaled pollutants from nearby peat or charcoal fires. Such a regimen obviously caused further worsening of the Archbishop's chronic asthma.

Cardano disagreed with the French doctors. He favored the hot theory, perhaps because he saw the utter failure of the cold theory approach. When Cardano treated the Archbishop, he decided that the cause of Hamilton's asthma was a high temperature of the brain. Cardano elected to purge the Archbishop's head and body of heat. A mixture of goat's milk, ship's tar, mustard, honey and blister fly was applied to the Archbishop's skull. Furthermore, he was instructed to regularly wash his head in warm water to which ashes had been added.

This regimen was followed by a cold shower and massage with cool dry cloths. Air-polluting peat and charcoal fires were removed from the Archbishop's carriage and rooms. The Archbishop was put on a strict timetable that mandated he sleep at least 10 hours a day. Perhaps most importantly, he was forbidden to sleep on his feather mattress, as Cardano believed that the feather mattress *"heated the spine and caused fluid matter to ascend to the brain."* Archbishop Hamilton benefited enormously from sound sleep, fresh air and escaping the smoky environment of his home and carriage. The removal of the peat and charcoal fires and his dust-mite-infested feather bed undoubtedly played a major role in his recovery. It is highly unlikely that Cardano made the connection between the Archbishop's asthma and an allergic reaction to his bedding as the discovery that specific allergens such as dust mites could trigger asthma was still centuries away. Cardano's approach to the treatment of asthma was the forerunner of proper environmental control and holistic medicine, as it addressed all aspects of the Archbishop's daily lifestyle. After the Archbishop's asthmatic condition dramatically improved, Cardano left Edinburgh after having spent 75 days with one very grateful patient.

## Renaissance Medicine

Beginning in the fourteenth century, the Renaissance or rebirth of science and culture began in Italy. The stagnant medical thinking of the Dark Ages was replaced by a revival in learning and scientific writing that gradually spread to Western Europe. In the era of da Vinci, Michelangelo and Descartes, medical researchers began to focus on the causes of respiratory diseases such as asthma.

The German physician Georgius Agricola (1494–1541) was the first to associate environmental pollution with pulmonary disease.

Agricola wrote a text on mining that made several references to occupational pulmonary disease caused by coal dust. In 1565 Leonardo Botallo (1519–1587), a Frenchman born in Italy who studied at the University of Pavia, described a group of symptoms (headache, sneezing and itchy nose) that occurred when roses bloomed. He called this condition rose catarrh.

> *"I know men in health who directly after the odor of roses have a severe reaction from this, so that they have a headache or it causes sneezing, or induces a troublesome itch in the nostrils that they can not for a space of two days, restrain themselves from rubbing."*

One of the more interesting Renaissance physicians was Jean Baptiste van Helmont (1577–1644), who came from Brussels. He was the first of many doctors in this era to write extensively on asthma. One of van Helmont's most accurate portrayals of asthma linked asthma to dust and seafood allergy. He described the case of

> *"A certain monk of the order of St. Francis who is busied in pulling down Houses or Temples. And forthwith as oft as any place is Swept, or the Wind doth otherwise stir up the Dust, he presently falls down, being almost choaked. This monk also had asthma when he eateth Fishes fried with Oyl for he presently falls down, being deprived of Breathing, so as that he is scarce distinguished from a strangled man."*

Van Helmont also described a man with seasonal catarrh and chest congestion (summer asthma), and noted that the man's mother and sister suffered from the same affliction. These early investigators failed to make the connection between wind-borne tree and grass pollen and summer asthma or rose catarrh. By the end of the eighteenth century, rose catarrh was thought to be an aristocratic disease, as it was most often diagnosed amongst the upper classes. This may be the first clue supporting the hygiene hypothesis, as the aristocrats of this era obviously led cleaner lives than the peasantry. The terms rose catarrh or "peach cold" were eventually replaced by the term "hay fever" at the end of the eighteenth century, when it was found that new-mown hay was a major cause of catarrh symptoms. This is a much more accurate name, as rose fever or rose catarrh has nothing to do with roses which just happen to bloom when grasses begin to pollinate.

In the seventeenth century, England's Sir Thomas Willis finally dispelled the erroneous anatomic belief that evil vapors traveled from the brain to the lung. Willis, who excelled in the description of various clinical conditions and human anatomy, is best known to students of anatomy for his description of the Circle of Willis, the arterial arrangement at the base of the brain. Willis wrote that the bronchial obstruction in the lungs resulted from thick and viscid humors, purulent matter, thickened blood, abscess, hard tumors or stones that were implanted in the airways. In 1674, Willis described the bronchospasm of asthma.

> *"Asthma is sometimes simple from the beginning that after some time, when the condition deteriorates, it may be concluded that in every inveterate Asthma to be a mixt affection, stirr'd up by the default partly of the Lungs ill fram'd, and partly by default of the Nerves and nervous fibres appertaining to the breathing parts."*

Willis believed that whatever caused the blood to boil, such as a violent motion of the body (exercise), anger (stress), excessive outside cold or heat, *"vini potus"* (strong wine and sex) or *"meriis Lecti calor"* (the mere heat of the bed), could trigger an asthma attack. Willis thought that nocturnal asthma could be explained by overheating of the blood by one's bedclothes. He advised his patients to sleep on a chair. Besides prescribing beer with wormwood as a morning drink, Willis was the first to treat asthma with an elixir of coffee prepared with sage.

The first English monograph on asthma, *A Treatise of the Asthma* by John Floyer, was published in London in 1698. Floyer, himself an asthmatic, classified asthma into two types, periodic and continued.

> *"When the Muscles labour much for Inspiration and Expiration or compression of the Bronchia… we properly call this a Difficulty of Breath, but if this Difficulty be by the Constriction of the Bronchia, 'tis properly the Periodic Asthma. And if the constriction be great, it is with Wheezing; but if less, the Wheeziness is not so evident."*

Floyer listed various asthma triggers, including exercise, weather changes, air pollution, tobacco, certain occupations, infections, the passions (emotions) and dietary factors. He advocated avoiding a "mucilaginous" diet and forbade the consumption of fish, legumes and milk, as he correctly believed that many foodstuffs thickened mucus or phlegm. Floyer vividly described his own nocturnal asthma attacks.

> *"I have omitted to mention this, that my Fits never seize me but in the Night, and then awake me with a Heaviness, and so grow worse and worse immediately. At first waking, about one or two of the Clock in the Night, the Fit of the Asthma more evidently begins, the Breath is very slow, but after a little time, more strait; the Diaphragme seems stiff, and tied or drawn up by the Mediastinum… The Asthmatic is immediately necessitated to rise out of his Bed, and sit in an erect Posture."*

## *The Eighteenth Century*

The most significant eighteenth-century asthma book was written by Benardino Ramazzini, a professor of medicine at the University of Padua in Italy. Ramazzini, widely recognized as the father of occupational medicine, drew attention to the irritant effect of organic dusts that caused both shortness of breath and hives among grain workers. He described the pulmonary consequences of many trades and professions, and reported cases of asthma in handlers of old mattresses and old clothing—both probably infested with dust mites. Due to advances in anatomy and neurology, a better understanding of the nervous system evolved during the eighteenth century. Some physicians overshot the mark. William Cullen went so far as to state that most diseases were caused by either too much or too little nervous tone, a pathologic condition that he called a "neurosis." Cullen considered neurosis to be an affliction of sense and motion that was not accompanied by pyrexia (fever) and that had no localized organic defect. Neurotic conditions were therefore considered to be functional as opposed to organic in nature. Diseases placed in this neurotic category included hysteria, tetanus, colic, epilepsy and asthma. Cullen's model of neurosis persisted well into the twentieth century. Cullen was among the first physicians to realize the potential for near-fatal and fatal asthma attacks.

> *"A feeling of breathing, returning at intervals, with a sense of straitness in the breast, respiration performed with a wheezing noise at the beginning of a paroxysm, a distressing cough, sometimes more, but towards the end easy and free, often with a copious discharge of phlegm. The asthma, though often threatening immediate death,*

*seldom occasions it, and many persons have lived under this disease. In many cases, however, it does prove fatal; sometimes very quickly and perhaps always at length."*

## Sarah and James

The field of asthma and allergy took another step forward in the nineteenth century, when the term "immunology" came into being. Immunology comes from the Latin word *immunis,* a word used to describe Romans who were exempt from taxes, military service and civic duties. One approach to the treatment of asthma and hay fever involves the administration of allergy vaccines that program the immune system to become less allergic.

The origin of vaccination or immunotherapy dates back to the late eighteenth century, when vaccine therapy was pioneered by Doctor Edward Jenner (1749–1823). One of mankind's most deadly diseases in that era was smallpox, a highly contagious disease that

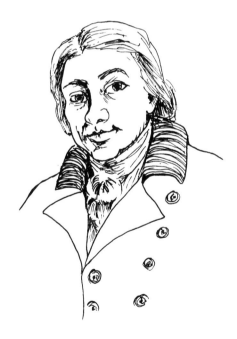

Edward Jenner

disfigured and killed tens of thousands of people each year. Jenner, an English physician born in Berkeley, England, grew up in an era where physicians either trained at prestigious universities like Oxford and Cambridge or took less desirable apprenticeships with apothecaries (pharmacists) or surgeons. This was the modern-day equivalent of the "town and gown" approach to medicine. At the young age of 13, Jenner, a country boy with no shot at Oxford or Cambridge, was apprenticed to a local surgeon. During his apprenticeship Jenner met a young farm girl who told him she was immune to smallpox because she had experienced cowpox, a similar, but milder disease, while she was growing up on a farm.

After completing his apprenticeship, Jenner moved to London to train with Doctor John Hunter, a prominent London surgeon. Under Hunter's tutelage, Jenner became a first-rate researcher and was widely published. In 1773, he returned home to open a country practice in Berkeley. Jenner again observed that cowpox infection appeared to protect individuals from smallpox. Jenner then theorized that deliberate exposure to cowpox might prevent smallpox. In 1793 he left practice to pursue his dream of curing smallpox. What follows is perhaps one of the greatest clinical experiments of all time.

In May 1796, Jenner treated Sarah Nelmes, a young dairymaid who had fresh cowpox lesions on her finger. On May 14, 1796, he took some fluid from Sarah's cowpox lesions and deliberately injected the cowpox fluid into eight-year-old James Phipps, who promptly developed a mild fever and a local lesion at the site of the cowpox inoculation. Six weeks later Jenner deliberately inoculated Phipps with smallpox and no disease developed. The Royal Society of Medicine promptly rejected Jenner's paper describing the results of this daring experiment. Jenner became the subject of scorn and ridicule. After collecting additional cases, he published his findings in a small book and coined the word "vaccination," a derivative of the Latin word *vacca* or cow. Once Jenner's vaccination techniques gained worldwide acceptance throughout the European continent and America, the death rate from smallpox quickly plummeted. Jenner received little or no personal gain for his discovery, and his personal finances suffered greatly. The English Parliament eventually voted him a princely sum of 30,000 pounds. Jenner, one of the truly great benefactors of humanity, retired to Berkeley, where he died in 1823.

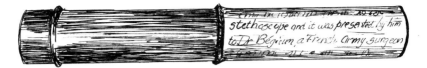

Laënnec's Stethoscope

In 1816, the great French clinician, Réné T. H. Laënnec (1781–1826), made an immense contribution to the nature and diagnosis of asthma and all respiratory diseases when he invented the stethoscope. Laënnec confirmed that bronchospasm was an essential component of asthma, and correctly noted that contraction of the bronchial smooth muscle fibers strangled the airway and prevented the entry of air into the lung. In 1852 an American physician, John Sweet (1808–1854), extended Laënnec's observations in his writings and lectures at the New York hospital.

> *"The spasms of the bronchii play a most important part in the paroxysm of chronic asthma...there can be no doubt that the bronchial inflammation is the principal inciting cause of the paroxysm...a very moderate exposure to cold and dampness, and even a mere change in weather...will irritate the bronchii to spasm."*

## Hay Fever

The discovery of pollen lodged in rocks millions of years old and in the graves of Neanderthals who lived in Iraq 50,000 years ago proves that man has been exposed to pollen since prehistoric times. In 1819, John Bostok (1773–1846), a native of Liverpool, England, and a graduate of the University of Edinburgh, wrote his classic description of his own hay fever and asthma, which he called *"summer catarrh."* Bostok suffered from nasal and eye symptoms in childhood, and in his teens developed asthma.

> *"About the beginning of every June in every year...a sensation of heat and fullness is experienced in the eyes...after this state of the eyes has subsided a general fullness is experienced in the head... producing fits of extreme violence... to the sneezing are added a further sensation of tightness in the chest, and difficulty of*

*breathing…a feeling of want of room to receive the air necessary for respiration. Since the attention of the public has been turned to the subject, an idea has generally prevailed, that it is produced by the effluvium from new hay, and it has hence obtained the popular name of the hay-fever."*

In 1831, John Elliotson (1791–1868), also a graduate of the University of Edinburgh, noted that some of the nobility have the highest order of hay fever, and he compiled a list of all the aristocrats who had the condition. An American, George Miller Bard (1839–1883), also believed that hay fever was a condition of the privileged classes when he wrote, *"Hay fever is a disease of the fashionable and thoughtful—the price of wealth and culture, a part of the penalty of a fine organization and indoor life."*

The connection between ragweed and hay fever was made by an American physician, Morril Wyman (1812–1903), who sniffed Roman wormwood, or ragweed pollen, to induce an attack of hay fever. In his lectures at Harvard Medical School and in his book, *Autumnal Catarrh,* Wyman correctly noted that this ragweed hay fever was unique to North America. At that time ragweed did not grow in Europe as it does now.

Charles Blackley (1820–1900), a British engraver and printer who entered the Royal College of Surgeons at the age of 38, was a general practitioner who researched his own asthma and hay fever. Blackley spent several years conducting experiments on himself, as he could not find any clinical subjects willing to suffer hay fever or asthma attacks. In those days there were no drug companies to fund clinical research studies and reimburse clinical subjects. Blackley's contributions were immense. He was the first researcher to link grass pollen to asthma and hay fever, which he called *"Catarrhus Aestivus,"* meaning hay fever or hay asthma. In his study of pollens Blackley designed and set up the first pollen-collecting devices to record daily pollen counts. He also rubbed pollen into his eyes and skin and noted the hive-like reaction that followed. This experiment was the forerunner of allergy skin tests. Lastly, Blackley's most important contribution was the observation that asthma and hay fever attacks had two phases—an early phase and a late phase response. As previously discussed, this classic discovery is the basic foundation of drug therapy in asthma and allergic disease in the twenty-first century.

In 1830, John Eberle made the first significant American contribution to asthma. His popular textbook, *A Treatise on the Practice of Medicine,* reviewed what was then known about asthma and listed atmospheric conditions, inhalation of offensive vapors and dietary indiscretions as triggering factors. Charles Turner Thackrah wrote one of the classic works on occupational medicine when he described coffee roasters who developed asthma only after being at their jobs for several years. Other occupations Thackrah associated with asthma included feather dressers, corn millers, snuff makers, flax spinners, dressers of cloth, rag sorters, miners, grinders, masons, machine workers and woodworkers.

In 1860, Henry Hyde Salter (1823–1871) of England provided the first accurate description of the causes and treatment of asthma. The author of one of the more popular nineteenth-century books on asthma, Salter was yet another physician who suffered from asthma himself. Salter was aware of the hereditary nature of this condition, and also stressed the role of emotions in asthma. He believed asthma was a form of *"perverted nervous action and exclusively, a nervous disease."*

The observation that asthma had psychological triggers may have been colored by Salter's personal experiences with hundreds of patients. Salter classified asthma into two main types: idiopathic or spasmodic and symptomatic. Although the pathway of allergy-induced asthma had yet to be discovered, Salter was among the first to point out that animal and vegetable particles of cats, rabbits, horses, wild beasts, guinea pigs, dogs, cattle, hay and grass could trigger asthma attacks. He believed a nervous reflux reaction to these substances triggered bronchospasm. Salter also listed a number of foods that could give rise to asthma attacks. Salter was certain that sleep favored asthma. He advised his patients to get out of bed at the very onset of an attack; realizing that this may be difficult, he emphasized *"but he must do it."* Salter knew that asthma was not only *"superlatively distressing"* but when it came to treatment, it was *"peculiarly and proverbially intractable."* Salter admitted *"the remedies for asthma are of very irregular and uncertain operation."* Salter was the first to focus on the concept of bronchial hyper-responsiveness, a theme that was to occupy investigators in the field of respiratory medicine for the next 200 years. Salter conveys the plight of a suffering asthmatic:

*"Paroxysmal dyspnoea [shortness of breath] of a peculiar character, generally periodic with intervals of healthy respiration between the attacks. It was not an uncommon disease and it is one of the direst suffering; the horrors of the asthmatic paroxysm far exceed any acute bodily pain; the sense of impending suffocation, the agonizing struggle for the breath of life, are so terrible, that they cannot even be witnessed without sharing in the sufferer's distress. Asthma never kills; at least I have never seen a case in which a paroxysm proved fatal and if asthma kills, it always does so by producing organic changes in the heart or lungs, or both."*

One of Salter's humorous anecdotes reminds me of my own experiences with my son.

*"Lately I meet with another case, in which I was told that when the asthmatic was a little boy, he found in his disease a convenient immunity from correction. 'Don't scold me,' he would say if he had incurred his father's displeasure, 'or I shall have the asthma,' and so he would: his fears were as correct as they were convenient."*

Armand Trousseau (1801–1867), one of the foremost French clinicians of his time, is yet another physician who suffered from asthma. He defined idiopathic asthma as a common condition that was rarely seen in hospitals and presented itself as paroxysms of dyspnea and oppression. Trousseau vividly describes the patient with a nocturnal asthma.

*"Thus, an individual in perfect health goes to bed feeling as well as usual, and drops off quietly to sleep, but after an hour or two, he is suddenly awakened by a most distressing attack of dyspnoea. He feels as though his chest were constricted and compressed, and has a sense of considerable distress; he breathes with difficulty, and his inspiration is accompanied by a laryngotracheal whistling sound. The dyspnoea and sense of anxiety increasing, he sits up, rests on his hands, with his arms put back while his face is turgid, occasionally livid, red, or bluish, his eyes prominent, and his skin bedewed with perspiration. He is soon obliged to jump off his bed, and if the room in which he sleeps be not very lofty, he hastens to throw his window open in search of air. Fresh air, playing freely about, relieves him. Yet the fit lasts one or two hours or more, and then terminates."*

Other patients with nocturnal asthma fared worse, for they may have been

> *"obliged to sleep in the most varied and sometimes the queerest attitudes. Sometimes, he can only find sleep by kneeling on his bed and resting his head on his knees, or by spending the night in an armchair, or by propping himself up in bed in the sitting posture; sometimes again, he can only sleep standing, resting on a piece of furniture or on the mantelpiece."*

Trousseau used traditional remedies such as a large flying blister pack to be applied to the whole chest immediately; ipecac, given in emetic (vomiting-inducing) doses; belladonna or atropine, followed by the administration of spirits of turpentine. For his own asthma, like Salter, he too smoked tobacco: *"I am not an habitual smoker, but I then had a cigar, and took a few puffs; in eight or ten minutes the paroxysm was over."*

After the British Army invaded India in the nineteenth century, the smoking of stramonium leaves was brought back to Western Europe as a treatment for asthma. Stramonium, a mild anticholinergic bronchodilating chemical extracted from the smoke of the burning leaves of the thorn apple tree, was the forerunner of the two anticholinergic drugs (Atrovent and Combivent) used today in bronchitis and asthma therapy. Trousseau stated that of all the remedies that have been tried in asthma, stramonium was the best. He pointed out, however, that not all asthmatics were relieved and,

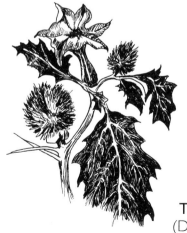

**Thorne Apple Tree**
(Datúta Stramónium)

in particular, habitual tobacco smokers seldom derived any benefit from stramonium treatment.

Trousseau employed herbal remedies for asthma, and recommended using the dried and pulverized roots of *Datura ferox*, another folk medicine from India. In Trousseau's opinion, asthma was *"a special and complete disorder, a manifestation, a peculiar form of a general complaint, having very variable local expressions, sometimes giving rise to paroxysms of dyspnoea, of oppression at the chest, to a curious kind of coryza, and to peculiar catarrhal attacks."* Strangely enough, Trousseau did not consider asthma to be potentially life threatening, as he described asthma as *"le brevet de longue vie"* or the certificate of a long life.

During the last three decades of the nineteenth century, more science was introduced to the understanding of asthma. The invention of the microscope allowed researchers to closely study the sputum or phlegm of asthmatic patients. Mucus viewed under the microscope revealed the presence of pointed crystals, called Charcot-Leyden crystals. These striking crystals were initially thought to cause an asthmatic attack by exerting a local mechanical irritant effect on the bronchial mucosa. This led one adventurous investigator to unsuccessfully attempt to reproduce asthma by introducing powdered glass into the airways of experimental animals.

In 1877, Paul Ehrlich, while still in medical school, discovered a white blood cell that had a striking affinity for the dye called eosin, and he named this unusual cell the eosinophil. When Ehrlich found high levels of eosinophils in the lungs of asthma sufferers, it became apparent that this fascinating cell was closely linked to asthma.

## The Twentieth Century

While the discoveries and observations of the nineteenth century set the stage, real advances in the fields of allergy and immunology did not begin until the twentieth century. The father of immunology is considered to be the Russian bacteriologist, Emil Adolph von Behring (1854–1917). In 1901, von Behring was awarded the Nobel Prize for his work with the Japanese physician Shibasauro Kitasato (1856–1931). These two investigators studied the immune response to tetanus and diphtheria. In 1890, they used the term "hypersensitivity reaction" to describe the reaction following immunization to

66

diphtheria and tetanus toxins. At the turn of the twentieth century, Sir Henry Dale (1875–1968) recorded the action of histamine on smooth muscle and defined the role of histamine in anaphylaxis or allergic reactions. Ultimately Dale was knighted for his contributions and shared the Nobel Prize in 1936. His important discovery of histamine set the stage for the identification of other mediators of inflammation.

The most famous physician in the world in the early part of the twentieth century was Sir William Osler (1849–1919). Born in Canada and trained at McGill University Medical School, Osler accepted an invitation to become the first Professor of Medicine at the newly formed medical school at Johns Hopkins University in Baltimore, Maryland. In the early days of this soon-to-be world-famous institution, there were few students to teach and Osler had ample time to write his medical textbook, *The Principles and Practice of Medicine.* This text ultimately became the most authoritative medical reference source for many decades. Unfortunately, Osler's discussion on asthma is quite brief. He astutely observed the similarity of hay fever and asthma: *"…these diseases have the same origin and differ only in site."*

Osler defined asthma as a neurotic affection, characterized by *"hyperaemia and turgescence of the mucosa of the smaller bronchial tubes and a peculiar exudate of mucin."* Unfortunately, Osler's use of the adjective, neurotic, left a stigma attached to asthma that persists even today. Osler accepted the prevailing views of his day that asthma could be induced by reflex influences from the stomach, intestines or genital organs, and that flatulence and passage of a large quantity of urine were premonitory sensations of asthma.

Osler added to the myth that asthma was never fatal, claiming that *"death during the attack is unknown."* He did emphasize that the asthmatic attack demanded immediate and prompt treatment with the usual range of sedative and antispasmodic medicines, such as belladonna, henbane, stramonium and lobelia, sometimes administered as cigarettes. Osler also recommended, *"Perles of nitrite of amyl broken on the handkerchief and a dose of spirits of chloroform in hot whisky."* Osler was of the opinion that more permanent relief was given by the hypodermic injection of morphia (morphine) or morphia and cocaine combined. Osler considered the use of compressed air in the pneumatic cabinet also beneficial, as were oxygen inhalations. His favorite asthma prophylactic was iodide of potassium, which he gave three times a day. Osler did not allow his patients to eat carbohydrates, because he believed they produced flatulence that induced asthma attacks. Coffee was also thought to be a more suitable drink than tea, but Osler did not list it as a remedy.

## A Specialty Is Born

Rapid discoveries in science and medicine in the early part of the twentieth century, leading to a greater understanding of asthma and allergic diseases, ultimately created the specialty of allergy and immunology. In 1901, two pioneer immunologists from the University of Paris, Paul Portier and Charles Richet, were asked by Prince Alfred of Monaco to develop a protective serum for vacationing bathers who were frequently stung by the Portuguese man-o-war jellyfish while swimming in the Mediterranean Sea. Prince Alfred was an amateur oceanographer, an avid scientist and a supporter of medical research.

While cruising on the Prince's ship in the Mediterranean Sea, Portier and Richet attempted to induce tolerance or immunity by injecting animals with the potent jellyfish toxin. Fortunately for man, Portier and Richet chose to use dogs in their early clinical trials. When the dogs received a second and subsequent injection of the jellyfish toxin, they experienced severe, often fatal reactions. Thus, instead of protecting the dogs against the jellyfish toxin, re-injection made the dogs more allergic to the toxin. Portier and Richet promptly coined the term anaphylaxis, which is derived from the Greek word *ana* (backward) plus *phylaxis* (protection), or "against protection." Richet was awarded the Nobel Prize in Medicine in 1913 for this important contribution.

Drs. Milton Rosenau and John Anderson, from the U.S. Public Health Hospital in Washington, D.C. (the forerunner of the National Institutes of Health), set about to study why some humans who received diphtheria or tetanus vaccine died immediately after a vaccine injection. Their research discovered that guinea pigs injected with antitoxins against diphtheria and tetanus prepared from horse serum developed acute allergic or anaphylactic reactions due to sensitization to the horse serum protein.

Clemens von Pirquet (1874–1929), an Austrian pediatrician, and his associate, Bela Schick (1877–1967), a Hungarian pediatrician, observed that many patients who were injected with diphtheria antitoxin derived from horse serum developed hives and asthma when they received a second and smaller dose of the antitoxin. Von Pirquet deduced that the immune system was producing antibodies to the injected antigen or horse serum, and he called this reaction a "hypersensitivity reaction." In 1907, von Pirquet suggested that the term anaphylaxis was not accurate, and he left his mark in medical history when he coined the term "allergy," a derivative of the Greek word *allos* or other and *ergos* meaning work or activity. Thus, the term allergy describes a changed state and altered activity to a foreign substance after a previous exposure to the offending substance.

In the following year, Alfred Wolff-Eisner (1877–1948) suggested that hay fever was an allergic or anaphylactic phenomenon when he described 90 asthmatic patients who developed an acute allergic reaction in the eye after a pollen suspension was dropped into the eye. In 1911, Drs. Leonard Noon (1878–1913) and John Freeman (1877–1962) from St. Mary's Hospital in London, introduced specific allergy skin testing, using an extract of grass pollen. The diagnosis of grass-pollen-induced hay fever soon led to attempts at specific desensitization by injecting patients with grass pollen allergen. Such desensitization injections are known today as immunotherapy.

In 1918, Doctor Francis Rackerman, a Boston physician, realized that not all asthmatics had skin sensitivity to tested allergens. He proposed a new classification of asthma based on skin-test responses, and introduced the terms intrinsic and extrinsic asthma. Patients with extrinsic asthma had positive skin tests, while those with intrinsic asthma had negative skin tests. In 1919, Maximilian Ramirez (1891–1946), an American physician, suggested that substances in the blood called anaphylactic or reaction antibodies might cause allergic reactions. In this fascinating paper, Ramirez described how a 35-year-old Greek waiter from New York City became sensitized to horsehair after he received a blood transfusion from a donor who was allergic to horses. After receiving the transfusion, the waiter suffered his first asthmatic attack during a horse carriage ride in Central Park. Ramirez correctly postulated that something in the transfused blood, possibly a protein or reaction antibody, was transfused into the waiter and made him allergic to horses.

This observation was followed up by experiments of two German physicians, Drs. Carl Prausnitz (1876–1963) and D. Heinz Kustner (1897–1963), who both suffered from allergies. Prausnitz had hay fever and Kustner was allergic to codfish. They were able to transfer their specific allergy to each other by injecting themselves with samples of their own serum. Thus, something in their serum was passively exchanged or transferred from one doctor to the other. This famous experiment became known as the passive transfer or the P-K reaction. The noted German-born allergist and immunologist Max Samter (1908–1999), who later emigrated to the United States, while an intern in Berlin first tested the response to inhaling histamine into bronchial tubes in 1933. Samter's work represented the first example of bronchoprovocation testing.

In 1923, the specialty of allergy took another major step forward when American physicians, A. F. Coca (1875–1959) and R. A. Cooke (1880–1960) refined the term "allergy" when they introduced the term "atopy" to describe a group of diseases characterized by abnormal reactivity to normally harmless substances. Atopy is dependent upon a hereditary predisposition to develop allergic diseases such as asthma, eczema and hay fever. Atopic or allergic individuals carried a sensitizing protein or antibody, which was labeled the "reaginic" antibody. Coca and Cooke founded the first allergy clinic in the United States at the New York Hospital in New York City which trained a whole new generation of allergy researchers who uncovered the mechanisms of the allergic-immune response.

Amazingly, the discovery of the true nature of this reaginic antibody took nearly six decades. In the late 1960s, Drs. S. Johansson (b. 1938) and H. Bennich (b. 1930) from Sweden found a unique antibody or immunoglobulin in a patient with multiple myeloma that they labeled IgND—ND being the initials of the patient with this newly discovered protein. IgND was found to be identical to the allergic or reaginic antibody. Subsequent studies found that patients with asthma and hay fever had very high levels of this antibody. Drs. Kimshige Ishizaka (b. 1925) and Teruko Ishizaka (b. 1926), Japanese-born American researchers at the Children's Asthma Research Institute in Denver, Colorado, also isolated the same antibody from a ragweed-sensitive patient. In 1968, Johansson's group met with the Ishizakas and, realizing that they had been studying the same antibody, agreed to call it immunoglobulin E or IgE antibody.

In addition, British researcher, D. R. Stanworth (b. 1928), independently discovered the same substance.

Once asthma and allergic diseases were recognized as having an allergic or true immunologic basis, research took on new dimensions. Investigators began searching for offending allergens, such as dust mites, animal danders, pollen grains, fungal spores, chemicals and drugs that could trigger asthma. Wilhelm Storm van Leeuwen (1882–1933) discovered that pollen grains and mold spores were common allergens. He correctly suggested that enclosing asthmatic patients in an allergen-proof chamber or taking them to high altitudes would reduce their allergy symptoms.

In 1928, R. A. Kern first speculated that certain mite insects could trigger asthma. However, it was four decades before Doctors F. Spieksma and R. Voorhorst from the University of Leiden in Holland identified the house dust mite as the major offending allergen in house dust. One important mediator, discovered in 1940, was a substance called slow-reacting substance of anaphylaxis, abbreviated SRS-A. Dissection of this SRS-A chemical led to the discovery of the asthma-inducing leukotriene chemicals, that eventually produced a whole new group of anti-leukotriene drugs in the 1990s.

Thus, from the time of Hippocrates, asthma theory has gone from the concept of evil humors flowing from the brain to the lung to highly sophisticated research discoveries in the fields of genetics, allergy, immunology and pharmacology. The important breakthroughs of the late twentieth and early twenty-first centuries in drug therapy, environmental controls and immunotherapy will be reviewed in the chapters devoted to those subjects.

# How Doctors **Diagnose** Asthma

# 5

**A**sthma is usually not a very difficult disease to diagnose. The major symptoms of asthma are cough, shortness of breath, chest tightness and wheezing. These symptoms are quite variable and are often triggered by the common cold; viral respiratory infections; vigorous exercise, especially in cold air; exposure to allergens when dusting or vacuuming or exposure to household pets. Other triggers include pollens, foods, chemicals and air pollutants. Symptoms often interfere with sleep. Wheezing is the cardinal symptom of asthma, and in one study of patients with a variety of heart and lung disorders, wheezing was named as the major symptom by more than 90 percent of patients with asthma.

## The Medical History

What happens during your first visit to a doctor or health-care provider for suspected asthma? First and foremost, the doctor should take a detailed medical history, often with the aid of a written questionnaire. The doctor will ask you to describe your symptoms, when they began, what makes them better or worse, and what medications relieve symptoms. He or she will inquire about seasonal patterns, smoking habits, effects of exercise or cold air and exposure to polluted air. The pattern of symptoms provides important clues. Seasonal flare-ups suggest pollen allergy, whereas year-round symptoms are more common with dust mite, cockroach and animal allergy. Nocturnal or early morning symptoms suggest allergen exposure in the bedroom—dust mites in a mattress or feathers and molds in a pillow. Headaches, nocturnal cough, throat clearing or foul breath may signal a chronic sinus condition. Frequent heartburn and indigestion suggests the presence of gastroesophageal reflux disease, or GERD. The doctor should inquire whether you have any other conditions closely associated with asthma, such as hay fever, eczema or allergic reactions to foods or drugs. He or she will want to know if you have repeated bouts of ear or sinus infections, nosebleeds or a loss of smell or taste.

The environmental history focuses on potential asthma triggers in your home, school and workplace. It should cover the age and location of the home, the type of heat and air conditioning system, the presence of a fireplace or wood burning stove, whether there is a basement, the use of central or room humidifiers and/or air conditioners and the proximity of nearby industry or sources of air pollution. The doctor will probably ask you to describe whether the home is damp, and report present or past water damage.

Additional questions should ask about the patient's bedroom, including the location of the bedroom, whether pets are allowed in the room, the type of pillow and mattress and whether dust mite-impermeable covers are used on the pillow, mattress and box spring of all beds in the room. The doctor should inquire about the presence of dust catchers such as stuffed animals, wall-to-wall carpeting, upholstered furniture, books and drapes. Further history should include questions about the school or work environment, and any other locations where the patient spends a significant amount of time. The doctor should also review the results of any previous treatment or tests, including skin tests, blood tests and X-ray studies.

## The Physical Examination

The next step in your office visit is the physical examination, which will focus on your skin, eyes, ears, nose, throat and chest. The doctor will look at your skin for signs of eczema or hives. Inflammation in your eyes may signify an underlying eye allergy or allergic conjunctivitis. Dark circles under the eyes, called "allergic shiners," or swelling in the nose are both telltale signs of allergic rhinitis or hay fever, often associated with asthma. The chest exam is the most important part of the physical examination. The doctor will rely on the stethoscope to detect wheezing and gauge the rate of air movement in and out of your chest. The doctor may ask you to take a deep breath or briefly exercise to make it easier to detect wheezing. An astute asthma doctor can often diagnose asthma by just looking at a patient's chest and observing what is called the barrel-chest deformity. When patients with chronic asthma constantly use their chest and rib muscles to move air in and out of their lungs, their chest wall is stretched to the limit, and it expands, giving the chest a barrel-like shape. In an asymptomatic patient, however, the physical examination may be completely normal. In those cases the history will yield critical information.

## Laboratory Tests

The next part of the evaluation involves laboratory testing. Commonly performed tests include a nasal or a sputum smear, where mucus from the nose or chest is examined under a microscope in the search for an excess amount of eosinophils, the telltale allergy blood cell. Eosinophils are the hallmark of asthma or an ongoing allergic reaction, and are increased in numbers in asthma and allergic diseases. Eosinophils usually comprise three to four percent of all white blood cells in your body. The level of eosinophils in your body, measured by a blood test called the total eosinophil count, often parallels the severity of asthma. Other diagnostic tests the doctor may order include a sweat test to rule out the possibility of cystic fibrosis, serum immunoglobulins to rule out an immunodeficiency disease, and intraesophageal pH monitoring or a barium swallow study to determine the presence of reflux or GERD.

## The IgE Test

One important blood test in your initial evaluation is the serum IgE test, which measures the amount of allergic or IgE antibody in your body. A high IgE level indicates that allergies may be playing an important role in your asthma. This test often helps to predict if an infant or a young child will ever develop allergies, as the IgE level may be elevated years before asthma or hay fever symptoms begin. The presence of asthma is closely related to the IgE level. A study of health and development in 562 children in New Zealand by Doctor Malcolm Sears disclosed that young boys had more asthma than girls, and the prevalence of asthma was directly related to the serum IgE level. No asthma was found in children with IgE levels less than 32 units, whereas more than one-third of those with high IgE levels had asthma. The higher the IgE level, the greater the chance that the child had asthma. Although a high serum IgE level is often seen in the allergic or asthmatic patient, a normal IgE level does not rule out allergy. Likewise, a high IgE level does not always predict allergic asthma.

## *Breathing Tests*

Pulmonary function studies, called spirometry or lung function tests, are breathing tests that measure your lung capacity. In a breathing test, you breathe into a closed tube connected to a machine which measures how much air you can expel from your lungs in one single breath (lung capacity) and how fast you can expel it (Figure 5.1). The key measurement in asthma is the amount of air you can blow out in one second. This is called the FeV1, or one second vital capacity. Measurement of the FeV1 is a more sensitive way to detect airway

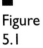
Figure
5.1

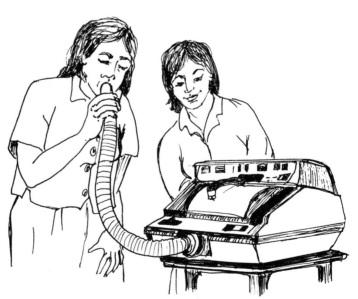

**Lung Function Test**

obstruction than the clinical history or the physical examination. Many patients are "poor perceivers" of their asthma symptoms. This means they are unable to sense airway obstruction until their lungs are functioning at a very low level. Thus, spirometry or lung function tests should be done in all patients in whom the diagnosis of asthma is being considered. The initial assessment of lung function helps to determine the severity of the asthma and outline an asthma treatment program. When the first set of breathing tests are abnormal, you may be asked to inhale a quick-acting bronchodilator drug and repeat the breathing test. If the second test shows more than a fifteen percent improvement in the FeV1, the diagnosis of asthma is almost a certainty. Follow-up measurements of lung function will reflect the progression of asthma and response to therapy.

Machines that measure lung functions range from relatively inexpensive devices or spirometers to sophisticated high-tech computerized equipment that records all facets of lung function. Any doctor that treats persistent asthma should use some sort of spirometer machine to diagnose and follow the progress of patients with asthma. The 1997 NIH asthma guidelines state "spirometry is the gold standard for the diagnosis and management of asthma."

## The Peak Flow Meter

It is now possible for people with asthma to monitor their own lung functions at home with small, inexpensive, portable pulmonary function devices called peak flow meters. These peak flow meters measure how fast you can expel air from your lungs. They are very helpful in detecting the early stages of an asthma relapse, and helping a person determine if substances in the home or workplace are triggering asthma. The peak flow meter plays a pivotal role in helping patients adhere to the new asthma guidelines' step-up and step-down approach to asthma drug therapy. The proper use of the peak flow meter will be thoroughly covered in chapter twenty-seven.

## Allergy Skin Tests

When the medical history, physical exam or blood tests suggest that allergens may be triggering asthma, skin testing is indicated. What are skin tests? In 1873, Doctor Charles Blackley discovered the cause of his own hay fever when he scratched a small amount of grass pollen on his skin and produced a small hive-like reaction at the test site. Amazingly, basic skin test techniques have changed very little since Blackley's century-old observation.

There are three basic types of skin tests: the prick or puncture, scratch, and intradermal test. In the prick test, the test antigen or allergen is placed on top of the skin, and the skin is pricked through the drop. In a scratch test, the skin is lightly scratched, and a drop of the test allergen is placed onto the scratched area. The weaker scratch or prick tests are done first, to minimize the chances of triggering a dangerous allergic reaction.

When the scratch or prick tests are negative, a stronger intradermal test is administered. In the intradermal test, allergen is injected beneath the skin with a very small needle. When you have an allergic or IgE antibody to the test allergen, the antigen combines with the IgE antibody and a wheal and flare reaction will develop at the test site. The flare refers to the redness, and the wheal is the white center in the middle of the redness. Actually, a small hive is produced. The size of the skin test often reflects the level of sensitivity to the testing substance.

The older scratch test method, often a traumatic experience, especially for young children, has been replaced by the prick test method, where several allergens can be tested at the same time. One such method, called the Multi-Test, allows a panel of several allergens to be lightly placed on the skin at one time with little or no discomfort or pain to the patient (Figure 5.2). Skin tests are most helpful in identifying allergies to inhaled substances like dust mites, molds, pollens and animals. A competent allergist can determine if allergens are playing a role in your asthma by performing 50 to 60 skin tests in one or two office visits. In young children you can get by with 10 to 20 tests.

Despite their ancient origins, skin tests are a quick and accurate way to determine the presence of allergy. As the clinical history is a poor predictor of skin test reactivity, I perform skin tests in all new patients with asthma. They are relatively inexpensive on a cost-per-test basis, and are very safe when carried out under the supervision of a knowledgeable physician experienced in allergy skin testing.

Figure
5.2

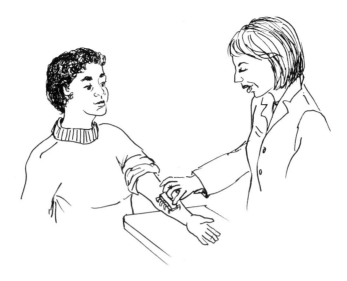

## *Allergy Blood Tests*

It is also possible to detect allergies with a blood test known as the radioallergosorbant or RAST test. In this test a small sample of your blood is processed through an analyzer to see if your blood contains allergic or IgE antibodies to a specific allergen. RAST tests are very helpful when the doctor cannot perform skin tests because of skin eruptions, undue fear of needles or if there is a chance of inducing an allergic reaction with the skin test, as may be the case in severe peanut or tree nut allergies. While allergy blood tests are helpful, they have three major disadvantages. They are not quite as accurate as skin tests, they are ten times more expensive, and the results are not immediately available.

Allergy skin and blood tests should be properly interpreted by an allergy specialist and correlated with your clinical history. A positive test does not mean that you are having symptoms to the test substance at the time of testing, as skin tests may be positive years before symptoms begin or remain positive long after allergy symptoms have subsided. The availability of allergy blood tests has created many abuses. Allergy walk-in centers and mail-order houses falsely promise their prospective customers a quick and easy diagnosis of allergic diseases. Such clinics and labs rarely correlate the results of allergy blood tests with a thorough history or physical examination. The end result is incompetent and expensive allergy care. One famous case illustrates the problems encountered with fraudulent allergy labs. In 1985, the FDA sent a sample of cow's blood to an allergy-testing lab in California that promised a quick and easy diagnosis of food allergy. The report that came back to the FDA from this physician-run lab stated that the cow was allergic to milk! The American Academy of Allergy, Asthma & Immunology has stated that indirect or remote evaluation of allergies by blood testing labs is not conducive to good patient care.

## X-ray Studies

A chest X-ray should be obtained in all patients with recurrent respiratory symptoms in order to rule out rare lung diseases and other potential causes of airway obstruction such as congenital defects or foreign bodies. The chest X-ray findings in asthma may vary from normal to lung overinflation with scattered areas of atelectasis or a collapsed lung. Chest X-ray findings may support the diagnosis of asthma in a child who is too young to perform lung function tests. Given the association between asthma and sinusitis, a sinus X-ray should be considered in patients who have a history of persistent rhinitis, nocturnal coughing, headaches or asthma that is difficult to control. In very young children a plain sinus X-ray may suffice. In older children and adults a limited sinus CAT scan has proven to be a better tool for the diagnosis of chronic sinus disease.

## Childhood Conditions That Mimic Asthma

Before concluding that a coughing or wheezing patient has asthma, the doctor should consider other conditions that mimic asthma. The three childhood conditions most often confused with asthma are viral bronchiolitis, foreign body aspiration and cystic fibrosis. The respiratory syncytial virus, or RSV, causes bronchiolitis, a viral infection of the bronchial tubes that strikes young infants. The second childhood condition commonly confused with asthma is foreign body aspiration. This problem is more likely to occur in toddlers who have *pica,* or a habit of placing everything they touch in their mouth. The foreign body, often a toy part or a piece of food, is inhaled into the lung and lodges in the windpipe or bronchial tubes, causing a wheezing condition that looks and sounds just like asthma.

Sometimes the wheezing will localize to one side of the chest, and the child does not appear to be very ill. This is not always an easy diagnosis to make, as many plastic toy parts and food particles, like peanuts, do not show up on a routine chest X-ray. Sometimes doctors must look directly into the bronchial tubes with an instrument called a bronchoscope to find and remove the foreign body.

Cystic fibrosis is a serious disease that induces chronic intestinal and pulmonary problems that may mimic asthma. Cystic fibrosis patients suffer from recurrent infections and pneumonia, often associated with wheezing. These victims are usually very sickly and underweight, and their chest X-ray shows excessive scarring from repeated bouts of pneumonia. When cystic fibrosis is considered as a real diagnostic possibility, the doctor should order a sweat test, as cystic fibrosis patients secrete abnormally high amounts of sodium and chloride, or salt, into their skin.

## Adult Diseases That Mimic Asthma

The two adult diseases often commonly confused with asthma are chronic bronchitis and emphysema. Sometimes all three of these conditions may co-exist in the same patient. Chronic bronchitis is a disease of heavy smokers that affects the large bronchial tubes. Long-term smoking causes inflammation of the bronchial tubes, leading to an overproduction of mucus and phlegm. The typical patient with chronic bronchitis is a heavy smoker who wakes up each morning and coughs up a great deal of phlegm. Sometimes these patients wheeze a great deal, making it difficult to distinguish bronchitis from asthma.

Emphysema is another disease of smokers that can be confused with asthma. Unlike bronchitis and asthma, where the bronchial tubes are the site of the disease, emphysema involves the lung's air sacs or alveoli. In emphysema, the alveoli are slowly destroyed. The lungs lose their capacity to exchange oxygen and carbon dioxide. People with emphysema gradually become very short of breath after minimal exertion. Emphysema, unlike asthma, is a permanent lung injury, as the air sacs do not regenerate once they are destroyed. As with bronchitis, some emphysema victims have an asthmatic component to their illness and may benefit from asthma drugs. In cases where the diagnosis is uncertain, emphysema can usually be distinguished from asthma by sophisticated breathing tests and chest X-ray studies.

Many patients with cardiopulmonary disorders gradually reduce their physical acitivity. They often complain of heavy breathing with exercise yet have normal lung function tests. Over time these patients gradually reduce their activities and become "cardiovascular deconditioned" or simply out of shape. Such patients may benefit more from an exercise program than an increase in their asthma medication schedule.

## *Vocal Cord Dysfunction*

Another emerging condition that may mimic asthma is VCD or vocal cord dysfunction. VCD is a condition caused by abnormal movements of the vocal cords during inspiration and expiration. Doctor Henry Milgrom, from National Jewish Hospital in Denver, Colorado, has found that a typical patient with VCD is often a single woman between age twenty and forty with significant psychological problems. These VCD victims are often mis-diagnosed with asthma for several years. Many patients have both asthma and vocal cord dysfunction.

Common complaints in VCD are wheezing, throat tightness, voice change and difficulty inspiring. Attacks are more common in daytime and often resolve quickly. These patients can usually hold their breath despite having severe shortness of breath and difficulty speaking. Symptoms are temporarily relieved when they are distracted. VCD patients often have a history of repeated bouts of severe airway obstruction that requires frequent emergency room visits, hospitalizations and oral cortisone drugs. Their chest X-ray is usually normal, and they do not respond to the common asthma medications. The diagnosis of VCD is best established by direct examination of the vocal cords during an acute episode. The treatment of VCD combines breathing exercises, speech therapy and intense psychological counseling.

One condition that may mimic asthma or even vocal cord dysfunction is the hyperventilation or "sighing syndrome." Such patients, usually young women, complain of shortness of breath, chest pain, lightheadedness, numbness and tingling in their extremities. Physical examination, lung function and exercise tests are normal and these patients do not respond to asthma medications. Measure of arterial blood gases may show a low level of carbon dioxide that indicates these patients are overbreathing. Treatment programs may include biofeedback and psychological counseling.

## The Specialty Visit

The early symptoms of asthma—chest congestion, coughing and wheezing—usually first come to the attention of the pediatrician, internist or family doctor. Many primary care physicians are capable of treating mild or even moderate asthma. However, when asthma complicates a patient's lifestyle by interfering with school or work, limiting exercise or causing frequent visits to the doctor's office or emergency room, the expertise of an asthma specialist may be required. Two types of doctors are experts in the care of asthma, the allergist-immunologist and the lung specialist or pulmonologist. These doctors have taken two to three additional years of medical training after completing a three-year residency in either pediatrics or internal medicine. The pulmonologist treats diseases like asthma, emphysema, bronchitis and tuberculosis, while the allergist specializes in the care of allergic or atopic disease like asthma, hay fever, food or drug allergy and allergic skin disorders.

Once you and/or your primary care provider decides you need to see an asthma specialist, you must choose between these two types of doctors. The asthma-allergy specialist is best at diagnosing and treating asthma when there is an allergic component to asthma or the patient has other allergic conditions. Pulmonologists are experts in managing patients with severe asthma, especially if they have coexisting pulmonary diseases like bronchitis or emphysema or have required repeated hospitalization or intensive care for asthma relapses. I frequently co-manage these patients with severe asthma. In this situation I take care of the patient outside of the hospital, while the pulmonary-intensive care specialist takes over when the patient requires hospitalized care.

## Advantages of Specialty Care

Numerous studies provide strong support for specialty care for patients with complicated asthma who are at risk for emergency room visits or asthma hospitalizations. Doctors Michael Mellon and Robert Zieger from the Kaiser-Permanente Medical Center in San

Diego, California, found a marked reduction in nighttime wheezing, asthma relapses and emergency room visits in patients referred to an asthma specialist when compared to patients who did not receive specialty care. Intensive outpatient asthma treatment programs, staffed by medical personnel skilled in the delivery of asthma care, improve outcomes and asthma control. Specialty care should be a two-way street. The asthma specialist does not usually need to take over total control of the patient, but should work closely with the primary care provider. Some patients only need to be seen by the specialist once or twice a year, at which time the asthma specialist quarterbacks the patient's asthma program. Such follow-up visits should include a letter to the primary care provider, who in turn can monitor a patient's progress and ensure compliance with the recommendations of the asthma specialist.

I prefer to evaluate new patients with asthma in two or three visits. Once the diagnosis of asthma has been established during the first visit, my nursing staff and I will present an asthma education plan to the patient or family. Such a program incorporates educational videos, asthma literature and hands-on instruction in the use of the peak flow meters and asthma inhalers. Implementation of an asthma action plan is extremely important. A detailed review of environmental controls is essential for patients with documented allergies to indoor and outdoor aeroallergens. Between visits, the patient is asked to monitor lung function with a peak flow meter. During the summary visit the doctor should review the results of lab tests, breathing tests, skin tests, medication programs, peak flow readings, and he or she should answer questions posed by the patient or family.

After the summary visit is concluded, I dictate a report for the referring or primary care physician and the patient or family. This report can then serve as a reference source for both the primary care provider and the patient or family when a review of the asthma action plan or treatment program is necessary. Such a report is especially helpful when a patient is away at school or is traveling and has to visit a hospital or doctor unfamiliar with the patient's clinical history and treatment program. In my summary report I classify asthma into one of the four new categories proposed by the new NHLBI Guidelines: mild intermittent asthma, mild persistent asthma, moderate persistent asthma and chronic severe asthma.

I will then list appropriate medications and their doses, and outline environmental controls that need to be implemented.

## The Managed Care Scene

In my first 20 years of practice most, if not all, complicated cases of persistent asthma were referred to asthma specialists for evaluation. Patients with mild to moderate asthma were usually co-managed by the primary care provider and the asthma specialist. More severe or difficult-to-manage asthma was closely followed by the asthma specialist. This pattern of asthma care dramatically changed once managed care medicine entered the health-care arena in the 1990s. In an effort to reduce costs, managed care organizations and insurers began limiting patient access to specialists. Managed care programs encouraged primary care providers to manage a wide variety of complicated illnesses, including asthma, diabetes, arthritis and cardiovascular and skin diseases. In some tightly managed care organizations, primary care physicians were economically penalized when they referred too many patients to specialists. No one will debate the fact that the "gatekeeper approach" has reduced the costs of medical care, at least in the short term.

In turn, specialty doctors and national organizations were asked to provide treatment guidelines to primary care doctors for many chronic diseases, including asthma. When one considers the vast array of asthma medications now available for the treatment of asthma, even asthma specialists, like myself, have difficulty keeping current and finding the right combination of asthma medications necessary to control a difficult patient with persistent asthma. The key to managing any chronic disease is patient education, which requires time on the part of the health-care provider.

A recent seminar that I attended at the Harvard School of Public Health noted that the average visit to primary care providers was seven minutes. Thus, while overworked primary care practitioners may have the knowledge and a proper set of guidelines at their disposal, they may not have the time to properly educate and care for patients and families with chronic asthma. One telephone survey of 12,385 primary care physicians found that one in every four physicians felt that the scope of care that they were asked to provide was greater than it should be.

Has the provision of asthma guidelines to primary care providers improved the quality of care? The jury is still out on this question. Provision of cookbook or recipe-type medicine is no guarantee of optimal patient care. Many studies have found that primary care providers do not always follow guidelines provided by specialty groups. While the managed care approach has reduced medical costs over the past decade, rationing of specialty care may be a penny-wise and pound-foolish approach. I am astounded by the number of new patients that I see who have had asthma for several years and have never seen an asthma specialist, despite the fact they have a lowered quality of life and have required repeated office visits or emergency room care for acute asthma.

Patients, families, employers and insurers are recognizing the value of specialty care. In the late 1990s American health-care consumers started to rebel against gatekeeper-rationed care. The pendulum is swinging back to easier access to specialty care. Many of my patients and families have switched to primary care doctors or insurance providers that allow open access to specialists. Many primary care physicians I deal with have embraced this trend in care, as they were not enthralled with insurers that forced them to care for sicker patients without specialty input. Numerous studies have shown the value of specialty asthma care in the managed care scene.

One study of 28,000 asthma patients in five managed care plans around the United States found that asthma patients treated by specialists had 37 percent fewer hospitalizations and 55 percent fewer emergency visits than patients treated by primary care physicians. Thus, specialty asthma care actually saved money for the insurance companies. Asthma patients treated by specialists were more likely to be using inhaled anti-inflammatory drugs and less likely to need rescue medications which means that their asthma was under better control.

In the largest reported study to date (Archives of Internal Medicine November 2001) to examine the outcome of patients with asthma in managed care plans, investigators from Johns Hopkins University surveyed 1,954 patients with asthma and 1,078 treating physicians enrolled in 12 managed care organizations. This mail survey assessed use of medications, cancelled activities, self-management knowledge, emergency visits, asthma attacks and overall satisfaction with asthma care. When asthma specialty care was compared to care delivered by generalists or primary care providers, outcomes were better for specialty care with regard to cancelled activities, hospitalizations, emergency visits and physical functioning. It should be noted that the patients surveyed had been hospitalized or had an emergency visit within the past two years. The results support the conclusion that many patients with more moderate to severe asthma cared for by internists and family practitioners would benefit from treatment by providers with more experience in treating asthma.

## Guidelines for Specialty Care

What are the current guidelines for referring a patient to an asthma specialist? The NIH expert panel report on asthma recommends specialty referral in the following situations.

▲ Difficulty maintaining control of asthma

▲ Frequent emergency room visits or life-threatening attacks

▲ Inability to meet the goals of care set by the primary care physician after three to six months of therapy

▲ Symptoms that are unusual or difficult to diagnose

▲ Severe hay fever or sinus disease

▲ Asthma requiring more intense asthma education

▲ Candidates for allergy injections

▲ Severe asthma requiring high-dose inhaled or oral cortisone (prednisone)

▲ Need for more than two bursts of oral cortisone in one year

▲ Young children with moderate to severe asthma who require daily long-term asthma therapy

A joint study between the National Jewish Center for Immunology and Respiratory Medicine in Denver, Colorado, and the John Hancock Mutual Life Insurance Company found that approximately 1,300 patients in Hancock's insured pool spent more than $28 million for asthma care. Approximately 200 of these asthmatics cost more than $100,000 a year. Such economic data has led insurers to take a closer look at asthma. The result has been the development of asthma education programs aimed at all the players in the asthma scene, including health-care providers, employers, patients and their families.

The key element to reducing asthma-related, health-care costs is teaching patients and caretakers to identify asthma triggers, know the early warning signs of asthma and develop asthma action plans that will reduce the need for expensive emergency visits or hospitalizations. One of the major ways to reduce asthma costs is to identify asthma sufferers at an earlier age. While asthma is a chronic condition, it is quite different from most other chronic diseases in that it starts early in life. Proper asthma care in infancy or early childhood may prevent the development of lifelong asthma.

## Choosing an Insurance Plan

Patients and families with asthma have to be very careful in selecting their health-care plan, especially when a chronic condition like asthma requires daily medications and frequent office or hospital visits. The two most important aspects in an insurance plan are coverage of prescription drugs and office visits to both the primary care provider and the asthma specialist. Before you sign up for any insurance plan, you should know the type of plan in which you are enrolling. Basically there are four types of insurance plans. The older-type plans, formerly known as fee-for-service or indemnity plans, allowed you to visit any hospital or doctor once you had paid a deductible fee, usually about 20 percent of the total cost of the plan, for the year. Due to the spiraling costs of health care, this type of plan has been replaced by managed care plans, such as Health Maintenance Organization (HMOs), or Preferred Provider Plans (PPOs). Such plans often set a fixed rate for care for the year for an individual or entire family, and are built around a network of primary care physicians and specialists. The primary care provider acts as a quarterback or gatekeeper who supervises the patient's total care and controls access to specialists. If you seek unapproved care inside or outside this type of plan, you may be responsible for some or all of the costs. The ideal plan for asthma sufferers and their families is one that provides coverage for peak flow meters, nebulizers, asthma drugs, emergency care, hospitalization and open access to specialty care.

# Diseases
## Associated
## with Asthma

# 6

**Y**our genetic makeup, and the environmental exposures that drive your immune system down the asthma-allergy highway, may also induce other allergic diseases, such as allergic rhinitis (hay fever), atopic dermatitis (eczema) and food and drug allergy. Two other diseases commonly associated with asthma that do not require the presence of asthma-allergy genes or environmental exposures to allergens are chronic sinus disease and gastroesophageal reflux disease, also known as GERD.

## Allergic Rhinitis

Allergic rhinitis, or hay fever, is a relative newcomer to the allergy stage. While the ancient Greeks described asthma and food allergy, there is no reference to hay fever until the tenth century, when Persian scholar, Rhazes, described the causes of the coryza that took place in the spring when roses were in bloom. The first case of hay fever was not reported until 1819. In the early twentieth century, hay fever was considered to be a rare illness of the upper class. Doctor John Morrison Smith described his own hay fever while still in medical school.

> *"I gradually recognized that it was not an ordinary cold and that the symptoms were much worse on the golf course or even during a nice day rowing on Loch Lomand. At first I did not know what I had, and neither did any other doctor I encountered in the next two or three years..."*

Just 70 years later, millions of people have hay fever or allergic rhinitis. The hygiene hypothesis is one possible reason for this meteoric rise in the prevalence of allergic rhinitis. While nearly eighteen million Americans have asthma, more than twice as many—approximately forty million people—suffer from allergic rhinitis. The prevalence of allergic rhinitis has followed the rise in asthma cases, and the incidence of allergic rhinitis has tripled over the past 20 years in most developed countries.

In America the total economic impact for allergic rhinitis is $4.5 billion and nearly 3.8 million missed school or workdays per year. The impact on quality of life is significant. Allergic rhinitis interrupts sleep and interferes with school and work performance. Sedating antihistamine that continues to be the mainstay of treatment in America contributes to diminished energy, mood disorders, learning problems, work injuries and automobile accidents.

There are two forms of allergic rhinitis—seasonal and perennial. Seasonal allergic rhinitis or hay fever is caused by seasonal exposure to tree, grass or weed pollens. Perennial, or year-round allergic, rhinitis, is triggered by exposure to dust mites, molds and animals parts. Allergic rhinitis is commonly linked with asthma, as more than 50 percent of asthmatics have allergic rhinitis. In one European Health Survey, 3,000 Swedish respondents with allergic rhinitis had five times more asthma than the rest of the population. Another survey found that 60 percent of Swedish schoolchildren with asthma also suffered from allergic rhinitis.

Some authorities believe that untreated allergic rhinitis leads to asthma. This concept has been difficult to prove, as there are few well-done population studies that have followed individuals with allergic rhinitis for several years. Doctor Guy Settipane has performed the best study in this area. Two decades ago, Settipane identified a group of freshman students at Brown University in Providence, Rhode Island, who had allergy problems and positive allergy skin tests. Settipane tracked these Ivy League students for 20 years after their graduation. Seven years after graduation, 71 percent of asymptomatic students with positive skin tests had developed allergic airway symptoms. Twenty years after graduation, 10 percent of the students with allergic rhinitis had developed asthma.

In a similar study in Italy, 40 percent of more than 500 students with allergic rhinitis developed asthma within eight years of follow-up. I used to believe that allergic rhinitis, even if untreated, did not cause asthma but simply preceded it. Now I am not so sure. Many authorities feel that allergic rhinitis and asthma are manifestations of the same systemic disease. This theory has raised an interesting question. Would aggressive treatment of allergic rhinitis, including administering immunotherapy or allergy injections, especially to young children, prevent the development of asthma? Several worldwide studies now underway will ultimately answer this very important question.

The major symptoms of allergic rhinitis are sneezing, itchy nose and eyes, and clear watery discharge. Patients with seasonal hay fever report symptoms during specific pollen seasons, while those with year-round or perennial allergic rhinitis complain when house dust mites, molds and household pets precipitate or aggravate their symptoms.

People who suffer from long-standing allergic rhinitis, especially children, can often be diagnosed just by looking at their facial characteristics and mannerisms. There is often a discoloration and

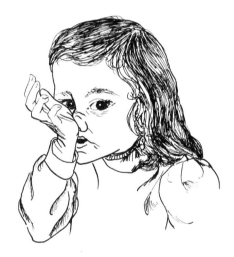

swelling under the eyes called "allergic shiners." When nasal obstruction persists, the typical open-mouth or adenoidal face is apparent. Frequent rubbing of an itchy nose results in the allergic salute, which produces a transverse "allergic crease" across the lower third of the nose. In allergic rhinitis, the mucous membranes inside the nose are often pale-bluish in color, as opposed to the typical red color seen in non-allergic rhinitis or the common cold. The treatment of allergic rhinitis includes antihistamines, decongestants and anti-inflammatory nasal sprays similar to those used in asthma, combined with proper environmental controls. In more persistent cases, allergy injections or immunotherapy may be indicated.

## One System—One Disease

Over the past three decades most allergy specialists tended to separate allergic rhinitis and asthma and consider them as two distinct conditions. Now there is renewed interest that they are one disease entity. The belief here is that these two conditions are part of a "united inflamed airway." Studies have shown that when these two conditions coexist in the same patient, symptoms are worse than when a patient has only allergic rhinitis or asthma. Does worse rhinitis trigger worse asthma or vice versa? Due to the fact that allergic rhinitis is now recognized as a global health problem that is increasing in prevalence and now affects millions of people worldwide, the World Health Organization has recently addressed this issue by publishing the Allergic Rhinitis and Its Impact on Asthma or the ARIA Guidelines. Such Guidelines will provide new parameters for the treatment of allergic rhinitis that will benefit patients who suffer from both asthma and allergic rhinitis.

## Atopic Dermatitis

The first sign that one has inherited the dreaded asthma-allergy genes often occurs in very early infancy, when babies develop an itchy skin condition known as eczema or atopic dermatitis. Eczema is a chronic skin disorder closely linked with asthma, allergic rhinitis and food allergies. When eczema develops before three months of age, the risk of developing asthma is significantly increased. Eczema is often accompanied with allergen sensitization and a high IgE allergic antibody level. Population studies have found that, like asthma and allergic rhinitis, the incidence of eczema has tripled over the past two decades. In some developed countries eczema now strikes one in every ten infants. Skin biopsies have demonstrated that eczema is a complex disorder involving many of the same inflammatory cells seen in asthma. Major eczema triggers include foods, aeroallergens and bacterial products. The symptoms of eczema include an itchy patchy skin eruption on the face, arms or legs, especially in the folds of the elbows and knees. As much of the skin eruption in eczema is self-induced by a scratching patient, doctors have labeled eczema as *"the itch that rashes."*

Conventional eczema treatment includes antihistamines to relieve itching, topical cortisone creams to control inflammation and antibiotics when secondary infection is present. Additional local measures include avoidance of irritants, dietary elimination of proven food allergens, skin hydration and skin moisturizers. Recent clinical trials have found a new immunomodulating agent, tacrolimus (Protopic), to be very beneficial when traditional eczema treatment fails. Protopic became available for the treatment of intractable eczema in early 2001.

## Chronic Sinus Disease

Chronic sinus disease is undoubtedly one of the most neglected diseases of our time. Figures from the United States Department of Public Health indicate that approximately 31 million Americans have sinus disease, causing 100,000 lost days from school and work. Sinusitis can be an important trigger of asthma in both children and adults, and its presence should be ruled out in any difficult-to-control asthma patient.

The sinuses are four paired air cavities surrounding the nose (Figure 6.2). Each sinus has a small opening, called an ostium, which allows secretions from the sinus cavity to drain into the nose. The

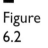
Figure 6.2

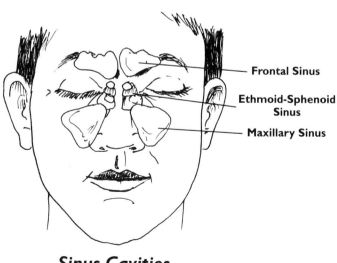

**Sinus Cavities**

varied functions of the sinuses include their role in smell and taste, voice quality and production of mucus. They also make our heads much lighter. If we did not have air-filled sinus cavities, our head would approximate the weight of a bowling ball. The linings of the sinuses contain many glands, which secrete mucus that is propelled from the sinus cavity into the nose by the sweeping action of hair-like structures called cilia. When the movement of mucus out of the sinus is impaired, mucus backs up and the sinus cavity becomes a fertile area for bacterial overgrowth. Sinus infections, therefore, most commonly accompany or follow a viral respiratory infection or the common cold. Predisposing factors to sinus infections include allergic rhinitis, deviation of the nasal septum (the bone between the two sides of the nose), nasal fractures, nasal polyps, cigarette smoke and pressure changes from flying, swimming and diving. Rarer illnesses that cause sinus infections include immune deficiency disorders and cystic fibrosis.

Several mechanisms have been proposed to explain why sinus infections trigger asthma. One theory is that sinus inflammation is transmitted to the lung by nerve reflexes connecting the upper and lower respiratory airway. Other experts argue that the asthma symptoms associated with sinus infections are a result of aspiration of mucus and postnasal drip into the lung. Finally, there is an emerging school of thought that chronic sinus disease and asthma may be one single disease syndrome that is triggered by inflammation in both the lower and upper respiratory tract. This theory is supported by the fact that inflammatory cells found in the asthmatic lung and in a swollen sinus cavity may be identical.

The symptoms of acute sinus infection are readily apparent. Patients complain of headache or pain and tenderness over the cheeks or above the eyes. They have a yellow-greenish or purulent nasal discharge and a constant cough. More subtle symptoms include nasal stuffiness and postnasal drip that may or may not be associated with a loss of smell and taste. Another common complaint in difficult-to-diagnosis sinusitis, especially in children, is foul breath—or as one mother aptly put it, a "dragon breath" odor. Pediatricians used to think that sinus infections were rare events in infants and toddlers, as it was assumed that their sinus cavities were not very well developed. This has been shown to be untrue, as infants and young children do have sinus cavities that can easily become infected at any age.

Difficult-to-control asthma patients should be evaluated for sinus disease. The diagnosis is made by taking a careful history, physical examination and X-ray studies. While plain sinus X-rays may be helpful in young children, in most cases plain sinus X-rays are useless and a sinus CAT scan is needed. Part of the difficulty in making the clinical diagnosis of sinusitis is that the signs and symptoms of sinusitis often overlap with many common childhood respiratory disorders, including the common cold or allergic rhinitis. Two features that distinguish sinusitis from viral upper respiratory infections are the length and severity of the symptoms. In allergic rhinitis the nasal discharge is usually watery or clear in color. Nasal congestion, cough and a thick yellow-green nasal discharge that lasts longer than 10 days increases the likelihood of a chronic sinus infection.

## Treatment of Sinus Disease

Once the diagnosis of sinusitis is apparent, appropriate treatment programs should include local or systemic decongestants, mucus thinners, topical cortisone sprays and nasal washings with salt water. Liberal amounts of fluid are recommended to thin out the thick mucus which may be blocking the narrow sinus openings. Antibiotics are essential in treating sinus infections. Sometimes it may be necessary to treat a sinus infection with antibiotics for four to six weeks. Patients who have several sinus infections a year that do not respond to appropriate medical management should be evaluated for potential sinus surgery. New sophisticated surgical techniques, such as endoscopic sinus surgery, offer hope to patients with chronic or refractory sinus disease. Results with the newer high-tech sinus surgical procedures are much better compared to older, more primitive and invasive sinus surgery.

In a study at the UCLA School of Medicine, 48 children with bad sinus disease and asthma were aggressively treated for their sinus disease. After five weeks of treatment, 38 of these children stopped wheezing and were able to discontinue all their asthma medicine. Similar results were observed in adult studies in Washington, D.C., and St. Louis, although adults were more likely to require surgery to control sinus disease. Not all asthma specialists agree that sinusitis can worsen asthma. Doctors at the Hospital for Sick Children in Toronto, Canada, found that 31 percent of 138 children with asthma had abnormal sinus X-rays, but they did not find the majority of bad sinuses in the worst asthma cases. They felt that the abnormal sinus X-ray was a reflection of allergy and inflammation associated with asthma.

The important point about all these sinus studies is that individuals with asthma and coexisting sinus disease may be completely unaware that they have sinusitis. Their symptoms may only include a mild postnasal drip or a nagging cough. I have seen many patients with "silent sinus disease," whose only complaint was bad breath in the morning. Astute doctors should closely question their patients about sinus symptoms and obtain a sinus CAT scan when they suspect the presence of hidden sinus disease.

## Gastroesophageal Reflux Disease

Ingested foods and beverages are transported to the stomach and the rest of the intestinal tract by the esophagus or food pipe (Figure 6.3). The junction between the esophagus and stomach is guarded by a muscle or sphincter that prevents food and stomach acid from being regurgitated back up into the esophagus. However, in some individuals this sphincter does not completely close and food and stomach acid flows back up or refluxes into the esophagus, resulting in indigestion and heartburn. Anyone who has overindulged in a fancy restaurant has experienced reflux. When reflux symptoms persist on a regular basis, the condition is called gastroesophageal reflux disease or GERD.

Figure
6.3

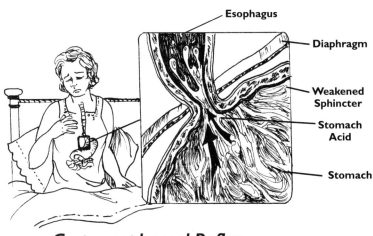

**Gastroesophageal Reflux**

96

Asthma specialists have long suspected that there was a strong link between reflux and asthma. Reflux symptoms are nearly twice as common in people with asthma. Several studies found that nearly 50 percent of patients with asthma suffered from acid reflux that could trigger asthma symptoms. Many of the patients in these studies denied having any reflux symptoms whatsoever. Why are asthmatics more prone to reflux symptoms? They may have a nervous system abnormality that reduces the pressure gradient between their esophagus and stomach and allows stomach acid to easily reflux back up the esophagus. Overreaction by the diaphragm—the large muscle that separates the chest cavity from the abdomen—may also promote reflux. Lastly, some asthma medicines such as theophylline lower the pressure in the esophagus sphincter and trigger reflux symptoms.

While it is now well established that asthmatics have more reflux than non-asthmatic patients, it is still not clear if reflux triggers asthma or if asthma triggers reflux. The literature on this issue is conflicting. If reflux triggers asthma, adequate control of reflux should improve asthma symptoms. Many clinical trials show modest improvement in asthma symptoms, but little or no improvement in lung functions, with anti-reflux therapy. Such treatment includes antacids, antihistamine drugs that block the release of stomach acid and drugs called proton pump inhibitors that lower the production of stomach acid. Dietary and lifestyle restrictions in reflux therapy include avoiding fatty and acidic foods, minimizing caffeine and alcohol intake, eating smaller meals, not eating before bedtime and elevating the head of one's bed.

Patients with severe reflux who do not respond to aggressive medical management may require a surgical procedure, called fundoplication, where the muscle between the esophagus and stomach is tightened by placing a band around the junction of the esophagus and stomach. The results of reflux surgery are difficult to evaluate, as most studies have serious design flaws. University of Washington researchers studied 90 patients with reflux who were randomly assigned to receive the anti-ulcer drug cimetidine, a placebo drug, or undergo reflux surgery. After six months, all three groups had fewer asthma symptoms, particularly those who received cimetidine and surgery. When cimetidine was discontinued, many patients relapsed. Over a long-term follow-up period, the surgically treated group improved the most. This and other studies imply that reflux plays a significant role in asthma and doctors should not ignore the co-existence of heartburn and indigestion in patients with asthma.

Anyone who suffers from moderate or persistent asthma should be considered a potential reflux victim, especially if they complain of heartburn, frequent burping, indigestion, or coughing and wheezing during or after eating. The difficulty in diagnosing reflux is that many patients have asymptomatic or "silent" reflux, which requires special diagnostic tests. Such tests require the insertion of a tube into the esophagus and measuring the amount of acid regurgitated back up into the esophagus.

This is called pH monitoring. A special X-ray study, called a barium swallow, involves the swallowing of a radioactive dye to see if the dye is refluxed from the stomach back up into the esophagus. When confronted with an asthmatic with reflux symptoms, it makes more sense to initiate a trial of anti-reflux therapy than immediately ordering a pH study or a barium swallow. Patients with moderate to severe asthma who have persistent reflux symptoms deserve a three-month trial of reflux therapy, as it has been shown that two to three months of reflux treatment may be needed before asthma symptoms improve.

# Common Asthma **Triggers**

# 7

## *The Aeroallergens*

**M**any people believe that all bouts of asthma are triggered by exposure to aeroallergens. This is a total misconception, as there are hundreds of other potential asthma triggers, ranging from indoor and outdoor aeroallergens, chemicals and air pollutants, beverages and food products, viral and bacterial infections to adverse psychosocial factors (Table 1).

**Table 1.** Common Asthma Triggers

▲ Aeroallergens

- House dust mites
- Cockroaches, rodents
- Molds
- Pollens
- Animal allergens

▲ Air pollutants

▲ Chemicals and foodstuffs

▲ Viral and bacterial infections

▲ Psychosocial factors

The best understood of all asthma triggers are the aeroallergens in our indoor and outdoor air that set off an allergen-antibody reaction when inhaled into your nose or lung. Aeroallergens, such as house dust mites, feathers, molds, insect parts, pollens and animal allergens have several common characteristics. They must be small and light enough to remain airborne over long periods of time, and only a brief exposure to tiny amounts of allergen will induce symptoms in the sensitized individual. Airborne allergens can be found anywhere—indoors, outdoors, at home, at work, at school or at play. Pollen and mold allergens fluctuate with the seasons, while perennial allergens such as house dust mites, cockroaches and animal allergens may be present in our indoor air on a year-round basis. Most aeroallergens can be identified with standardized allergy skin and blood tests.

## House Dust Mites

House dust has been recognized as an important asthma trigger for centuries. Indoor dust is not quite the same as outdoor dust. Outdoor dust or just plain dirt is a simple non-specific irritant. Indoor house dust is an incredibly complex mixture of dust mites, cotton fibers, cellulose, mattress parts, animal hairs, mold spores, dead insects, discarded food particles and bacteria. Seventy percent of all allergic asthmatics are sensitive to house dust, and for many it is their only significant allergy.

House-dust-mite-allergic asthmatics usually cough or wheeze shortly after arising in the morning, or during the dust season, which in northern climates coincides with the heating season—late fall to early spring. Warm, heated indoor air creates turbulent air currents throughout the home that increase the circulation of dust particles. Dust levels tend to be much higher in older homes, and in carpeted dwellings heated with forced-hot-air systems.

In 1964, two Dutch scientists, Drs. Spieksma and Voorhorst, startled the world of allergy research when they discovered that a microscopic-sized arthropod, the house dust mite, was the major allergen in house dust. Dust mites are tiny, sightless, eight-legged insects that look like creatures from a late-night horror film. These mites are members of the Arachnid insect family. Unlike their spider and tick cousins, they are not visible to the naked eye, and they do not bite or transmit any diseases. What is even more frightening than the

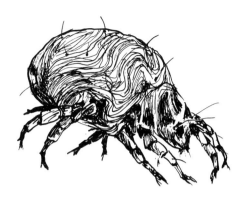

House Dust Mite

mite's appearance is its living and eating habits. House dust mites live in bedding, carpets, upholstery and other textiles, where they feed on human skin scales, fungi, bacteria and various human secretions. There are thousands of different species of mites, but so far only a few are known to cause allergic reactions. One species, *D. farinae,* does well in prolonged dry weather, while the other major allergy-inducing mite species, *D. pteronyssinus,* thrives in damp humid environments.

The dust mite's favorite food is your very own human skin scales. Mites are no dummies. To get closer to their cherished food supply, mites congregate in mattresses, rugs and stuffed furniture. The distribution and abundance of dust mites is not uniform. Houses next door to each other of the same design can have vastly different mite population density and species composition. Nobody knows the exact numbers of mites in a given mattress or a carpet. Each mite would have to be removed and counted individually—an impossible task considering that the average mattress probably contains two million mites!

Dust mite populations fluctuate from season to season. In temperate regions mite populations are highest in late summer and autumn and lowest in winter. Larger mite populations are found in damper climates than dry ones. The optimal growth condition for the dust mite is a warm, humid environment. This explains why dust mites thrive in damp homes, especially in carpeted basements. Mites die when the temperature falls below 50 degrees, or when humidity levels are kept at less than 50 percent. Due to the dry air at higher altitudes, house dust mite allergy is less common among people living in continental interiors or mountainous regions like Colorado than residents of low-altitude maritime locales like Boston. A dormant or a dead mite is still an allergenic mite, as the mite's feces and body parts are the real triggers of your allergy symptoms. The key symptoms that help to identify mite-sensitive patients are sneezing and wheezing in the morning, onset of symptoms while vacuuming or making beds and feeling better outside the home.

In the last 30 years major changes in housing design have produced energy-efficient homes and buildings with insulated, double-glazed windows, central heating and low rates of outdoor air exchange. Such alterations in housing design resulted in warmer, damper homes—a more favorable domestic microclimate for the dust mite. This change in our home environment has been cited as one of the major reasons for the asthma epidemic.

Most of the world's population resides in cities located on or near the coastline at altitudes less than 100 feet above sea level. Studies in Australia and France have found lower dust mite levels in homes in inland and mountainous regions. This finding nicely explains why so many of my patients who live near the ocean do well when they visit or move to the mountainous regions of northern New England. My son's asthma improved dramatically when he left our home in Marblehead, a seacoast town north of Boston, to attend college in the mountains of northern Vermont.

## Risk Factors for Asthma

Innovative studies have shown that allergens are significant risk factors for patients with allergic rhinitis and asthma. Let me explain what the term risk factor means. Allergists can accurately assess the severity of any hay fever season by counting the number of pollen grains in air. We know that a prolonged period of dry, windy weather at the time of tree, grass or ragweed pollination leads to high pollen counts that will trigger symptoms in millions of hay fever sufferers. Thus, a high pollen level is a "risk factor" for people with hay fever. Likewise, the level of molds in the air is a risk factor for mold-sensitive patients.

Doctors have long suspected that a positive skin test to the dust mite, molds or dog or cat allergen, combined with an environmental exposure to these allergens, was a risk factor for people with allergic rhinitis and asthma. Until recently, allergists could not correlate the level of exposure to indoor allergens to the severity of asthma symptoms. Times have changed. Immunologists have developed precise methods to measure the amounts of indoor allergen in our homes and public buildings. A large body of evidence proving that exposure to indoor and outdoor allergens is a major risk factor for asthma has been gathered from all parts of the world. Doctor Susan Pollart and her colleagues at Travis Air Force Base in northern California looked at annual asthma epidemics, which occur in May, the peak of the grass pollen season in California. Pollart found that 90 percent of patients coming to the emergency room for acute asthma care during the grass season had high levels of IgE antibody to grass pollen.

Doctor Thomas Platts-Mills reviewed exposures and sensitization to the house dust mite allergen in children from Virginia admitted to the hospital with asthma. He found that the majority of these children were exposed and sensitized to dust mites, and that continued exposure to high levels of house dust mites increased their risk for a re-admission for asthma. Doctor J. Korsgaard found that the presence of significant amounts of dust mites in Danish homes was a sevenfold risk factor for the development of asthma. In other words, subjects who lived in dust-mite-infested Danish homes were seven times more likely to have asthma than those who lived in mite-free homes. In New Zealand, dust mite exposure was the most important allergen associated with asthma.

Exposure to *Alternaria* mold has been shown to be a risk factor for sudden respiratory arrest and asthma deaths in the United States. Several studies from Northern Europe have detailed the risk factors posed by household pets, especially cats. A study done in Boston, Massachusetts, found doctor-diagnosed asthma to be more common in homes with high levels of cockroach allergens. House dust mite sensitivity is important in childhood asthma, as once sensitized, children are continually exposed to high levels of these small allergen particles from bed, carpeting and household furnishings.

New Zealand has one of the highest incidences of asthma in the entire world. In one study of 11,000 patients, one in every four New Zealanders had bronchial hyperreactivity or signs of asthma. Doctor

Ann Woolcock postulated that the increase in the frequency and severity of asthma in New Zealand was related to the local customs in this sheep-producing nation, which boasts four million citizens and seventy million sheep. Virtually every infant in New Zealand has a sheepskin rug that serves as a daytime bed. Thus, infants who spend most of their waking hours lying on these most perfect of all dust mite breeding grounds can become sensitized to dust mites at a very early age. Woolcock also studied children who resided in different climatic areas of New South Wales, Australia. Symptoms were assessed via a detailed questionnaire, and bronchial hyperreactivity was measured by inhalation challenge tests. Children who had one or more positive skin tests had more wheezing, hay fever, eczema and bronchial hyperreactivity. Most allergic children were allergic to dust mites, cat dander, weeds, grass and molds. Sensitivity to dust mites had the strongest correlation with asthma in all three Australian climates. This Australian study mirrored a study done in England, which found that exposure to house dust mites in early childhood increased the likelihood that children would develop asthma at a later age.

## Cockroach Allergy

Cockroach allergy is another latecomer to the allergy scene, as it was not recognized until 1967. The two most common cockroach species in the United States are the American and German cockroaches. The German cockroach is a small insect—approximately three-quarters of an inch in length—that infests kitchens and bathrooms. The larger and more easily visible American cockroach is more likely to be found in factories, schools, hospitals and public buildings. German cockroaches are important asthma triggers in older urban dwellings.

Seldom seen during the day, cockroaches enter the home at night. Like teenagers, they head for food sources for a late night snack, and congregate on kitchen floors and cabinets. Cockroach allergen, present in the saliva, feces, skin shedding, and the dead bodies of the insect, are relatively large particles that only become airborne after significant air disturbance. Thus, unlike animal allergic patients, cockroach-sensitive individuals may not develop asthma immediately after entering a cockroach-infested home.

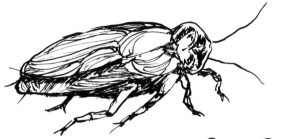

German Cockroach

The quantity of cockroach allergen that becomes airborne during vacuum cleaning is in the same range as has been reported for dust mite allergen. Cockroach activity has a seasonal pattern that usually peaks in the summer months. While dust mite and cat allergy might be considered a self-inflicted wound of suburbia and more affluent asthmatics, cockroach allergy is a pestilence visited upon the urban and rural poor. Hypersensitivity to cockroaches is highest in the uninsured and low-income populations in the United States. Nearly 40 percent of patients attending a New York City allergy clinic had positive skin tests to cockroaches. In Chicago, 60 percent of asthmatics had high levels of IgE antibody to cockroach allergen and 50 percent had positive bronchial challenges to cockroach. Cockroach allergy is found around the world, especially in subtropical or tropical climates. In Taiwan and Marseilles, France, six in every ten asthmatics are skin-test positive to cockroach.

Cockroach allergy may present early in life. In Chicago's Cook County Hospital pediatric allergy clinic, one in every four children under age four had cockroach allergy, and for many it was their only allergy. The National Cooperative Inner City Asthma Program found that children living in urban dwellings with cockroach infestation had more emergency room visits and hospitalizations for asthma. In this inner-city study, 85 percent of the homes surveyed had detectable levels of cockroach allergen. Cockroach exposure during the first three months of life was identified as a major risk factor for the development of asthma in an urban study in Boston.

## Mold Aeroallergens

Molds or fungi are tiny plants lacking roots or stems that reproduce by releasing mold spores into the surrounding air. Indoor molds grow in damp, musty areas like cellars, garages, bathtubs, shower stalls, laundry rooms and home humidifiers. Outdoor molds prefer the warm, moist, shady confines of mulch piles, black soil, gardens and fallen leaves. Molds survive by digesting small amounts of decomposing foods or vegetable matter. A typical example of mold growth is the fungus you see on stale bread or cheese. Mold that grows on aging foods is far less dangerous than the mold that grows in your bathroom, wet basement or garden. Molds reproduce by releasing small spores into the air, creating airborne allergens similar

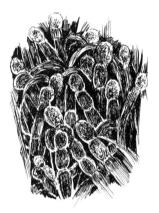

Mold Spores

to pollen. Mold-allergic patients sneeze or wheeze after inhaling mold spores. There are tens of thousands of mold species, and only a few experts in the world are able to identify all of them. Under the microscope, mold spores look like golf balls without a name or logo.

Molds are everywhere in nature, including soil, decaying wood and leaves. Molds need four things to grow: food, air, proper temperatures and water vapor. Since molds eat just about anything and air is everywhere, the best way to inhibit mold growth is to control temperature and humidity. Molds thrive on garbage cans, houseplants, shower stalls, basement walls and damp floors. Some molds reproduce when it rains, while others release their spores during the dry period that follows a rainy spell.

In temperate climates molds start to release their spores in early April or May. Outdoor mold levels usually peak in July or August. Mold symptoms may last until the first freeze or snowstorm. Molds are present year-round in the semitropical and tropical climates. The most intense exposure to molds in the United States occurs in the summer in the Midwest farm belts. When the ground freezes in early winter or it snows, outdoor molds cease to be a major problem. The most common asthma-inducing molds in North America are *Alternaria, Penicillium* and *Cladosporium.*

## Animal Allergens

A variety of domesticated animals live and work closely with humans either as household companions, farm animals or in research labs. It is estimated that over a hundred million domestic animals reside in the United States, with dogs and cats being the most popular household pets. Tens of thousand of farmers and laboratory workers are exposed to animal allergens such as cows, chickens, horses, pigs, rodents, rabbits and guinea pigs. Animals raised for fur production like mink, fox and raccoon are also recognized as occupational risks. Bird allergens can cause asthma and a special form of pneumonia.

## Dog Allergy

Dog ownership is common—there are approximately 50 million dogs in the United States. Studies have shown that approximately 35 percent of people with asthma are allergic to dogs. In a Los Alamos, New Mexico, survey 67 percent of asthmatic children were found to be allergic to dogs, and 62 percent were sensitized to cats. While dog allergen is found in homes and public places that do not house dogs, allergen levels are 250 times higher in homes where dogs reside. In homes that do house dogs, the highest allergen levels are found in carpets. The highest concentration in homes without a dog is found in upholstered living room furniture, suggesting that dog allergen is carried from home to home via the dog owner's clothing.

While there is some debate as to what part of the dog contains the most allergen, most allergen comes from skin scales and fur. Despite the claims of many dog breeders, there is no such thing as a non-allergenic dog or species. Even "hairless breeds" have significant amounts of allergen in their dander and skin. There is no evidence that longhaired dogs are more allergenic than shorthaired dogs.

I can offer some personal experience in this area. Both my oldest son and I are allergic to dogs. Many years ago an Old English sheepdog was brought into our home on a trial basis. Needless to say, this dog and the several other sheepdogs that followed became a permanent fixture in our family. Interestingly enough, neither my son nor I were very sensitive to this particular dog, while we would have problems visiting friends or relatives where other breeds resided. We would also entertain guests with dog allergy who had little or no problems in our home. I am not touting the Old English sheepdog as a non-allergenic breed, but in my experience there does seem to be a breed-to-breed or dog-to-dog difference. This observation probably relates to the fact that some dogs produce more airborne dog allergen than others.

One French investigator studied the allergen output from 141 dogs to determine if there were any differences between males and females, long and shorthaired dogs, and castrated or intact dogs. No significant differences in allergen levels were noted in these dogs. However, dogs who had dry skin or seborrhea had much higher levels of dog allergen, suggesting that aggressive skin care in dogs with skin problems may lower allergen output. In my own experience poodles, schnauzers and some of the wire-haired terriers appear to be less sensitizing than shorter haired breeds like boxers, Dalmatians and Labrador retrievers.

## Cat Allergy

Cat allergy is a very common affliction. It is estimated that nearly three percent of the United States population, or 10 million Americans, are allergic to cats. According to a survey by the American Pet Product Manufacturers Association, approximately one in every three American homes now houses a cat or cats. That adds up to 28 million homes with an average of two cats per home, or roughly 60 million cats! Thanks to big strides in veterinary medicine, the average cat now has a lifespan of 20 or more years. It was once thought that the cat dander was the prime source of cat allergen. It is now known that the major sources of cat allergen are the proteins produced in the cat's saliva and sebaceous glands that attach to the cat's dander and hair.

Many patients may not develop allergy or asthma symptoms for several years after a cat has been introduced into their home. The average exposure time needed to develop nasal allergies to cats is about two years, and for asthma it may be up to four to five years. The main in-home reservoirs of cat allergen are carpets, especially wall-to-wall carpeting, upholstered furniture and bedding.

A French study found that male cats produce more allergen than female cats, and that the castration of males significantly lowers levels of cat allergen. These studies forewarned that castrated cats still produce enough allergen to affect most cat-allergic individuals. More work is needed in this area before castration can be recommended as an environmental control measure. Cat allergen is found everywhere, even in places where a cat has never resided, as cat allergen is carried from place to place on the cat owner's clothing.

Studies have shown that 50 percent of cat-allergic people have never owned a cat, attesting to the fact that cat allergen is a very powerful allergy and asthma trigger. Two of my five children and I are extremely sensitive to cats, yet we have never kept a cat in our home. Public buildings and the school setting are the most likely setting of cat allergen exposure.

A study in Sweden, a country with cold, dry climate with little house dust mite or mold problems, found a strong link between asthma and sensitization to household animals, especially cats. The authors linked the growing number of indoor pets with the increasing incidence of asthma in Sweden. Most children in northern Sweden who were allergic to cats did not keep cats in their own home. The amount of cat allergen in Swedish classrooms was directly proportional to the number of students and teachers with cats at home. While it is yet to be determined whether the amount of cat allergen in the school environment is high enough to trigger allergies or asthma attacks, this Swedish study suggested cat-allergen control needed to be considered in the school setting, especially for allergic children who do not maintain pets in their own homes.

In Chicago Children's Hospital Asthma Clinic, children with positive skin test to cats were three times more likely to have severe asthma. A similar survey at high altitude (7,200 feet) in Los Alamos, New Mexico, where home concentrations of dust mites are very low and outdoor air pollution is negligible, found extremely high levels of cat allergen in all homes possibly because most cats in Los Alamos remained indoors at night due to the threat of coyotes. A higher incidence of asthma was strongly associated with allergy to indoor allergens, especially cat allergen.

All asthma caretakers know that the "asthma season" begins in the fall shortly after children return to school. In the past the increase in the number of acute cases of asthma seen at this time of the year was attributed to weather changes, heating systems being turned on in the home and viral respiratory infections. Swedish researchers may have found another reason why children start to wheeze when they go back to school. They studied 10 children with mild asthma who were not exposed to animals in their home. These animal-allergic children were symptom-free weeks before they returned to a school setting where there were significant concentrations of dog and cat allergen. One week after these children started school, analysis of secretions from their noses and lung showed a dramatic increase in inflammatory or allergy blood cells. Thus, asymptomatic Swedish children with mild asthma had signs of inflammation in their airway one week after returning to classrooms infested with animal allergens, suggesting that exposure to animal allergens in the school is a major risk factor for asthma.

In a New Zealand study, where 62 percent of all students lived with a cat, investigators collected samples from school carpets and student's clothing. Large amounts of cat allergen were found in the school carpets and on the students' clothing. Wool and polyester garments carried more cat allergen than cotton clothing, possibly due to more frequent laundering of cotton garments. Girls' clothing carried more cat allergen than boys' clothing, possibly because girls spend more time indoors. When cats were kept out of their bedroom, students carried lower levels of cat allergen. High levels of cat allergen were found in school carpets where the children sat for several hours a day. These studies imply that sensitization to cat allergen is an evolving public health problem, in which exposure in the school setting may unknowingly sensitize susceptible children or trigger asthma attacks in patients who do not keep cats in their own home. This may be a solid reason for new school construction or renovations to avoid carpeted surfaces in school classrooms.

## Cat Asthma

Over the past several years the growing number of new asthma patients who are allergic to cats has impressed me. In many cases cat allergen is their major asthma trigger. I like to call this form of asthma—"cat asthma."

A typical story of cat asthma is one where a cat is brought into the home, and on close questioning it becomes apparent that the patient began to have asthma symptoms a year or two after a cat was introduced into the home. At first, most of these patients will deny that the cat is bothering them, despite the fact they have a positive skin test to cat allergen. When I press the issue, they will admit that close contact with the cat will induce sneezing or itchy eyes. When I ask, "What happens when the cat licks you?", the answer is, "Oh, I get itchy and break out in welts." Upon further questioning, patients with cat-asthma will admit that their asthma worsens when they return home from school, work or vacations. They note substantial improvement when they leave home for any extended period of time.

I am totally convinced that exposure to cat allergen in people born with allergy-asthma genes is a bad news combination. Cat allergen, the most powerful of all antigens, is remarkably stable. It may remain in the environment long after a cat is removed from the home. I used to think that the most allergy-provoking part of the cat was its hair or dander, but some studies imply that one of the most allergenic parts of the cat is its saliva. Cats constantly lick their bodies and cover themselves with this potent allergen, which is then deposited on rugs, beds and furniture throughout the home.

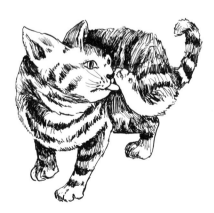

Cat allergen, being the smallest of all inhaled allergens, penetrates very deep into the lung. I cannot overstate the importance of cat allergy and asthma. Some of my more dramatic "asthma cures" are the result of cats finally being removed from the home environment.

I am currently in the process of reviewing my experience with cat asthma over the past 30 years. Preliminary data reveals that the number of cases of cat asthma has dramatically increased in the past decade. If these early observations hold up, one may ask why then is there an increase in cat asthma? The answer to this question may be quite simple. There are more cats in more American homes than ever before. Inflation, economic pressures and the cost of decent housing mandate that many families have two breadwinners. When both parents work, acquisition of a family dog is out of the question, as there is no one around to take the family pooch out for his much-needed midday walk. A growing number of single adults prefer a low-upkeep pet that does not require walking or exercising. In fact, once inside, many cats never leave the owner's home or apartment.

While I have no national statistics at my fingertips that prove that the cat population is increasing, every veterinarian I ask assures me their cat practice has nearly tripled in the last decade. Cat care comprises up to 80 percent of many veterinary practices. One recent survey estimated that cats now outnumber dogs 71 to 58 million. Thus, one of the reasons for the asthma epidemic may be due to the fact that there are more cats in more homes of more individuals at risk for developing cat asthma.

## Laboratory Animal Allergy

Laboratory workers exposed to mice, rats, guinea pigs and other laboratory allergens have a nearly 30 percent rate of allergy symptoms. The most sensitizing animals are rats, mice and rabbits. The most important source of allergen is the urine of the laboratory animal.

## The Pollen Allergens

Trees, grasses, weeds and flowering plants all reproduce by producing pollen, the male sperm of the plant kingdom. Insects and wind currents transfer pollen from plant to plant. Pollens from trees, grasses and weeds are light enough to be blown through the air and easily inhaled. The heavier pollens of flowering plants, like roses, and privet hedges, that are carried about by low-flying insects, are much less allergenic than the wind-borne pollens.

Hay fever sufferers and allergic asthmatics are exposed to three major pollens each calendar year, namely tree, grass and weed pollens. In the southerly regions of the United States, tree pollination starts in February or March, while trees in the more northern areas of the United States do not pollinate until April or early May. Grass pollinates after the trees in late May or early June. The ragweed plant releases its pollen in late summer and early fall. The severity of any pollen season varies from year to year. The factors controlling pollination are air temperature and weather patterns. Cold, damp, rainy weather minimizes pollination, while hot, dry, windy weather accelerates it.

## Ragweed Allergy

Some of the more potent hay fever and asthma-inducing pollen in the East and Midwest comes from the ragweed plant family. Members of the ragweed tribe include sunflower, cocklebur, goldenrod, and dandelion. Flowering plants like goldenrod and dandelion do not usually cause hay fever symptoms. Ironically, the scientific name for the ragweed plant means *Ambrosia*, or food of the gods. In reality ragweed is an ugly, coarse, hairy, tiny-flowered plant that has a noxious odor. Before North America was widely settled, ragweed only grew along riverbanks and flood plains. Ragweed does not grow well in virgin lands, mountains, forests, wetlands or swamps. When America was developed and the soil was cultivated, the hardy ragweed plant was widely dispersed. As a result, ragweed plants thrived in the poorest of soils like vacant lots and roadside areas.

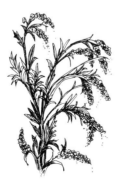

Ragweed

Ragweed starts to pollinate in mid-August, when the days become shorter and evening temperatures drop below 60 degrees. Thus, unlike the spring tree and summer grass pollination that starts in the south and proceeds in a northerly direction, ragweed pollination begins in the north and moves south. In most areas, ragweed pollination lasts for four to six weeks. Allergists used to think that ragweed victims only sneezed or wheezed when the plant was pollinating. Patients who continued to have symptoms in October and November were thought to be allergic to molds or house dust. Thanks to studies done at the Mayo Clinic, we now know that particles from dead ragweed plants can remain in the air long after the plant stops pollinating. These plant particles can trigger sneezing and wheezing well past the first killing frost.

## *Latex Allergy*

One particular form of allergy that has become much more common in the past decade is latex allergy. Latex is a natural rubber product derived from the rubber tree, *Heavea brazilienis,* found in South America, Africa and Southeast Asia. Latex is a common component of many medical supplies, including surgical gloves, stethoscopes, catheters, syringes and tubing. It is used in thousands of consumer products, such as gloves, balloons, condoms, shoes, pacifiers and rubber tires. Due to the increasing threat of infectious diseases, including AIDS and hepatitis B, the use of latex products has exploded, especially in the health-care industry. It is now estimated that between 10 and 15 percent of all health-care workers are sensitive to latex allergen.

Clinical symptoms of latex allergy may range from mild skin rash (hives or contact dermatitis) to sneezing, itchy eyes, asthma or a full-blown, life-threatening anaphylactic reaction. Allergic and asthmatic individuals are more prone to developing latex allergy. Latex allergy sufferers also have a higher incidence of allergy to certain foods, including chestnuts, hazelnuts and some tropical fruits, as these foods share common properties with the latex allergen. Allergists used to think that individuals who sneezed or wheezed when they put on powdered latex gloves were allergic to the talc or powder that is released into the air when the gloves are put on or snapped off. We now know that the talc powder carries the latex protein into the air. For this reason, many latex-allergic patients have fewer symptoms when they use non-powdered gloves. In most cases latex allergy develops after repeated exposure.

Latex allergy can be diagnosed by the clinical history or by performing blood or skin tests. The only real treatment for latex allergy is avoidance of the offending allergen. All health-care providers, especially dentists, surgeons and obstetricians, need to be made aware of latex allergy, as inadvertent encounters with latex allergen during dental and surgical procedures and labor and delivery have resulted in severe anaphylaxis or allergic reactions, including tragic fatalities. Most, if not all, hospitals and health-care facilities now provide non-latex gloves and latex-free environments for their patients and employees.

# Air **Pollution** and Asthma

# 8

Growing concerns over the asthma epidemic have led researchers to reexamine the role of air pollution in asthma. Atmospheric air pollutants come in several forms, including gases, aerosols and small particles or particulate matter. Air pollutants vary in size from invisible, virus-sized molecules to easily seen, large, raindrop-size particles. Outdoor air pollutants arise from factories, power plants and the internal combustion engines of motorized cars, trucks and buses. It is not surprising that outdoor and indoor air pollutants trigger asthma. When air pollutants are

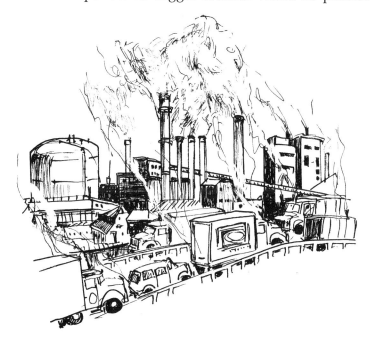

inhaled into the lung, they can trigger an inflammatory response similar to that seen from inhaled aeroallergens.

Three major pollution episodes between 1930 and 1950 highlight the detrimental effects of air pollution on health. In December 1930, the heavily industrialized Meuse Valley in Belgium experienced a severe air pollution episode that affected several hundred people and caused 60 deaths. A similar event took place in Donora, California, in October 1948, where thousands became ill and 18 people died. The worst of all air pollution episodes occurred in London in 1952, when air pollution killed more than 4,000 people in a two-week period. All of these air pollution disasters were associated with colder weather, little wind and a temperature inversion that trapped polluted air near the ground. Most of the people who died during these air pollution disasters had preexisting cardiovascular or respiratory disease.

One report from Japan linked air pollution to asthma. An unusual number of American servicemen and their families developed asthma while stationed at a military base in Yokohama, Japan. After they were transferred out of this base, their asthma rapidly improved. This problem, labeled "Yokohama Asthma," was more likely to occur in the fall or winter months during periods of heavy smog. This report, and others like it, point out that while levels of outdoor air pollutants may be highest in the summer, air pollution episodes that occur in colder weather are more dangerous to individuals with preexisting lung disease. An Environmental Protection Agency study in Seattle, Washington, found that the number of emergency room visits for asthma was higher when wood stoves are utilized on colder days when particulate air particles were higher. The four major outdoor air pollutants in our outdoor air are ozone, nitrogen dioxide, sulfur dioxide and particulate matter.

## Ozone

Ozone is the by-product of the interaction of sunlight and automobile exhaust fumes. Excess ozone creates smog, or the brown haze that permeates our atmosphere on the lazy-hazy days of summer. Ozone is a big problem for asthmatics residing in areas like

Los Angeles, California, where there is abundant sunlight and heavy automobile traffic. Ozone is a colorless gas with both good and bad qualities. The presence of ozone 10 to 30 miles up in our stratosphere protects life on earth by screening out the sun's harmful ultraviolet rays and thereby minimizing dangers from the sun, including skin cancer. Ground-level ozone, on the other hand, is a direct irritant to the eyes, nose, throat and lungs. Ozone production varies by season. The lowest concentrations occur during winter months, higher levels in spring and peak levels in the summer. The ground-level ozone level that usually peaks in the late afternoon is directly proportional to atmospheric conditions and concentrations of exhaust emissions from motorized vehicles powered by fossil fuels.

Most asthmatics will tell you that they wheeze more during hot, humid weather. Studies show that high ozone levels lead to more hospitalizations and emergency room visits for asthma, and this risk is much greater in cigarette smokers. There is evidence that many people who are continuously exposed to high levels of ozone become increasingly tolerant to it. In one study, Los Angeles residents who were exposed to the highest levels of ozone in the United States tolerated more ozone exposure than visitors from Montreal, Canada, where ozone levels are much lower.

Several investigations have examined the effects of ozone on respiratory health in children. An increase in respiratory symptoms and a decline in lung function have been observed with high levels of ozone exposure. A certain genetic make-up may predispose one to develop inflammation and lung scarring after ozone exposure. Ozone and other air pollutants may adversely affect individuals who carry this gene. Someday people with the "ozone gene" will be easily identified at an early age. Those who carry this gene could then be advised to live in areas or regions of the world where ozone levels are low.

## Nitrogen Dioxide

Nitrogen dioxide arises from the burning of fossil fuels in power plants and automobile exhaust emissions. Nitrogen dioxide levels are directly proportional to the number of cars, buses and trucks on the road and, like ozone levels, peak during the late afternoon rush hour. Unlike ozone, nitrogen dioxide is also an important indoor air pollutant, as it is a by-product of cigarette smoke, gas stoves and indoor kerosene heaters. Nitrogen dioxide levels are higher in homes with poorly ventilated gas cooking and heating appliances. Nitrogen dioxide also plays a role in workplaces such as bus garages and ice skating arenas. Several investigators have demonstrated that nitrogen dioxide levels are related to the frequency and duration of respiratory illness in children. This applies to outdoor as well as indoor exposure. Furthermore, people with allergic asthma have an increased response to inhaled allergens after a nitrogen dioxide exposure.

## Sulfur Dioxide

Sulfur dioxide, a by-product of fossil fuel combustion in heavy industry, is more bothersome to people with asthma in cold, dry air versus warm, moist air. Sulfur dioxide gas is emitted into the air by coal-fired power plants, refineries, smelters, paper pulp mills and food processing plants. The United States Environmental Protection Agency (EPA) considers sulfur dioxide a serious widespread outdoor air pollutant. People with asthma are especially sensitive to very low concentrations of sulfur dioxide—as little as one part per million. The combination of exposure to cold air and a high sulfur dioxide level has an additive effect.

## Particulate Matter

Particulate matter is the term that refers to air particles arising from diesel or gasoline combustion, wood stoves, industrial smokestacks and all other types of fuel combustion. Particulate matter is the most complex of all pollutants regulated by the Environmental Protection Agency. The EPA considers particulate matter to be one of the two major air pollutants—the other is ozone. Seventeen of 20 of the world's largest mega-cities (cities with a population of more than 10 million people) have levels of particulate matter that exceed the maximum level recommended by the World Health Organization. When particulate levels are high, asthmatics have increased medication use, low peak flow readings and more hospital admissions and emergency room visits. A survey in Salt Lake City, Utah, found that a rise in particulate matter levels on cold days decreased peak flow readings and increased medication use in asthmatics. High levels of particulate matter were associated with an increase in bronchitis and croup in five German cities. A new study shows that particulate air pollution is a killer. Doctor Jonathan Samet from Johns Hopkins University assessed five outdoor pollutants—ozone, carbon monoxide, sulfur dioxide, nitrogen dioxide and particulate matter in 30 U.S. counties inhabited by 50 million Americans from 1987 to 1994. This survey found that the daily death rate was higher on days when particulate matter counts were elevated.

One form of particulate matter that is receiving increased attention is diesel exhaust particles. Pollen grains and other allergens can attach themselves to diesel particles and essentially fly with the wind. In some large cities, 70 percent of particulate matter comes from diesel exhaust fumes. In Munich, Germany, poor breathing tests in asthmatics were directly related to the volume of traffic. Many cities are considering limiting the volume of diesel-powered vehicles. Good luck to them. Diesel engines are almost indestructible—the average diesel engine can go one million miles!

A high incidence of dust mite allergy has been found in neighborhoods with diesel air pollution. Japanese children who live near major highways have a higher level of cedar tree allergy versus those living in the forest, even though the cedar pollen levels were the same in both locales. Citizens of England who live close to the busy motorways have a higher incidence of respiratory problems, including asthma. The closer they live to the motorway, the greater the likelihood of having asthma. The level of diesel particles rise dramatically in the autumn, a time when asthma admissions also peak, suggesting that in some cities asthma admissions may be directly related to the level of diesel exhaust particles.

## Epidemic Asthma

Several cities throughout the world have experienced sudden epidemics of asthma. One dramatic example of epidemic asthma is found in the city of New Orleans, where hundreds of people with asthma often seek emergency care at local hospitals during a single day. This "New Orleans Asthma" was thoroughly investigated by

Doctor John Salvaggio of Tulane University. Salvaggio found that New Orleans asthma epidemics occurred on damp fall days when temperature and humidity levels were low and ragweed counts were high. The asthma epidemic begins when a fast-moving cold air mass enters New Orleans and triggers a sudden drop in temperature. Similar asthma outbreaks have been reported in New York City, Philadelphia, Los Angeles and Donora, Pennsylvania.

## Barcelona Asthma

Doctors in Barcelona, Spain, recorded 26 asthma epidemics from 1981 to 1987. One outbreak that affected several hundred individuals led to more than one thousand emergency room visits within just a few days. At first, medical detectives (epidemiologists) suspected that high levels of nitrogen dioxide were triggering the Barcelona asthma epidemic. Additional detective work uncovered the fact that these asthma outbreaks occurred when large cargo ships were unloading soybean in Barcelona's harbor, and soybean dust was blown throughout the city. High barometric pressure and low winds apparently triggered the release of tiny soybean particles. Once bag filters were placed on top of the soybean storage silos, the Barcelona asthma epidemics stopped. This clever piece of investigation points out the need to constantly monitor air quality, particularly in urban areas located near grain or soybean plants.

## Guidelines for Air Pollution Alerts

People with asthma who reside in areas subjected to thermal inversions, air pollution alerts and asthma epidemics should monitor daily reports on weather and air pollution alerts. The following guidelines should be observed during air pollution alerts:

▲ Avoid unnecessary physical activity

▲ Avoid smoking and smoke-filled rooms

▲ Avoid dust and other irritants

▲ Avoid people with colds or the flu

▲ Stay indoors and use air conditioners

▲ Know your asthma medicines

▲ Exercise in the early morning, before pollution levels peak

▲ Run or cycle on less-congested roadways

▲ Travel or vacation in pollution-free areas

▲ Follow air pollution alerts via newspapers, radio or TV

▲ Take additional medicine during air pollution alerts

## Indoor Air Pollution

Thanks to the efforts of the Environmental Protection Agency, we now know that indoor air pollution poses more of a public health problem than outdoor air pollution. Common indoor pollutants include microscopic-sized particles such as bacteria, yeast, house dust mites, molds, animal parts, pollens and tobacco products. Air pollutants are also emitted from electrical appliances, hair dryers and wood, coal and gas burning stoves and fireplaces. Additional sources include perfumes, colognes, household cleaners, deodorants and hair sprays.

While numerous studies have defined the risks posed by indoor aeroallergens such as house dust mites and animal parts, the hazards of indoor pollutants from gas stoves, wood stoves and fireplaces are poorly defined. Indoor combustion sources produce a mixture of respiratory irritants, including nitrogen dioxide, aldehydes, acids and particulate matter. Fortunately, research efforts on air pollution has shifted to studying indoor air pollution. The EPA has found that air pollutants may be 100 times higher inside versus outside the home. Since Americans spend nearly 90 percent of their lives indoors, the threat that indoor air pollutants now pose is greater than outdoor air pollutants.

The most damaging indoor air pollutants are invisible to the naked eye. Scientists measure the size of an air particle in microns. A micron is one millionth of a meter, or approximately .000036 inches. Larger, heavier particles (over eight to ten microns in size) are not inhaled into the lung. Particles from three to eight microns in size are often trapped in the mouth and nose. Particles less than three microns in size are the most dangerous, as they are more easily inhaled and deposited deep in the lung. When one considers that one single cubic foot of air in our indoor environment may contain up to one million particles, it is obvious that our respiratory tract is incredibly efficient at filtering out air particles.

## Smoking Parents

The risk for asthma posed by environmental tobacco smoke (ETS) is firmly established. Over the last 15 years, there has been a steady accumulation of evidence that parents, especially mothers, who smoke in the home, increase the risk of repeated respiratory infection and asthma in their children. A National Health Survey of 4,331 children found that if a mother smoked more than one-half pack of cigarettes per day, the risk of a child developing asthma was 2.6 times higher in the first year of life. Similar numbers came out of a study in Tucson, Arizona, where children of mothers who smoked more than 10 cigarettes a day were 2.5 times more likely to develop asthma than children of non-smoking mothers.

Another study looked at 120 children of allergic parents. If one parent smoked, the risk for developing asthma was four times normal, and if both parents smoked, the odds increased nearly five times. Children born to pregnant mothers exposed to passive smoke during their pregnancy have a greater chance of developing asthma. It is estimated that the exposure to ETS causes 8,000 to 26,000 new cases of asthma per year. Children with asthma who are exposed to secondhand smoke are more likely to die of their disease. ETS exposure is closely linked to bronchitis and pneumonia in children. There are now nearly 100 such studies, proving the high risk of asthma for infants and young children when they are exposed to ETS.

There is additional evidence that active cigarette smoking in adolescents and young adults also poses a risk for asthma. What are the mechanisms by which ETS exposure worsens asthma? Infants born to smoking mothers have smaller airways than infants of non-smoking mothers. Infants with small lungs are more likely to wheeze during a viral respiratory infection. Smoking accelerates mucus production and airway inflammation. Common sense dictates that asthmatics should not smoke. Yet nearly one in every four asthmatics does smoke. Smoking asthmatics do not respond as well to asthma medications. They greatly increase their chances of developing chronic bronchitis or crippling emphysema. ETS exposure is potentially the most preventable risk factor for asthma. It is encouraging that the ban on smoking in public places in affluent countries has reduced exposure to ETS in the community. Unfortunately, the home is still the primary location for ETS exposure for children. Infants and children need to be protected from exposure to ETS in their own homes. Eliminating exposure to ETS reduces the incidence of serious respiratory infections in early childhood and may prevent asthma. It is essential that the medical community develop public health strategies that focus on pregnant women and smoking parents to prevent early ETS exposure to pregnant mothers and infants and children.

## The Sick Building Syndrome

Modern-day construction methods employ energy-efficient building techniques to control fuel costs. Eighty-five percent of all new homes and buildings are energy efficient. People who live and work in these structures rarely breathe fresh outdoor air. In most newer office buildings employees cannot open their office windows. This problem is not confined to new structures. Older apartment and office buildings are being remodeled with new energy-efficient conservation methods. Heated or cooled air that is recycled through a closed system of air ducts may trigger a controversial set of symptoms called the sick building syndrome. Victims of the sick building syndrome experience headaches, frequent colds, sinus infections, nausea, eye irritation, skin rashes and asthma.

Attack rates for asthma may approach 70 percent in some buildings. The sick building syndrome, also called building-related illness, is thought to be due to continuous inhalation of stale, recycled, contaminated air. Industry, governmental agencies and medicine have been slow to respond to the hazards posed by indoor air pollution. While Congress has appropriated millions of dollars for the study of air pollution, until recently less than 10 percent of air pollution expenditures was earmarked for indoor air studies. The National Institute of Occupational Safety and Health recommends that office ventilation systems provide outdoor air circulation at a minimum rate of 20 feet per minute per occupant in smoking areas, and five feet per minute in non-smoking areas. There are no standards for home ventilation rates. Asthmatics who are victimized by a sick building often require alterations in their environment. In some cases job relocation may be the only solution. One way to find out if you are living or working in a contaminated environment is to measure the level of carbon dioxide in the air. If the carbon dioxide level is high, it means that the heating or cooling system is not circulating enough fresh air. Building managers often shut down the fresh air intake to control heating or cooling costs. Simply increasing the intake of fresh air into the system will solve a lot of problems when office windows cannot be opened.

## *Hot Air Heating Systems*

The typical forced-hot-air heating system in a home or office building recycles air through vents after it has been warmed or cooled by an oil- or gas-fired furnace or heat exchanger. Low costs entice builders and developers to install hot air systems in new homes, apartments and condominiums. Hot air systems pose a serious threat to asthmatics, as their vents constantly recycle dust, mold, pollen, bacteria and animal parts throughout the dwelling.

The allergic asthmatic living in a home heated by forced hot air must take some special precautions. The system should be properly filtered and maintained. Avoid using central humidifiers that tend to become infested with molds. Family room and bedroom air vents should be covered with cheesecloth or fiberglass filters. In some cases it may be necessary to seal off the ducts and install supplemental electric heat. Hot air systems should be vacuumed or professionally cleaned before the start of each heating season. Sometimes I find it necessary to advise a sick asthmatic to move out of a rented home or apartment with hot air heat. Tenants who feel they are at the mercy of a tight lease or rental agreement usually have no problem breaking their lease after I write a letter to their landlord stating that their present environment poses a significant health hazard.

## Wood and Coal Stoves

The ancient fossil fuels, wood and coal, are man's oldest source of energy. Wood and coal combustion produces more toxins and air pollutants than oil or gas combustion. The devastating effects of coal combustion were brought to light in the Great London Smog Epidemic of 1952, when 4,000 people died after inhaling the toxic products of burning coal. In communities where wood stoves are used, wintertime air inversions trap wood smoke and produce a ground-hugging layer of contaminated outdoor air pollutants, particles and toxins that aggravate asthma. A typical wood stove produces up to 80 pounds of unburned material per cord of wood. Each day a wood stove emits as much carbon monoxide as an automobile does on a 50-mile trip.

The most damaging microscopic-sized wood smoke particles are inhaled deep into the lung. Children who live in homes heated by wood or coal stoves have more colds, bronchitis and asthma than children who reside in homes heated with gas or oil-fired furnaces. The energy crunch of the early 1980s created a resurgence in the use of wood and coal as a primary energy source. Fifty percent of Northern New England homes were heated in part with wood or coal. Twenty percent of all homes in Vermont were heated by wood in 1986. Virtually every new home in Northern New England now has a wood stove.

In 1986, the Environmental Protection Agency estimated that 15 million homes were heated with wood, and predicted that one million homes a year would convert to wood or coal as a primary heat source. While these estimates were downgraded in the 1990s due to the slackening of the energy crisis, the energy crunch of the twenty-first century has led to another resurgence in the use of wood and coal stoves.

Many communities have taken a close look at the harmful effects of wood and coal stoves. Vermont's Environmental Conservation Agency found that 65 percent of the pollutants in Vermont air on cold winter days came from wood-burning stoves. Vail, Colorado, implemented aggressive measures to control the wood smoke that creates a blue haze over the town on cold winter mornings. Vail building codes allow only one wood stove per dwelling, and coal stoves are prohibited. All wood stoves must be equipped with catalytic converters to reduce air pollution by burning recycled smoke at higher temperatures. Amherst, Massachusetts, passed a law that requires one occupant of every home to obtain a license to run the wood stove. When an improperly managed stove puts out too many pollutants, Amherst officials can fine the homeowner. Telluride, Colorado, officials will not issue a new stove permit unless the builder can persuade two other residents to give up their wood stoves. Many communities forbid the use of wood or coal stoves during air pollution alerts and regulate that these stoves be equipped with catalytic converters, much like automobiles. Most of these new laws do not affect ordinary fireplaces. Wood stoves should not be converted to coal, since coal smoke is more hazardous than wood smoke. When a coal stove is an absolute necessity, only hard coal, or anthracite, should be burned.

There is no question that wood and coal stoves can aggravate asthma, but convincing stove owners is another matter. Families who save hundreds of dollars a year in heating costs are understandably reluctant to give up their stoves. I usually recommend turning the stove off for three to four weeks on a trial basis. If asthma improves while the stove is off, or recurs when the stove is turned back on, the stove should be permanently shut down.

## Controlling Indoor Air Pollution

How does one address air quality within your own home? Doctor Rebecca Bascom, Chief of Pulmonary Medicine at Penn State University, has outlined a five-step, walk-through approach to evaluate the major areas in your home.

**Step 1.** Look at the overall structure of the home. The home may be too tightly insulated, preventing the exchange of fresh air. While such a home has lower heating and cooling costs, indoor air pollutants are easily trapped. Make sure combustible appliances like gas stoves, furnaces and hot water heaters are professionally installed and vented to the outdoors. If you are building a new home or remodeling your kitchen, consider installing an electric stove.

**Step 2.** Look at things inside your home. New rugs, furniture or flooring may emit gas or chemicals months after they are installed. Many European countries do not allow occupants of new buildings to enter the structure for several months after construction has been completed.

**Step 3.** Evaluate activities in the home. Eliminate indoor smoking. Minimize use of aerosol and spray can products. Avoid personal products with strong odors or scents. Avoid using pesticides within the home.

**Step 4.** Evaluate how air moves in and around your home. Doctor Bascom quotes an old adage, "The solution to pollution is dilution." A regular supply of fresh air is essential for good indoor air quality. Houses heated or cooled with central air systems are of particular concern. Make sure that air conditioning systems are checked and are free of excess condensation and molds. Filters should be changed on a regular basis. Hot air heating ducts should be professionally vacuumed and cleaned annually. Poor maintenance of these systems encourages the build-up of dust particles, mold and bacteria.

**Step 5.** Determine how water and humidity moves in and around your home. Water vapor in the air produces what is known as humidity. Humidity levels above 50 percent provide an ideal growth environment for dust mites, molds and bacteria. Control indoor humidity levels, especially in damp basements, with properly functioning air conditioners or home dehumidifiers. Condensation on heating or air conditioning ducts is usually a sign of excess humidity. Insulation of these ducts may be necessary. An instrument called a hygrometer, sold in home improvement outlets or hardware stores, can measure indoor humidity levels.

## Warm Days, Cool Nights and Thunderstorms

The fact that asthma relapses have a seasonal variation has been recognized since the time of Hippocrates, who noted that asthma was more common in the autumn months. Studies in both northern and southern hemispheres show that there are two seasonal peaks in asthma cases. First, there is a moderate rise in the late winter–early spring that declines in the summer, only to be followed by a stronger peak in the fall or early winter. I used to think most asthma emergency visits or hospitalizations were triggered by viral or respiratory infections. This may be wrong. In my experience, asthma relapses and admissions are commonly seen in the months characterized by warmer (for New England) days and colder nights, especially on days characterized by a mid-afternoon temperature of 60 or so degrees Fahrenheit. In the late afternoon or early evening, these comfortable daytime temperatures can rapidly plunge down to the low forties or high thirties. I believe this rapid and wide swing in outdoor temperature is an important risk factor for some people with asthma. Many of my patients or parents of asthmatic children relate that asthma is much worse on the days when this late afternoon–early evening temperature change is most extreme. Savvy emergency room nurses know that these are the evenings, especially Halloween night, when the emergency room will be busy treating wheezy trick-or-treaters.

A study from Israel supports this relationship between sudden weather changes and asthma relapses in children. Asthma relapses were closely associated with late afternoon weather changes in data collected for three years in Israeli children hospitalized for acute asthma. It appears that the airways of asthmatics are particularly sensitive to the rapid air-cooling that occurs in the late afternoon or early evening. Changes occurring in the autumn are more likely to trigger asthma, especially when cold air masses rapidly move into an area.

Mini-asthma epidemics have been linked to thunderstorm activity in England and Europe. In 1997, British researchers tracked phone calls made after thunderstorms and found a tenfold increase in calls to doctors for asthma care immediately after a thunderstorm. Australian researchers may have found the answer to thunderstorm asthma. Thunderstorm asthma may be caused by high winds sweeping up pollen and concentrating it into a narrow downdraft of air at ground level. In one asthma epidemic in Wagga Wagga, Australia, the level of grass pollen activity increased four to twelve-fold during thunderstorm activity. Those asthmatics affected by thunderstorms should go indoors or take their preventative asthma medicines when such storms are approaching their areas, especially during the pollen seasons.

# Food Allergy
## and
## Asthma

# 9

While early medical historians lacked a basic understanding of immunology, they were able to objectively describe reactions to foods. For example, the medical word for hives or urticaria comes from the Latin word, *urtica*, or nettle. Greek and Roman physicians recognized that when people ate or handled nettle, a stinging herb, they developed an itchy, raised rash or hives. Hippocrates recorded that many people were intolerant of milk and cheeses. *"Cheese does not harm all men alike, some can eat their full of it, while others come off badly. If cheese were bad for human consumption, it would have hurt all."*

In the first century, Titus Lucretius Carus (96–55 B.C.), the distinguished Latin poet and philosopher, wrote *"What is food for some may be fierce poison for others."* In other words, one man's meat is another man's poison. Avicenna (980–1037) warned about the potential dangers of certain foods. He understood that food reactions varied according to previous exposure, and few foods could be universally proscribed. *"Thus, a food which is often used, though injurious to a certain degree, may be more appropriate for a given individual than a food which he does not often take."* In 1808, Robert Willan (1757–1812), described several patients with hives (urticaria) and swelling (angioedema). He vividly depicts a reaction to a tree nut in his patient, Doctor Thomas Winterbottom, who had eaten a small amount of almonds.

> *"Symptoms were soon followed by an edematous swelling of the face, especially of the lips and nose, which were very hot and itchy. There was at the same time an uneasy tickling sensation in the throat...the tongue likewise became enlarged...soon after going to*

131

*bed an eruption took place over the whole body of spots nearly as large as a sixpence."*

Willan noted that only certain foods (including mushrooms, seafood and almonds) induced this response in certain individuals. After Alfred Wolff-Eisner's (1877–1948) description of anaphylaxis in 1906, serious research into food allergies began. Once the concept of food allergy was accepted, many reports came forth, including reactions to eggs, oatmeal and nuts.

## *Food and Chemical Triggers*

Foodstuffs, beverages and chemical additives can trigger asthma and allergic reactions. Throughout our lifetime, the average human being consumes five to six thousand pounds of foodstuffs and chemical additives and several thousand gallons of beverages. Normally our intestinal tract and digestive system are incredibly efficient organs that separate the helpful from harmful foods and beverages. However, in a small percentage of individuals, ingested foods and beverages trigger an allergic reaction. While more than 200 foodstuffs can cause an allergic reaction, most reactions are caused by the "big eight;" peanuts, tree nuts, fish, shellfish, milk, eggs, wheat and soybeans.

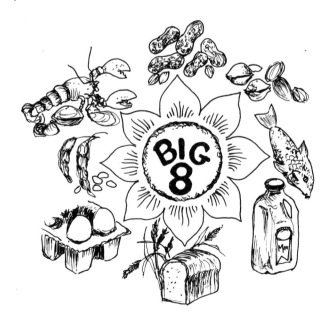

A recent survey found that between one and two percent of adults are allergic to peanuts or tree nuts, and another two percent of adults are allergic to other foods, especially fish and shellfish. These numbers add up to about seven million Americans having food allergies. The incidence of food allergy is highest in infancy and early childhood, presumably due to immaturity of the gastro-intestinal tract's immune system. Six to eight percent of children under age four have one or more food allergies. Most children will outgrow their food allergy by age 10, when the prevalence of food allergy approaches adult levels.

Children with eczema have a much higher incidence of food allergy. Children who have eczema and food allergies are more likely to be allergic to milk, eggs, peanuts or tree nuts. Five percent of children with asthma have food allergies, and about one percent are prone to a severe food reaction. Asthmatics may be developing more food allergies, but while food allergy can cause asthma, it is an uncommon and somewhat overstated asthma trigger.

In one of the earliest studies to employ a placebo-controlled food challenge, Doctor Charles May of the National Jewish Hospital in Denver, Colorado, tested 38 children with severe asthma and found 11 children had positive challenges to foods, but their symptoms were primarily gastrointestinal. None of the children in May's study developed asthma or respiratory symptoms. A subsequent study by Doctor Alan Bock found that foods could trigger asthma. Twelve of 68 food-allergic children with asthma wheezed within 12 hours of a food challenge.

Researchers in Montpelier, France, found that two of 25 food-allergic patients developed asthma on direct food challenges. In a larger comprehensive review of 1,000 double-blind, placebo-controlled food challenges at the National Jewish Hospital, it was found that one percent of children exhibited asthma as a sole response to blind food challenges. Nearly one in every four American families has altered their dietary habits because of the perception that one or more members of their family suffer from a food allergy. While some surveys imply that 25 percent of the population has a food allergy or an adverse food reaction, only one in every 10 food reactions is a true immunological reaction driven by the allergic or IgE antibody response.

## Killed by a Kiss

The diagnosis of food allergy requires a careful medical history followed up by allergy skin or blood tests. Unfortunately, there is a wide discrepancy between the perceptions of patients and physicians regarding food allergy. Food allergy is often erroneously blamed for a variety of conditions, including asthma. When food does induce asthma, the most common inciting foods are peanuts, tree nuts and shellfish. The time between food ingestion and the onset of wheezing is usually quite brief—minutes to hours. In the majority of cases, the amount of food required to induce symptoms is quite small. Sometimes merely inhaling odors from a cooking food, or being exposed to airborne peanut particles in an airplane will cause wheezing or an allergic reaction.

In her excellent book, *The Allergy Bible* (Readers Digest Publications 2001), Linda Gamlin describes how food-allergic patients can be killed by a kiss. Gamlin described a young man with fish allergy who required emergency care after being kissed by his girlfriend who had just eaten mackerel. In another incident, a peanut-allergic child experienced a severe allergic reaction after he was kissed by his aunt who had just eaten some peanuts.

When foods do trigger wheezing, patients will often experience other allergic symptoms, such as swelling or edema, hives, shock and even complete cardiovascular collapse. When hives are the only symptom, the food reaction is usually mild. When lung, heart and blood vessels are involved, or if the throat closes up, the allergic reaction becomes a severe, life-threatening medical emergency called anaphylaxis. When the clinical history reveals a severe, life-threatening or anaphylactic reaction, skin testing may be dangerous, as it could trigger an acute allergic reaction. Blood or RAST testing is the preferred method for detecting the offending food in such cases. Skin testing to foods is not as accurate as skin testing to airborne allergens. A positive skin test to a food does not always indicate the presence of food allergy, as studies have shown that only 40 percent of patients with a positive skin test react to a food challenge.

Most children who are allergic to eggs, cow's milk, soy and wheat outgrow their food allergy and become tolerant of these foods by age three or four. Unfortunately, allergy to peanuts, tree nuts or shellfish is not always outgrown. A recent study in England found that only 20 percent of school-aged children who had a peanut reaction in infancy became tolerant to peanuts later on in childhood. Those children who did outgrow their peanut allergy had smaller skin test reactions to peanuts, and were less likely to have eczema or asthma. Skin tests are one way to determine if a child has outgrown a food allergy. A negative test is a good indicator that a food allergy has resolved. Sometimes a food allergy skin test remains positive long after the food allergy is outgrown. This is called a false positive skin test. In these cases a careful food challenge may be the only way to determine the presence or absence of a food allergy. Sometimes food allergy starts in adulthood, especially fruit and vegetable allergy. Most allergic reactions to fruits and vegetables are mild and not life-threatening events.

## Anaphylaxis—Yet Another Epidemic

Food allergy can trigger severe, life-threatening reactions, especially in patients who are allergic to peanuts or tree nuts. It is estimated that 200 patients die per year in the United States from fatal food reactions. Four independent studies from the United States and England looked at emergency room records to determine the cause of severe allergic reactions that required an emergency room visit. The leading cause by far for this type of emergency visit was a food allergy, which accounted for one in every three visits. Food allergy has not been spared by the asthma-allergy epidemic. There is a growing concern about the rising incidence of severe allergic reactions to foods, which has paralleled the rise in asthma and other allergic diseases. The type of allergic reaction that is generating the most concern is life-threatening anaphylaxis.

The initial reports of anaphylaxis date back to Egypt in 2641 B.C. Ancient Egyptian hieroglyphics from that time depict the Pharaoh Menes dying from a wasp sting. Despite this historic and graphic depiction of anaphylaxis, the first reports of human deaths from anaphylaxis did not appear in the medical literature until 1895, when fatalities to diphtheria vaccinations with extracts derived from horse serum were described. The next wave of anaphylactic deaths occurred after the introduction of injectable penicillin in the 1940s.

Today the most common causes for anaphylactic reactions are foods, aspirin-like drugs, antibiotics and stinging insects. The modern definition of anaphylaxis describes a rapid, generalized and often

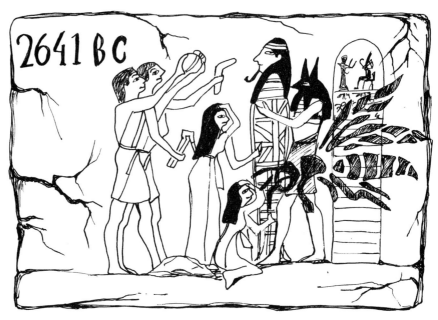

Pharoah Menes

unanticipated immunological, usually IgE-mediated, event that occurs after exposure to an allergen in a previously sensitized person. Anaphylaxis is sometimes confused with the term "anaphylactoid reaction," which produces similar symptoms but lacks a history of prior exposure to the offending substance and a true allergic or IgE-mediated allergen cannot be identified. The best example of an anaphylactoid reaction is the person who reacts to injected contrast media or an X-ray dye, even though they have never been previously exposed to this dye.

Anaphylaxis is more frequent and more severe in adults, especially women. Severe food reactions are more likely to occur in atopic or allergic people who are better allergic antibody or IgE producers. Anaphylaxis can strike the skin, gastrointestinal tract, respiratory and cardiovascular symptoms (Figure 9.3). Skin symptoms of anaphylaxis are facial flushing, itchiness, excess sweating, hives (urticaria) and swelling (angioedema). Gastrointestinal symptoms include nausea, vomiting, abdominal cramps and diarrhea. In severe cases cardiorespiratory symptoms cause dizziness, low blood pressure (fainting or collapse), swelling in the throat, shortness of breath, coughing and wheezing. Not all these symptoms have to be present, nor do they appear in any special order. In most cases anaphylaxis symptoms begin within minutes or one to two hours after exposure to the offending allergen. Sometimes the reaction may be delayed for several hours.

Figure
9.3

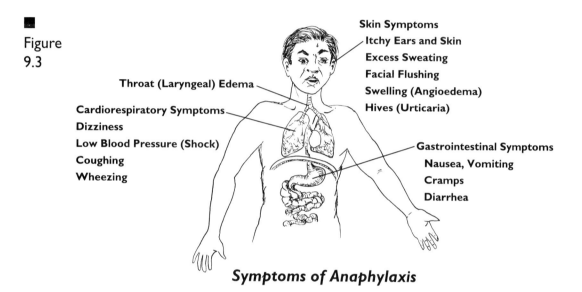

**Symptoms of Anaphylaxis**

One dangerous type of anaphylaxis is called biphasic anaphylaxis, where the victim has an immediate reaction that resolves with appropriate treatment and then recurs several hours later. The biggest danger of biphasic anaphylaxis is that patients may respond promptly to their initial emergency room treatment and be prematurely discharged, only to experience a second or biphasic reaction several hours after they have left the emergency room. The take-home message here for emergency room docs and nurses is that anyone who experiences a moderate to severe anaphylactic reaction should be observed in the emergency room for six to eight hours before being sent home.

## *Treatment of Anaphylaxis*

The treatment of choice in anaphylaxis is epinephrine or adrenaline, the hormone produced by our adrenal gland. There are few major risks to epinephrine. In my earlier medical career, in order to support my family of six children, I moonlighted in emergency rooms two to three nights a week. Most of the lives I saved were due to the use of epinephrine, one of the few true life-saving drugs in medicine. Epinephrine increases heart rate and blood pressure, constricts blood vessels and opens up narrowed airways. Minor side effects include a pounding heart, pallor, dizziness, tremors and headache. In the clinic or hospital setting, epinephrine is given by injection. Automatic epinephrine injector kits are available for use in the home, at school or in public places. The best kit is the EpiPen, which is easy to use and carry. The safest and most effective place to inject the EpiPen is the outer thigh.

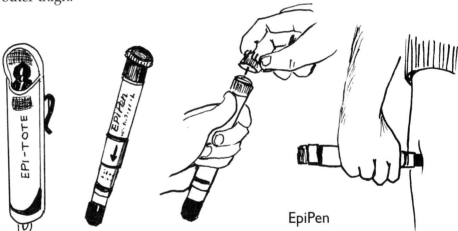

EpiPen

Anyone who experiences symptoms of an allergic or anaphylactic reaction should take Benadryl, an antihistamine; self-administer the EpiPen and immediately proceed to the nearest hospital. You should carry extra epinephrine on trips or while camping, boating, golfing or engaging in activities where immediate medical care is not readily available.

For further information on anaphylaxis, I suggest you contact Media Works in Canada. Media Works has produced an excellent video and booklet for anaphylactic victims and their families.

Kimberly Curran, a video producer and mother of a child with severe peanut allergy, initiated this work. These materials are sponsored by the Anaphylaxis Foundation of Canada and endorsed by the Canadian Society of Allergy and Clinical Immunology Allergy. Contact Media Works @ P.O. Box 64, Cobourg, Ontario Canada K9A 4K2. Phone 905-373-9324 or www.mediaworkstudio.com

## A New Threat—Asthma and Food Anaphylaxis

The frequency of severe, life-threatening and fatal reactions to foods in patients with asthma has risen dramatically over the past two decades. Tragically, the majority of these fatalities occur in children and young adults with asthma who were fully aware of their preexisting food allergy. Case studies have found that most near-fatal or fatal anaphylactic reactions due to foods occur in asthmatics who are severely allergic to peanuts, tree nuts or shellfish. After accidental ingestion of the offending foods, these unfortunate individuals did not take or were not given the proper emergency care that could have saved their lives. Such care includes prompt administration of epinephrine (EpiPen), Benadryl and immediate transport to an emergency facility.

Doctor John Yunginger from the Mayo Clinic has collected seven cases of fatal food anaphylaxis. One case involved a peanut-allergic Brown University student who died shortly after she ingested chili laced with peanuts in a local restaurant. Her needless death received national attention and led to congressional hearings that addressed the issues of menu disclosure and food labeling. The other six fatal cases occurred in children and young adults after accidental ingestion of pecans, peanuts or seafood. There were several common features in these seven preventable deaths. All but one occurred away from the home in local restaurants. Every patient had asthma and a history of a prior allergic reaction to the offending food. Only one patient was carrying a potentially life-saving epinephrine kit.

Doctor Hugh Sampson, director of the Jaffe Food Allergy Institute at Mount Sinai Hospital in New York, described six fatal and seven near-fatal anaphylactic food reactions in children age two to seventeen years. Once again all near-fatal and fatal events took place in children and young adults with asthma. All 13 cases had a history of a previous reaction to the food, and every victim accidentally ingested the offending food. Symptoms in these children included tingling, flushing, itching, hives and swelling, air hunger or wheezing, abdominal cramps, vomiting and in fatal cases cardiovascular collapse. Most of the fatal reactions did not develop hives or swelling, which could have served as a warning sign of impending disaster. Some of the fatal cases experienced immediate oral symptoms (itchy mouth) followed by a lulling quiescent period and then major respiratory collapse. None of the patients who experienced fatal reactions received epinephrine immediately after the onset of their symptoms, whereas all of the survivors received epinephrine within five minutes after developing symptoms. The most common triggers were peanuts, tree nuts and seafood.

Thirty-two cases of fatal food reactions were reviewed in the Journal of Allergy and Clinical Immunology in January 2001. Most patients were adolescents or young adults. Only three patients were less than ten years of age. All but one had asthma, 90 percent of deaths were due to peanut or tree nut ingestion, and all but one of these patients were aware of a preexisting peanut or tree nut allergy. The two deaths to fish and milk ingestion occurred in younger children. Only three patients had their EpiPen available. The following two cases typify fatal food anaphylaxis:

*Case 1. BF was a nine-year-old male with asthma and nut allergy who was given some peanut candy by a classmate in school. Ninety minutes later he went to the nurse's office complaining of abdominal pain. Unfortunately, the school nurse was not aware of his peanut allergy. Within twenty minutes he began to vomit and have difficulty breathing and three hours after ingesting the peanut-laced candy he died in a local emergency room.*

Clearly this was a preventable death, which points out the need for education of all caretakers of children as well as the need to administer epinephrine immediately after the signs and symptoms of a food reaction begin, even if the symptoms are mild in nature.

*Case 2. AF was a 32-year-old female with chronic asthma and a history of peanut and nut allergy since childhood. Her asthma was considered to be moderate in severity as she experienced four to five relapses per year that required prednisone. She had no prior history of emergency room visits or hospitalizations for asthma. In June 1990, while driving her car and eating a Danish that contained a hidden nut, she began to wheeze and she drove herself to a local emergency room where she was treated with epinephrine, Benadryl and Solumedrol (a cortisone drug). She improved rapidly and was discharged in about two hours. This proved to be a mistake. On the way home, her asthma recurred. She drove back to the emergency room, collapsed in the parking lot and was found in acute respiratory arrest. She was immediately admitted to an intensive care unit, placed on a respirator and subsequently recovered. Over the next four years her asthma was relatively stable. In January 1994 while dining at a mall restaurant she ordered a dish with pesto sauce, which according to her waiter did not contain any nuts. Tragically, the pesto sauce contained hidden walnuts and she immediately experienced a severe anaphylactic reaction and arrived in the local emergency room in a comatose state and died several days later.*

The take-home message of this heartbreaking case is that waiters don't prepare your food, and food-allergic patients should ask to speak with the restaurant manager or even the chef before ordering foods that may contain hidden food allergens. Patients must be taught to read menus and food labels and to be very vigilant in restaurants where cross contamination or spatula carryover may occur.

## Exercise-induced Anaphylaxis

One unique form of anaphylaxis is called exercise-induced anaphylaxis. In 1980, Doctors Albert Sheffer and Frank Austin, researchers from Harvard University, described a group of adolescents and young adults who during or shortly after exercise felt warm and itchy, developed hives or swelling, or experienced cardiovascular collapse. Additional symptoms included wheezing and stomach cramps. This reaction was more likely to occur in young athletes during vigorous exercise in warmer weather. Sheffer and Austin labeled this syndrome exercise-induced anaphylaxis.

In 1983, Doctor Jordan Fink from the University of Wisconsin reported additional cases of young athletes with exercise-induced anaphylaxis. Fink's patients related that they only experienced symptoms when they ate certain foods prior to exercising. The most common foods that predisposed them to exercise-induced-anaphylaxis were celery and carrots. Many subsequent reports have described many other foods, including fish, nuts and wheat, that are capable of triggering exercise-induced anaphylaxis. It is postulated that people with food-related, exercise-induced anaphylaxis have a subtle or unrecognized allergy to certain foods that only manifests itself when the offending food allergen is rapidly absorbed during or after exercise. The treatment of exercise-induced anaphylaxis is quite basic. First, if it is food-related, one must avoid the triggering food before exercising. It may also be helpful to avoid exercising in warmer weather. Allergy skin tests, especially with fresh foods, often help identify the offending food. Victims of exercise-induced anaphylaxis should not exercise alone, and should always carry an emergency, self-injectable epinephrine kit.

## Oral Allergy Syndrome

Allergy specialists have long been aware that many of their patients with hay fever or pollen allergy complain of an itchy mouth, tongue or lips after eating fresh fruits and vegetables, like apples, pears, peaches, celery, carrots and members of the melon family. Yet they have no problems with cooked foods, such as apple pie, canned fruits or heated vegetables. Heating or cooking a food often denatures the allergenic part of the food. Any given food may contain 10 to 30 proteins, of which only a few act as an allergen. Some food allergens have a striking resemblance to pollen and latex allergens. This observation helps to explain why some pollen and latex-sensitive individuals experience an itchy mouth or throat when they eat these fruits and vegetables, especially in their raw state. For example, people with tree pollen allergy may have difficulty eating raw apples, pears, peaches or raw carrots or celery.

Ragweed-sensitive individuals experience symptoms after eating melons or bananas. Latex-allergic patients may react to chestnuts, bananas, avocado and kiwi fruit. This cross-reactivity is due to a shared enzyme, called a chitinase, that protects plants and fruits against insects. Latex comes from the sap of the rubber tree, and the tree is laced with this enzyme to protect it from insects. This syndrome has been labeled the Oral Allergy Syndrome. Fortunately, it is usually a mild reaction localized to the mouth or tongue. Treatment is simple—avoid the offending food, especially in its raw or uncooked state.

## *Treatment of Food Allergy*

Once a specific food has been identified as an asthma or allergy trigger, the treatment is avoidance. Patients with asthma and food allergy should be aware that most foods belong to a food group or a food family. An allergy to one member of a specific food family often means that ingestion of other members of the same food family will cause an allergic reaction. For example, if you are allergic to lobster, a member of the crustacean family, you are quite likely to experience an allergic reaction when you eat other crustaceans like crab or shrimp. Can the lobster-sensitive person eat fried clams or scallops? The answer is usually yes.

Unfortunately, many doctors have forgotten their basic biology. When confronted with a patient with a crustacean allergy, they recommend avoiding all forms of shellfish or seafood. This is unnecessary, as shellfish like clams, oysters and scallops belong to the mollusk family, and do not usually cross-react with crustaceans. In other words, the patient with lobster allergy may not be allergic to clams, oysters or scallops. Properly performed skin or RAST tests may help sort out food allergies. Food-sensitive asthmatics should not experiment with food groups without the approval of their doctor or allergy specialist. They should also consult their physician, nutrition center or local library for a complete list of foods and food families.

Patients and families with peanut allergy often ask if they can eat other nuts, like walnuts or pecans. Likewise, patients with tree nut allergy want to know if they can safely ingest peanuts or peanut butter. Believe it or not, peanuts are not true nuts. They are members of the legume vegetable family that includes peas, soybeans and beans. On the other hand, true nuts such as walnuts, almonds and pecans belong to the tree nut family. Doctor Hugh Sampson has helped answer these questions. He conducted an extensive survey of children with peanut and tree nut allergy and found that one in every three peanut-allergic patients were sensitive to tree nuts. The bottom line is that one can never predict when the peanut-allergic patient will become tree nut allergic and vice versa.

Thus, it is best for a peanut-sensitive or tree-nut-sensitive person to avoid all forms of peanuts and tree nuts. Sampson's survey also found that 30 percent of tree-nut-allergic patients experienced an accidental ingestion of tree nuts, and more than half of peanut-allergic children had two or more accidental encounters with peanuts within five years of their first peanut reaction. The modes of accidental ingestion included hidden ingredients in processed foods, cross-contamination of foods, sharing food with friends, skin contact with peanut butter in classroom and day care centers, and hidden foods in restaurants, especially Asian restaurants.

People with asthma and peanut or tree nut allergy should avoid most if not all packaged foods. An unpublished FDA study found that only half of 85 candy, ice cream and baked good food plants in Wisconsin and Minnesota were checking to see if the ingredients on their labels matched the ingredients in the foods. Half of these FDA-surveyed plants were turning out foods that contained allergens not listed on their label. Many factories used the same utensils that were supposed to be used in allergen-free foods when making foods with peanuts or eggs. One in every four FDA-sampled foods contained undisclosed peanut allergen. Several important points to remember in preventing food allergy include:

- Educate younger siblings, baby sitters, nannies and grandparents
- Keep epinephrine (EpiPen) kits available everywhere, especially in remote locales—golfing, boating and hiking
- Maintain a peanut- and tree-nut-free home
- Special precautions in the day care and school settings include separate eating tables, no food swapping or trading eating utensils, and the washing of hands, tables and toys after eating
- Encourage teachers and school nurses to develop an action plan for food-allergic children. Families and health-care providers must partner with parents, staff and school nurses in food-allergy education.
- Allow responsible students to carry their own EpiPen
- Do not discriminate or isolate these students, as they are fully protected by federal disability laws

## Food Allergy and Anaphylaxis Network

I strongly urge any patient or family affected by food allergies to join the Food Allergy and Anaphylaxis Network or FAAN. This excellent, proactive national organization provides support and educational materials for food allergy sufferers and their families. FAAN's many publications include allergen-free recipes, timely alerts when processed foods become contaminated with food allergens, booklets, videos and a well-thought-out School Allergy Program. FAAN also publishes a bimonthly newsletter for its members. Food Allergy News for Physicians is distributed to 10,000 pediatricians throughout the country. In December 2000, FAAN launched a new e-newsletter for teens called Food Allergy News for Teens. Patients can sign up for this newsletter through FAAN's Web site. FAAN is also working closely with the Federal Aviation Association and lobbying for placement of self-injectors of epinephrine in commercial aircraft emergency medical kits. They are also encouraging Emergency Medical Services to allow all EMTs to administer epinephrine. The total cost of membership in FAAN is only $24 per year. For additional information contact FAAN at 10400 Eaton Place, Suite 107, Fairfax, VA 22030-2208. Tel: 1-800-929-4040 or 703-691-3179. Fax: 703-691-2713. www.foodallergy.org

## The Peanut Allergy Answer Book

My good friend and colleague, Doctor Michael Young, has written a very informative resource book for parents of children afflicted with peanut and tree nut allergy—*The Peanut Allergy Answer Book* (Fairwinds Press 2001). The easy-to-read, question-and-answer format helps relieve the anxiety and frustration often associated with food allergy and anaphylaxis. Young's collection of illustrative cases helps to explain the up-to-date scientific information for those who want to learn more about peanut allergy. I highly recommend this book to all my patients, parents, caregivers and health-care providers who deal with peanut or tree nut allergy.

## Sulfite-induced Asthma

If you read the labels on foods and beverages you purchase in your local supermarket, you are fully aware that thousands of agents are added to the foodstuffs we consume on a daily basis. Such additives

145

include preservatives, stabilizers, conditioners, thickeners, colorings and flavorings. It is somewhat amazing that despite the widespread use of food additives, relatively few of these chemicals trigger asthma or other allergic reactions. One of the few additives that may trigger asthma is the sulfite chemical metabisulfite. Sulfites have been used for centuries to preserve raw potatoes, seafood and fresh vegetables. The Romans were the first to discover that sulfites prevented wine from turning into vinegar. Ingestion of large amounts of sulfites by normal individuals is usually quite safe. Not so for those susceptible asthmatics, in whom sulfites may trigger severe asthma attacks. Sulfite sensitivity is rare in children, and mainly occurs in adults with persistent asthma.

From 1980 to 1998 the FDA received over one thousand reports of severe sulfite reactions, of which 12 were fatal episodes. More than 90 percent of these sulfite reactions occurred away from home in restaurants. The FDA and National Restaurant Association have responded to the threat of sulfite sensitivity by developing training programs and handouts for food manufacturers, restaurant personnel and consumers. In 1986, a partial FDA sulfite ban prohibited the use of sulfites in restaurants, supermarkets and salad bars. The FDA required labeling disclosure when the sulfite concentration exceeded 10 parts per million and prohibited sulfite use on raw fruits (except grapes) and vegetables. Since then the incidence of sulfite reactions has dropped dramatically—to about ten a year. It appears that restaurant chefs may have been using too much sulfite on salad bar fruits and vegetables.

The exact incidence of sulfite-sensitive asthma is unknown. Drs. Donald Stevenson and Ronald Simon, of La Jolla, California, estimate that five to ten percent of all adult asthmatics may be sulfite sensitive. If their figures are correct, there may be 500,000 sulfite-sensitive asthmatics in the United States. At first I doubted these estimates and thought sulfite asthma was a rare problem. But now that I am looking for it, I find so-called "Restaurant-Induced Asthma" is not all that uncommon. Fresh shrimp and some factory-prepared foods, like mashed potato flakes or fried potatoes, still contain sulfites, as do most beers and imported wines. If you can drink beer or wine, you are not sulfite sensitive, as most domestic and imported beers and wines contain sulfites. It is really up to the consumer to be aware of the potential sources of sulfites. (See Table 9.2.)

## Table 9.2. Foods and Beverages That Contain Sulfites

▲ Wine, beer and cider    ▲ Avocados

▲ Fruit drinks    ▲ Corn sweeteners

▲ Fresh shrimp    ▲ Salad bars

▲ Potatoes, French fries    ▲ Dried fruits, grapes

▲ Beet sugar    ▲ Baked goods

Sulfites are also used in the manufacture of many drugs, including some asthma aerosols. There are very few well-documented case reports of sulfite-drug reactions. Nevertheless, sulfite-sensitive asthmatics should avoid drugs that contain sulfites. The only valid test for sulfite sensitivity is a challenge test, where the subject swallows or inhales small amounts of sulfite under controlled conditions while doctors monitor vital signs and lung functions. Challenge tests can be dangerous, and should only be done under careful supervision in a hospital setting.

Several other food additives and colorings have the reputation of inducing asthma, including tartrazine or FD&C Yellow Dye Number 5. This dye, a derivative of coal tar, is commonly used to color foods, like margarine, yellow. Tartrazine is widely avoided by many people with asthma. This is unnecessary, as the threat of tartrazine allergy is grossly overrated. Similar concerns have been raised about other food additives and chemicals, including sodium benzoate, BHA and BHT. Tests in large asthmatic populations have failed to implicate these chemical additives as important asthma triggers.

## MSG-induced Asthma

Individuals with MSG, or monosodium glutamate, sensitivity usually experience facial flushing and a generalized tingling sensation after consuming MSG. Since Chinese foods frequently contain large amounts of MSG, this condition is commonly known as the "Chinese Restaurant Syndrome." In the early 1980s a possible association between MSG and asthma was raised, as several studies described patients who developed asthma-like symptoms after ingesting Chinese food. Since MSG is a widely used dietary supplement (we normally ingest one gram of MSG per day), the possibility that MSG might play a major role in asthma was raised.

In 1999, doctors from the Scripps Research Institute in La Jolla, California, studied this issue. They carefully challenged 100 asthmatics with MSG, and none of these patients developed asthma symptoms or had any change in their lung functions. Many patients who thought they were sensitive to MSG were found to have gastroesophageal reflux disease, or anxiety or depression that caused them to overstate their fear of MSG products. Doctor Raif Geha of Harvard University challenged 130 patients who thought they were sensitive to MSG with a large test dose of MSG and found only a low level of MSG sensitivity. On the basis of these studies and my own professional experience, I do not consider MSG to be an important asthma trigger.

## *Alcohol-induced Asthma*

In contrast to MSG, many of my patients with asthma relate that ingestion of beer, wine or grain alcohol frequently triggers sneezing, nasal congestion or wheezing. Wine, especially red wine, is a more frequent offender than beer or grain alcohol. In a survey in Western Australia one in every three asthmatics noted that alcoholic drinks worsened their asthma. Wines were the most frequent offenders, with a response time of less than one hour. Wine-induced asthma that was mild to moderate in severity was more common in women. I used to think that alcohol-induced asthma was due to the sulfite preservatives added to alcoholic beverages to prevent spoilage, but it was always a puzzle why not all alcoholic beverages triggered asthma.

It appears Japanese investigators may have come up with the answer to this observation. Alcohol-induced asthma in Japanese people has been well documented, as more than half of asthmatic patients from Japan will wheeze after consuming alcohol. Japanese researchers found that many Japanese have a genetically determined enzyme defect that prevents the breakdown of acetaldehyde, a by-product of alcohol. This enzyme defect is more common in people of Asian descent. It is postulated that accumulation of high levels of acetaldehyde triggers the release of histamine from mast cells, which leads to bronchospasm and wheezing. Japanese researchers recently published a small study on 13 patients that provides some hope for patients who enjoy imbibing beer or wine, as they demonstrated that pretreatment with antihistamines often blocked alcohol-induced asthma.

## Summary

The only effective treatment for food- or chemical-induced allergy or asthma is avoidance and patient and family education. When indicated, the treatment of choice is an inhaled asthma rescue drug, immediate use of epinephrine and prompt transport to a local emergency room. One preliminary study done at the National Jewish Hospital in Denver evaluated the effect of allergy (peanut) shots in a small group of severely peanut-allergic children. This study showed promise until the study subjects developed a high rate of systemic or allergic reactions. Futuristic biotech research in food allergy is now focusing on several other ways to treat food allergy, including anti-IgE therapy and allergy injections with highly purified and less allergenic proteins. Such research may one day lead to a "prevention or cure" for food allergy.

# Infections
and
Asthma

# 10

The first association between infections and asthma was made in the flu epidemics of 1957 and 1958. One report depicted how an outbreak of a flu infection in a Boy-Scout camp led to relapses of asthma in 27 asthmatic children. The second report described a similar asthma epidemic in a girls' camp in Canada. These important reports stimulated interest on the role of respiratory tract viruses as precipitants of asthma in both children and adults. The current literature on this subject is conflicting. Some investigators feel asthma relapses are frequently associated with infections; others believe that naturally acquired viral and bacterial infections have a protective effect. Proponents of the hygiene hypothesis argue that the lack of infections in infancy and early childhood may be playing a major role in the emerging asthma epidemic.

## Viral Infections

There is no doubt that the most important asthma trigger other than an aeroallergen is a viral infection or the common cold. As laboratory identification of viruses is notoriously difficult and time consuming, virus particles were not discovered until the early part of the twentieth century. The discovery of influenza virus in 1937 was followed by the discovery of parainfluenza virus, enterovirus, adenovirus and RSV virus in the 1940s and 1950s. In the 1960s the common cold viruses, rhinovirus and coronavirus, were isolated. Today more than 240 viruses are capable of causing a common cold. A virus is a living biologic particle that has the ability to invade a specific cell and use the metabolic machinery of the invaded cell to duplicate itself. Viruses are actually parasites. They cannot survive on their own, but must live off the chemicals of the invaded cell. All viruses are composed of a core surrounded by a protein shell. Every virus has the ability to enter a host cell, duplicate itself and form more viral particles that are then released into the surrounding tissue. Once inside a cell, viruses use the cell's enzymes and metabolic machinery to reproduce proteins and building blocks required to duplicate itself. The final stage in the life cycle of a virus depends on its ability to be transmitted from one victim to another.

Viruses that cause respiratory symptoms are transmitted through touching, coughing or sneezing. Infected secretions from infected individuals contain various-sized droplets. Larger droplets settle on handkerchiefs, hands and other surfaces. Smaller droplets remain airborne and are inhaled into the nose and lower airways, where they cause infection. In the absence of transmission from person to person, most respiratory viruses are so fragile that their particles are quickly degraded, and they become noninfectious. Fortunately for mankind, the AIDS virus is a very fragile virus that does not survive long outside the invaded cell. The common cold viruses are somewhat more stable and more easily transmitted. The typical symptoms of a common cold include mild systemic upset, fever, fatigue, joint pains, nasal discharge or blockage, sneezing, sore throat and coughing.

## *Viral Infections in Childhood*

Common childhood viral infections are among the most potent of all asthma triggers. One study found that four out of every ten hospitalizations for childhood asthma were caused by a common cold virus. Different viruses strike different age groups. Infants and children are more susceptible to the RSV virus and mycoplasma infections. Adult asthmatics are more likely to be infected with the influenza or rhinovirus group. There are recent clues as to why patients with allergies and asthma are prone to repeated colds and asthma relapses. Some allergic individuals are more likely to produce an allergic or IgE antibody to certain viruses. Doctors also know that the common cold is more likely to be transmitted by hand-to-mouth contact than by droplets produced by coughing or sneezing. Many children and adults with asthma and allergies have an itchy nose that they constantly rub. (See page 91.) This easily recognizable habit, dubbed the "allergic salute," is a very effective way to transfer viral particles from hand to mouth, explaining why so many asthmatics get one cold after another. Upper respiratory tract viruses cause nasal congestion, which leads to long periods of mouth breathing. Air inspired through the mouth is not subject to the warming and humidifying that occurs in the nose, and may trigger bronchospasm in the same way that cold and dry air precipitates exercise-induced asthma.

Wheezing in children has traditionally been divided into two classes: wheezy bronchitis precipitated by a viral infection, and classic asthma. Epidemiological studies that looked at asthma attacks provide evidence for virus involvement. In one study done in London, England, the asthma hospital admission rates were analyzed for 11 years. There was no association between admission rates and changes in weather or aeroallergen exposure. The peaks of asthma admissions coincided with the beginning of school terms when children were exposed to viruses in their classrooms. Respiratory viruses were associated with one in every four episodes of wheezing in London schoolchildren.

Another study compared the contribution of respiratory viruses and aeroallergens in asthma relapse in 169 children over two years of age. There was no association with aeroallergens. In nearly one-third of these children, a respiratory virus was identified at the time of the asthma exacerbation, the most common being RSV and rhinovirus. A prospective study of 32 young children admitted to the National Jewish Hospital found that one-third of wheezy episodes in the first year of life were associated with a viral infection. The most common asthma-triggering virus was RSV.

## RSV Infection

RSV or respiratory syncytial virus is a viral infection of infants and young children that triggers nearly 100,000 hospitalizations a year, costing $300 million. RSV outbreaks usually occur between October and May, with a peak in January and February. The most severe RSV infections occur in young infants, especially premature infants with underlying lung problems. RSV is a highly endemic disease, as nearly 100 percent of all children will experience at least one RSV infection by two years of age. Re-infection with RSV is very common. Half of all children infected during their first year of life will be re-infected with RSV in their second year of life. The RSV re-infection rate is even higher in infants attending day care centers. The most common symptoms of an RSV infection are fever, wheezing, coughing and chest congestion. RSV illness is called bronchiolitis. In older children and adults bronchiolitis may be a milder disease, often presenting as a simple cold or bronchitis-like illness.

What is the link between RSV and asthma? Several decades ago, researchers who followed a group of children with RSV-bronchiolitis found that more than half of these RSV victims had further episodes of wheezing, and were twice as likely to develop asthma later on in childhood. At first it was thought that the RSV virus might trigger several years or even a lifetime of asthma. Now it appears that the RSV virus itself does not trigger asthma unless it attacks infants or young children with other asthma risk factors, such as a high IgE level, eczema or food allergies, a family history of allergy or asthma, or exposure to tobacco smoke.

In addition, some viruses, like RSV, have the ability to trigger the formation of IgE antibodies, and that may trigger asthma in genetically predisposed individuals. Finally, the interactions that occur when individuals are simultaneously exposed to both allergens and viruses are being explored. In children presenting to an emergency room with acute episodes of airway obstruction, the combination of allergy and a viral illness has been found to be a larger risk factor than either of these two factors alone.

## New Developments

A recent international roundtable looked at the association between RSV and reactive airways disease or asthma. The seminar suggested that the different responses to RSV infection in both animals and man are genetically determined. The long-term prognosis of RSV bronchiolitis appears to be directly related to the severity of the initial RSV infection. It still remains unclear whether RSV contributes to the development of asthma and allergies. Milder cases had no special risk for asthma, whereas severe cases (hospitalized infants) were more likely to be wheezing several years later. Post-RSV wheezing lasting several years after an RSV infection could not be linked to a family history of allergy. The ability of RSV to produce a mediator called "substance P" may predispose affected children to airway hyperreactivity. The direct interaction of RSV with certain T-cells may also determine the outcome of RSV infection. Viral researchers have been trying to develop an RSV vaccine for decades. In the 1960s, RSV-vaccinated infants who later contracted RSV had more severe disease than usual, and tragically some RSV-vaccinated infants died. At the present time there is no licensed vaccine for the routine prevention of RSV. A monoclonal antibody drug is now available to modify or lessen the severity of RSV bronchiolitis, but the approximate cost of $5000 per month will make it somewhat prohibitive for routine use in infancy.

## Adult Studies

Under certain circumstances adult viral infections favor the development of asthma. Adult hospital admission rates for asthma are highest when children return to school, mirroring the trends seen in childhood asthma. This explains why many adults develop asthma for the first time in their lives after a simple viral respiratory infection. Such respiratory infections may also reactivate latent asthma that had been present in childhood. Taken together, these observations strongly support the concept that the airway response to viral infections and allergens may share common pathways.

The clinical manifestations of the upper and lower airway response to viral and bacterial infections are dependent on multiple factors including age, sex, family history, and allergen and passive smoke exposure. The interrelationship between virus infections, allergic disease, sinus infections and asthma is especially intriguing. The anecdotal evidence supporting the link between respiratory viral infections and episodes of asthma in adults is less well established. Few studies have tested the concept that viral infections trigger acute asthma in adults.

## Mycoplasma and Chlamydia Infection

Interesting research by Doctor Richard Martin from National Jewish Hospital in Denver, Colorado, discovered that 60 percent of the asthma patients he studied harbored mycoplasma bacteria in their lungs. Martin initiated this study after he found this *mycoplasma* bacteria in the lungs of a 24-year-old woman with severe lifelong asthma who dramatically improved after she was placed on the antibiotic clarithromycin. Over the next five years she took this antibiotic on a daily basis and was able to stop oral prednisone and resume normal day-to-day activities. Doctor Martin then postulated that patients with persistent asthma might be chronically infected with *mycoplasma* bacteria.

This story is not unlike the discovery by two Australian physicians, who found that their patients with chronic peptic ulcer disease were infected with a bacteria called *Heliobacter pylori.* Doctor Martin is now conducting a five-year study to determine if chronic *mycoplasma* infection causes asthma. This theory brings up an intriguing question. Would aggressive antibiotic therapy in infants with a high risk profile for asthma block the onset of asthma?

Another type of infectious agent, *Chlamydia pneumonaie,* may play a role in asthma. *Chlamydia pneumonaie* is a new and unusual human pathogen discovered in 1986. *Chlamydia* is a unique organism that strikes both birds and humans and causes a variety of infections, including bronchitis and pneumonia. One form of the bird-borne *Chlamydia* disease can induce a severe form of pneumonia in humans called psittacosis. *Chlamydia* also causes blindness (trachoma), infertility and chronic urinary tract infections. Most human *Chlamydia* infections are low-grade infections that can go undetected for months or years.

Some researchers believe that chronic infection with *Chlamydia* may be linked to asthma and COPD. Doctors can test for *Chlamydia* and, when indicated, administer appropriate antibiotics. These findings need additional research before asthma specialists recommend widespread use of antibiotics in all patients with chronic asthma. However, I believe that a six- to eight-week trial of an appropriate antibiotic is indicated in patients with severe persistent asthma, as it may be years before we have a valid answer to the question of whether or not chronic bacterial infections, such as *Mycoplasma* or *Chlamydia,* cause asthma.

## New Theories

The hygiene hypothesis proposes that exposure to naturally acquired infections or even parasites in infancy and early childhood may protect against asthma. For the past 30 years I have been telling my patients that the existence of allergies predisposes them to the common cold. The evidence to support this statement is weak at best. Nevertheless, there is agreement among asthma specialists that pre-existing inflammation in the lung accentuates the effects of viral infections.

University of California investigators inoculated allergic subjects with a nasal allergen before deliberately infecting them with a common cold virus. They expected to prove that a pre-existing allergy would worsen the effects of the common cold. Much to their surprise they found just the opposite. Pre-exposure to an offending allergen delayed the onset of cold symptoms and reduced the duration of the cold. Thus, pre-existing allergy may in some way protect against or reduce the symptoms of the common cold. At the present time there is no final answer as to the protective or harmful role played by viral, bacterial or parasitic infections in asthma. It is probably a two-way street. In other words, certain viral infections like the common cold and RSV may lead to asthma, whereas other naturally acquired infections may actually prevent allergy and asthma.

# Drug Therapy
## in Asthma

# 11

## *History of Asthma Drugs*

**T**he history of asthma drugs is worth reviewing, as asthma therapy has a rich tradition in medical folklore. Popular mythical remedies have included rubbing tomato paste on the chest, sleeping with Chihuahua dogs, taping pennies to the forehead, eating chicken livers or medicinal herbs and smoking asthma cigarettes and cigars. Fortunately, today's more rational approach to asthma drug therapy is based on important discoveries in the twentieth century. The modern asthma guidelines divide asthma drugs into two major categories—the relieving or bronchodilating drugs and the controlling or anti-inflammatory drugs.

The most effective group of asthma relieving drugs or bronchodilators are derived from adrenaline, the natural hormone produced by our adrenal gland. Adrenaline was found to relieve acute asthma in 1903. Amazingly, a century later adrenaline (or epinephrine) and its derivatives are still the first-line therapy for allergic reactions and acute asthma. In 1925, the oral bronchodilator ephedrine was introduced. Ephedrine, the first legitimate oral asthma drug, was actually discovered by observant Chinese healers more than 4,000 years ago. Ancient Oriental practitioners found that wheezing patients experienced marked relief after inhaling the burning leaves of a Chinese herb called *Ma huang*. When the active portion of this plant was isolated, it was named ephedrine, a derivation of the herb's Latin name, *Ephredus vulgaris.*

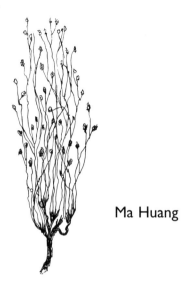

Ma Huang

Ephedrine is an effective but weak bronchodilator that belongs to the adrenaline group of drugs. *Ma huang* is now a common ingredient of many herbal preparations. Asthmatics living in the first half of the twentieth century deserve our sympathy, as there were few effective asthma drugs in that era. Doctors had to resort to ineffective and dangerous remedies such as smoking stramonium leaves and injecting morphine. In 1938, the asthmatic's outlook brightened somewhat when a new drug called theophylline was introduced. Ten years later another major breakthrough occurred when the cortisone drugs were developed and found to control severe asthma. From 1950 to 1970, doctors would rely on adrenaline-like drugs, theophylline, and oral cortisone, to treat asthma without any clue as to how or why these drugs actually worked to control asthma.

## New Breakthroughs

In the 1970s, American and European pharmaceutical companies launched aggressive research programs that produced spectacular breakthroughs in asthma therapy. New drugs developed in this era included safer and more effective bronchodilating or beta-agonist drugs, long-acting theophylline products and effective anti-inflammatory drugs like cromolyn and the cortisone aerosols. The 1990s witnessed the development of longer-acting beta-agonist drugs, more potent cortisone inhalers, and a new group of non-cortisone drugs called the antileukotrienes. Present-day asthma therapy now makes it possible for the health-care provider to precisely tailor asthma drugs to an individual patient's needs.

While breakthroughs in pharmacology research have made more effective asthma treatment a reality, these newer, more sophisticated and complicated treatment programs have made it more difficult for health-care providers to treat complicated asthma. Anyone who treats asthma must have the training and expertise to choose the right asthma program for the right patient. Any doctor or health-care provider who has not kept abreast of new developments in asthma drugs by reading medical journals or attending postgraduate courses has no business treating persistent asthma.

Asthma drugs have different effects on the early and late-phase asthma response. Bronchodilating or *relieving* drugs, like the beta-agonists and theophylline, open up or dilate the bronchial tubes. While these drugs prevent or relieve the symptoms of the early phase of asthma, they have little or no effect on the late phase or inflammatory response. The *controlling* or anti-inflammatory drugs like cromolyn, cortisone and the new leukotriene inhibitors do not relieve acute asthma symptoms. They prevent or control the late-phase inflammatory response. In the following chapters on drug therapy I will discuss the relieving or bronchodilating drugs, the anti-inflammatory or controlling drugs, and conclude with alternative and futuristic asthma drugs.

## *The Relieving or Bronchodilating Drugs*

Beta-agonist drugs stimulate a part of our nervous system called the sympathetic nervous system. Drugs that act directly on a receptor in the nervous system called the beta receptor are called beta-agonist drugs. The sympathetic system controls the tone of the bronchial tubes by counteracting the constricting impulses of the opposing cholinergic or bronchoconstricting system. The sympathetic system has three types of receptors, or signal boxes, that regulate heart rate, blood pressure and bronchial tone. The alpha receptor tightens muscles and increases the production of mucus. The beta-1 receptor increases heart rate and blood pressure. The beta-2 receptor is the bronchodilator receptor that relaxes smooth muscle and decreases mucus production. Older asthma drugs, like adrenaline and ephedrine, acted on all three receptors. When you got a shot of adrenaline or took an ephedrine pill, you stopped wheezing because of the drug's effect on the beta-2 receptor. However, stimulation of the alpha and beta-1 receptors caused tremors and an increase in pulse rate or blood pressure.

This led to the search for an ideal asthma drug, one which would selectively stimulate the all-important beta-2 receptor. Aerosol or inhaled drugs are preferred over oral preparations for several reasons. After a drug is swallowed, it is absorbed into the blood stream and circulates to all organs in the body. One must take a relatively large amount of drug to deliver a small dose to a selected target organ like the lung. The drug is also transported to other organs and causes unwanted side effects. For example, oral ephedrine works well in the lung, but the brain reacts to ephedrine with insomnia or tremors. The shortcomings of oral drugs prompted researchers to look for drugs that could be delivered directly to the lung. This quest led to the development of asthma aerosols that could be inhaled into the lung and produce a faster onset of action while minimizing side effects.

The first drug to be successfully used as an asthma aerosol was adrenaline, a relatively weak bronchodilator with a brief duration of action. Adrenaline also caused an increase in blood pressure and heart rate, as it stimulated both the alpha and beta-1 receptor. This primitive asthma aerosol is still available in a popular over-the-counter (OTC) drug called Primatene Mist. The next asthma aerosol to be developed was isoproterenol, a more powerful drug than adrenaline. This drug, sold under the brand names of Medihaler-Iso and Isuprel Mistometer, was the most widely used asthma aerosol from 1950 to 1970. Like adrenaline, it had a short duration of action and a tendency to increase heart rate and blood pressure.

## The Beta-2 Agonists

In 1961, English investigators announced the discovery of a new beta-agonist drug, called metaproterenol or Alupent. This new product was a more selective beta-2 agonist that lasted longer and was less likely to increase blood pressure or heart rate. Over the next 20 years, many other effective beta-2 agonist drugs would be developed, including terbutaline (Brethine), bitolterol (Tornalate), pirbuterol (Maxair) and albuterol (Proventil or Ventolin). Albuterol is now the most effective and widely used short-acting broncho-dilator. In addition to reversing acute asthma, albuterol can prevent and relieve exercise-induced asthma. In 1992, salmeterol (Serevent), a longer-acting beta-agonist drug with a 12-hour duration of action, became available. The newest long-acting beta-agonist, formoterol (Foradil), became available in 2001.

Beta-agonist drugs are administered by mouth, by injection, intravenously or by inhalation. The preferred route of administration is by inhalation or aerosol due to a rapid onset of action and lesser risk of side effects. Short acting beta-agonists are front-line drugs for relieving acute asthma and preventing exercise-induced asthma. Due to their limited duration of action, they are not well suited for maintenance bronchodilator therapy. The best drugs for daily maintenance beta-agonist therapy are the long-acting beta-agonists. In most instances, beta-agonists are administered via a metered dose inhaler or MDI. Patients who experience difficulty using inhalers benefit from using spacers or holding chambers that lessen the need for coordination between actuation of the inhaler and breathing in the medicine. Sometimes young children and older adults will require a nebulizer to administer their beta-agonist drug.

## *Side Effects of the Beta-agonists*

Potential side effects of the beta-agonists include an increase in heart rate and blood pressure and a transient fall in blood oxygen levels in patients with acute asthma. This fall in oxygen level is not considered to be an important problem, but oxygen levels should be monitored when treating acute severe asthma. Other common side effects of beta-agonist therapy are jitteriness or tremors—the result of stimulation of the skeletal muscle beta-1 receptor. The two most commonly used over-the-counter inhalers that contain epinephrine, Primatene and Bronkaid Mist, continue to sell millions of canisters per year. Both these drugs increase pulse rate, raise blood pressure and cause tremors. They also have a very short duration of action—about 20 minutes. The other risk of these inhalers is that they lull asthmatics into a false sense of security that delays relapsing patients from seeking medical care as doctors have no way to monitor refills or excess use of the OTC products.

The Montreal Protocol, which limits the release of Freon into the earth's atmosphere, will eventually spell the doom of the OTC Freon-propelled inhalers. Once these Freon-propelled inhalers are banned, new OTC products will have to submit new drug applications to the FDA. This should give the FDA an opening to carefully scrutinize OTC inhalers that have many more side effects than newer beta-agonists. It seems unlikely that they will pass muster. Most companies producing these products will be unwilling to risk the millions of dollars needed to develop new OTC products.

## Long-Acting Beta-agonists

Over the past 10 years selective beta-agonists with a longer duration of action have come into play. Currently, there are two long-acting compounds available, formoterol (Foradil Aerolixer) and salmeterol (Serevent). These drugs are administered via a metered-dose or dry powder inhaler. Formoterol and salmeterol have a bronchodilating effect of over 12 hours, and are more potent than albuterol. Doctor Ann Woolcock studied poorly controlled asthmatics taking inhaled cortisone drugs and found that adding salmeterol (Serevent), while not increasing the daily dose of the inhaled cortisone drug, had better results—less nighttime wheezing, improved pulmonary function tests, less need for rescue medication—than doubling the daily dose of their inhaled cortisone.

There is no doubt that the introduction of long-acting beta-2 agonists represents a significant milestone in asthma therapy. It is now generally agreed these drugs are indicated in patients who fail to respond to inhaled cortisone drugs alone. However, some studies have shown that daily use of a long-acting beta-agonist may mask inflammation and delay one's awareness of worsening asthma. Thus, anyone using a long-acting beta-agonist needs to also take an inhaled cortisone drug on a regular basis. GlaxoSmithKline's new drug, Advair, a combination of an inhaled cortisone (Flovent) and a long-acting beta-agonist (Serevent) promises to be a beneficial product for patients who require both of these asthma drugs.

## Third-Generation Beta-agonists

A new form of beta-agonist has been developed. Through clever pharmacology, research chemists have been able to alter the basic structure of the older beta-agonist drug albuterol. This new compound, levalbuterol (Xopenex), possesses desirable broncho-dilating characteristics, yet has eliminated the undesirable side effects like tremors and increased heart rate. This third-generation beta-agonist drug has been shown to have an excellent safety record and duration of action of up to eight hours.

## The Beta-agonist Debate

The debate over the role of the inhaled beta-agonist drugs in asthma is a long and controversial one, dating back to the late 1960s when asthma mortality increased in England and Wales. British investigators found that the increase in asthma deaths in England followed the introduction of a potent beta-agonist drug, called Isoproterenol Forte. In 1967, the United Kingdom issued a warning on this product. Sudden and unexplained asthma deaths in young people were tied to excess use of this beta-agonist aerosol. After Isoproterenol Forte was removed from OTC sales, asthma mortality rates significantly declined. Were these asthma deaths due to a direct effect of the drug itself or did overuse of the beta-agonist create a false sense of security and thus lead to a deadly delay in seeking medical care? Thirty years later this question remains unresolved.

In 1979, an editorial in *Lancet*, England's leading medical journal, stated, *"there is a growing realization that pressurized aerosols were probably not the main culprit in the asthma epidemic of the 1960s and poor asthma treatment and a delay in seeking medical care was the main cause of asthma mortality."* In the early 1980s, another asthma mortality epidemic in young asthmatics was reported in New Zealand. These reports implied that overuse of the beta-agonist drugs played a role in asthma deaths, particularly when taken with theophylline. The New Zealand Asthma Mortality Study Group thoroughly reviewed 271 asthma deaths and could only identify nine cases where excess use of beta-agonists triggered an asthma death. This report emphasized the risks of under-utilization of treatment and a delay in seeking appropriate treatment during relapsing asthma.

However, many asthma specialists disagreed with these conclusions. Doctor Neil Pearce from Wellington, New Zealand, proposed that that introduction of a long-acting and more potent beta-agonist, fenoterol, was the cause of the New Zealand asthma death epidemic, as the increase in asthma deaths coincided with the introduction of fenoterol to New Zealand. Doctor Malcolm Sears added additional fuel to this fire in December 1990. Sears's well-designed, placebo-controlled study evaluated 64 asthmatics for six months. One group took their inhaled beta-agonist (fenoterol) on a regular basis; the other group used it strictly on as-needed or on-demand basis. The as-needed or on-demand group had fewer bouts of nighttime asthma, less need for prednisone, lower bronchial reactivity and better peak flow rates than patients who used their beta-agonist on a regular basis. Doctor Sears concluded that round-the-clock inhalation of a beta-agonist drug was associated with poorer control of asthma compared to patients who only used their inhaler on demand or only as needed. One attractive explanation for the poor asthma control in the round-the-clock users was that patients using beta-agonists on a regular basis experienced higher exposures to allergens and asthma triggers. Sears strongly recommended that inhaled beta-agonist drugs should be used only on demand to relieve acute asthma and that the practice of regular round-the-clock inhalations of beta-agonists should be discarded.

Sears's paper generated heated discussions within the medical profession. Experts pointed out that the findings of this study should not be applied to all beta-agonists, as fenoterol was a much more potent beta-agonist than the shorter-acting beta-agonists like albuterol. Another study linking beta-agonist drugs to asthma deaths appeared in the *New England Journal of Medicine* in February 1992. This Canadian survey by Doctor Walter Spitzer of McGill University examined the medical records of 12,031 asthmatics who took asthma drugs between 1978 and 1987. Spitzer found that the 44 patients who died from asthma used twice as many inhalers as those who did not die from asthma. Patients using two inhaler canisters per month were more than twice as likely to die from asthma.

There were several possible explanations for the association between beta-agonist use and asthma deaths. Patients with severe asthma are more likely to use more asthma inhalers, beta-agonists have an adverse effect on the cardiovascular system, or beta-agonists may open up the airways too much and increase bronchial hyperreactivity. Lastly, over-reliance on beta-agonists misled patients into thinking their asthma was under control, which delayed seeking proper asthma care. The editorial that accompanied this article pointed out the control group probably had less severe asthma than those who died from asthma, and if patients with asthma become overly fearful of beta-agonist inhalers, emergency rooms would soon be flooded with patients with acute asthma. The first drug such patients will receive in the emergency room will be an inhaled beta-agonist!

Critics of this report pointed out that many Canadians were using fenoterol (Berotec), a drug not available in the United States. This is the same drug that alarmed investigators in New Zealand in the 1980s. Concerns generated by this report created justifiable anxiety among asthmatic patients and their families. The two major allergy organizations in the United States, the American College of Allergy, Asthma & Immunology and the American Academy of Allergy, Asthma & Immunology, issued press releases stating that there was not enough data to justify sweeping changes in the use of beta-agonist drugs. Doctor Edward O'Connell from the Mayo Clinic, then President of the American College of Allergy, Asthma & Immunology, stated that doctors have been successfully and safely using beta-agonist drugs to treat asthma for more than 10 years. The FDA revisited this issue at a special hearing in December 1992 and concluded that more studies were needed before recommending any changes in beta-agonist dosing guidelines.

The beta-agonist debate raises one important question. Should asthmatics take beta-agonist drugs on a round-the-clock or only on an as-needed basis? I believe the answer to this question falls into a gray zone. Inhaled beta-agonist drugs are still the most effective drugs for relieving acute asthma attack and preventing exercise-induced asthma. Many asthma care providers, including me, now recommend using inhaled beta-agonists only on an as-needed basis in stable patients with normal peak flow rates. Patients with unstable asthma and wide fluctuations in peak flow rates may require regular use of bronchodilators, particularly in the morning or at bedtime. The best drug in this situation is the long-acting beta-agonist salmeterol (Serevent), combined with an asthma-controlling drug.

## The Theophylline Drugs

In 1859, an article in Scotland's *Edinburgh Medical Journal* stated, "One of the commonest and best reputed remedies of asthma, and one that in many cases is more effective than others, is strong tea or coffee." Unfortunately, this sage advice was ignored for more than 50 years, until German and American research teams set out to determine why asthmatics stopped wheezing when they drank strong tea or coffee. In 1888, the disclosure that caffeine was a mild bronchodilator led to the discovery of the caffeine-like drug theophylline. Boehringer and Sons began industrial production of theophylline in Germany at the turn of the century. Initially, American doctors were slow to accept theophylline, until a 1938 report in the *Journal of the American Medical Association* noted that patients with asthma experienced marked relief after receiving an intravenous injection of a form of theophylline, called aminophylline. Oral forms of theophylline were then developed. However, theophylline had many drawbacks, including a bitter taste and a tendency to cause nausea and vomiting. This problem was partially solved when chemists added other drugs to the theophylline drugs to improve its taste and reduce side effects.

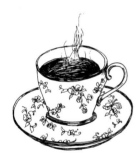

## The Three-In-One Drugs

In 1940, the *New England Journal of Medicine* published a report by Doctor Ethan Allen Brown that transformed asthma therapy. This report cited Doctor Brown's success in clinical trials with a new oral medication called Tedral, a combination of three drugs in one tablet—theophylline, ephedrine and phenobarbital. This combination drug and others like it became the backbone of outpatient asthma therapy for the next 30 years. These drugs had several disadvantages. Doses of each individual drug could not be increased separately. For example, patients requiring a higher dose of theophylline also had to take more oral ephedrine, a potent stimulant that caused insomnia, tremors and heart palpitations.

Today these outdated fixed-combination drugs would not receive approval from the FDA. The glaring deficiencies of the combination drugs were ignored until 1972, when Doctor Elliot Ellis from National Jewish Hospital in Denver urged doctors to use theophylline as a single drug that allowed each patient's dose to be individualized. These efforts sparked another revolution in asthma therapy, leading to the development of pure, more effective theophylline compounds. Within a few years the fixed combinations became obsolete. The first single theophylline preparations were short-acting drugs that only lasted a few hours. Innovative alterations in theophylline tablet and capsule design produced longer-acting drugs that allowed once or twice-a-day dosing. Children metabolize, or use up, theophylline much more rapidly than adults. A 50-pound child may require more theophylline on the basis of body weight than a 200-pound adult. Smokers need more theophylline than non-smokers, and elderly asthmatics often require less theophylline. After researchers developed a simple blood test, called a theophylline blood level, to determine if patients were taking too little or too much theophylline, doses could be precisely tailored to individual needs for the first time in asthma therapy.

## *Theophylline Interactions and Side Effects*

Different drugs prescribed for different medical conditions may interact when they combine in the body. For example, when an asthmatic on oral theophylline develops an infection and requires the antibiotic erythromycin, the combination of both theophylline and erythromycin may cause significant problems. When these drugs are taken at the same time, erythromycin slows down the rate at which theophylline is metabolized, which in effect doubles the amount of theophylline in the body. Thus, a normal dose of theophylline acts like a double dose when taken along with erythromycin. This drug interaction in effect causes a theophylline overdose. Many other drugs interact with theophylline, including the ulcer drug cimetadine (Tagamet) and blood pressure-migraine medicine propranolol (Inderal). Some viral infections also double the effect of theophylline.

Long-term use of theophylline is usually no more hazardous than the daily consumption of tea or coffee. About one in every ten patients may develop nausea, loss of appetite or vomiting. Some children become hyperactive or develop learning problems, as theophylline has been found to decrease attention span and concentration in some patients. Additional theophylline side effects include headache, insomnia and jitteriness. Most of these side effects are due to the caffeine-like properties of theophylline. Patients who cannot tolerate coffee or tea cannot usually take theophylline. As one of my theophylline-intolerant patients aptly stated, "When I take theophylline, I feel like I've overdosed on coffee." The minor theophylline side effects that occur soon after starting treatment often subside after a few days of therapy, or are eliminated by taking the drug with food or after meals. Sometimes a dose reduction is necessary, and occasionally theophylline must be discontinued altogether. Fortunately, the major toxic reactions caused by high blood theophylline levels—vomiting of blood, mental confusion, and seizures—are rare.

Theophylline therapy continues to have its ups and downs. Once the first-line drug or mainstay of asthma therapy in both the doctor's office and the emergency room, theophylline has been relegated to the third or fourth line of asthma defense. The reasons for this demotion are twofold. Theophylline has many side effects and a narrow dosing range between effectiveness and toxicity. Secondly, the availability of safer and more effective asthma medications like inhaled cortisone, long-acting beta-agonists and the new leukotriene modifiers have pushed theophylline to the back of the bus. Should theophylline be kicked off the bus altogether? My answer to this question is no. Theophylline is an effective drug for patients with stubborn nocturnal asthma. Once-a-day theophylline drugs may be quite helpful in elderly patients with mild asthma. Theophylline may also turn the tide in severe asthma that is unresponsive to inhaled cortisone drugs, long-acting beta-agonists and the leukotriene modifiers.

I would not be surprised if theophylline actually makes a comeback in the next few years. Recent studies have shown that low-dose theophylline has anti-inflammatory activity. One asthma guru, Doctor Peter Barnes from London, has stated that theophylline drugs are more effective in severe asthma than the new leukotriene modifiers. To minimize side effects, theophylline treatment should be initiated with low doses, and the final dose should be carefully adjusted. Patients on maintenance theophylline therapy should have their blood level monitored once or twice a year. I usually maintain a theophylline blood level between five and ten. Such a level minimizes the chances for a drug interaction due to viral illness or the presence of another drug that may produce a theophylline level over 30, the level at which most major toxic reactions occur.

## The Anticholinergic Drugs

Bronchial tube smooth muscle tone is kept in balance by the opposing actions of the sympathetic and parasympathetic nervous system. The bronchodilating drugs that act on the sympathetic side of the scale have been reviewed. What about drugs that block the opposing or cholinergic system? This system is the excitatory part of the nervous system, and any drug that acts here would have to inhibit or block this side of the nervous system. In fact, these so-called anticholinergic drugs have been used for centuries to treat asthma.

Derivatives of belladonna and stramonium were first used as burning powders and asthma cigarettes and cigars. R.R. Schiffman recognized the potential of atropine-like drugs 70 years ago, when he advocated smoking Schiffman's Asthma Cigarettes for the treatment of asthma. These cigarettes were derived from the leaves of the thorne apple tree which contained stramonium, an atropine-like drug. Naturally the risks of inhaling stramonium leaves far outweighed any potential benefit of these asthma-inhibiting cigars or cigarettes.

Atropine, the first cholinergic drug to be synthesized, is routinely given to patients prior to surgery to dry up mucus secretions during anesthesia and surgery. A renewed interest in the potential benefit of anticholinergic drugs in respiratory diseases like asthma led to the development of an inhaled cholinergic drug, called ipratropium bromide (Atrovent). Inhaled ipratropium bromide owes its safety to the fact that it is poorly absorbed. While it is not as potent a bronchodilator as the beta-agonist drugs, it may be helpful in asthmatics that produce a lot of mucus or have chronic bronchitis from cigarette smoking. It can also be used to treat acute asthma along with a short-acting beta-agonist to help get asthma under control more quickly. One product that combines both ipratropium and albuterol (Combivent) is very helpful in asthmatics with chronic bronchitis and excess mucus production.

# The **Controlling**
Drugs

## 12

The last chapter reviewed the role of the *reliever* drugs or bronchodilators in asthma; now we will move on and discuss the asthma-*controller* drugs. These drugs do not relieve acute asthma. They reduce and control airway inflammation that helps to prevent acute asthma and should be used in all cases of persistent asthma.

## *Cromolyn Sodium*

Cromolyn sodium or Intal was the first asthma controller drug to be developed. It is a rather unique preparation discovered by the unconventional and courageous investigational techniques of Doctor Roger Altounyan. Doctor Altounyan, a brilliant English scientist and lifelong asthma sufferer, became interested in a derivative of an Egyptian herbal plant called khellin. Altounyan suspected that khellin might have an anti-asthmatic effect, as it was a muscle relaxant used in ancient times to relieve intestinal colic. While studying khellin, Altounyan volunteered to be a human guinea pig. He deliberately inhaled derivatives of khellin to determine if they could block his asthma attacks.

Several years and approximately 2,000 asthma attacks later, Altounyan isolated a safe and effective asthma-preventing compound that he called cromolyn sodium or Intal. Since cromolyn did not dissolve well and was poorly absorbed by the intestinal tract, Altounyan figured out a way to get the cromolyn powder into the lung. Drawing on his World War II RAF flying experience, Altounyan developed an ingenious propeller-driven device called the Spinhaler to deliver the powder into the lung (Figure 12.1). This device was the forerunner of today's dry powder inhalers. As a result of Altounyan's efforts, cromolyn or Intal and its offspring, Nedocromil, are used worldwide.

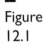

Figure
12.1

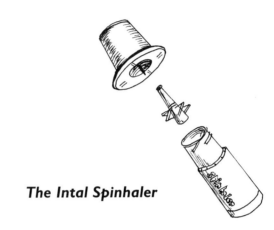

**The Intal Spinhaler**

## Clinical Trials with Cromolyn

Cromolyn has a unique mode of action. It does not relieve but actually prevents asthma. In some way that is not fully understood, cromolyn inhibits the release of mediators from the mast cell. Cromolyn is capable of blocking both the early and late phases of the asthmatic response. Cromolyn has been subjected to more than a thousand clinical trials throughout the world. The largest American study reviewed its effects on 252 patients from several asthma centers. Seventy percent of these study patients improved. More importantly, 50 percent of those patients who needed oral cortisone to control their asthma were able to taper or discontinue their oral cortisone drug. In 1970, I participated in a 54-patient study of cromolyn at the Children's Hospital Medical Center in Boston. Two-thirds of our study patients improved, and nearly one-third became symptom-free.

After I entered practice in 1970, like many other asthma specialists I was only able to obtain cromolyn for my patients from pharmacies in Canada, because it was not released for general use in the United States until 1973. Initial fears that this relatively unknown powder could harm the lung were unfounded, as were the theoretical concerns that cromolyn, being an anti-allergy drug, could injure the immune system. There are a few isolated case reports of hive-like skin rashes. I have never seen a skin rash or any significant side effect from cromolyn, which I have used for nearly 30 years in hundreds of patients. Cromolyn side effects are very rare. It may be the safest drug in all of medicine.

## Who Benefits from Cromolyn?

Cromolyn works best in children and some adults with mild persistent allergic asthma. It prevents asthma triggered by an animal exposure or exercise. Sometimes cromolyn will relieve a stubborn case of hidden or cough variant asthma that does not respond to other asthma medicines. Cromolyn should not be used to treat acute asthma. Because cromolyn does not work as well in more severe or non-allergic asthma, pulmonary specialists are less enthusiastic about this drug. Cromolyn must be given three to four times a day on a regular basis. It is important to give cromolyn a fair trial—a positive response may not become apparent for three to four weeks.

When cromolyn was first introduced in 1973, asthma doctors were taught that it was a "steroid-sparing" drug, which meant that it would allow their sickest patients to stop using steroid or oral cortisone drugs. Thus cromolyn was initially employed in severe asthma, where it was less likely to have an effect. As a result of experiencing treatment failures in severe asthma, many asthma specialists stopped using cromolyn altogether and it temporarily fell into disfavor.

Additional experience with cromolyn found it to be a valuable drug in treating mild persistent asthma, especially in young children. The original cromolyn capsule and Spinhaler were too complicated as delivery methods for many infants and young children. In 1982, an Intal solution that could be administered by a home nebulizer became available. This Intal solution represented a major advance in asthma therapy for infants and young children with chronic asthma. In 1986, the developers of cromolyn went one step further when they released an Intal metered-dose inhaler. Cromolyn is not just an asthma drug. It is also an effective spray for nasal allergies or hay fever sold over-the-counter under the brand name—Nasalcrom. Victims of allergic eye diseases often respond to a cromolyn eye formulation, called Opticrom. The newest cromolyn drug, nedocromil or Tilade, does not offer any therapeutic advantages over Intal or cromolyn.

## The Cortisone Drugs

Before we discuss the role of the cortisone drugs in asthma, we must review the function of our adrenal gland. The adrenal gland, a small gland located behind the kidneys, produces three types of cortisone hormones. The first group, the mineralocorticoid hormones, regulates the body's salt balance. The second group, the anabolic steroids, controls growth, muscle mass and sexual features. The third group, the glucocorticoids, regulates levels of sugar, fat and protein in the body, and fight inflammation. This anti-inflammatory effect makes cortisone drugs the most effective of all asthma medications.

Even though all three cortisone compounds are made in the adrenal gland, the corticosteroids used in the treatment of asthma have no anabolic effect (they do not increase hair growth or muscle mass), and they have little effect on the body's salt balance. Corticosteroids act on virtually every cell and gland involved in asthma, including the mucus glands, macrophages, smooth muscle cells, mast cells, T-cells or lymphocytes and the eosinophils.

After cortisone was chemically isolated from human adrenal glands in 1948, the results of early clinical trials in asthma were spectacular. The sickest asthmatics stopped wheezing for the first time in years. Doctors thought that the cure for asthma had finally arrived. This initial enthusiasm for cortisone quickly waned when it became apparent that daily oral cortisone use over a long period had devastating side effects, including adrenal gland suppression, slow wound healing, excess weight gain, easy bruising, brittle bones (osteoporosis), eye cataracts and growth retardation in children. Eventually it was discovered that many of the unacceptable side effects of daily dosing with oral cortisone could be avoided by taking cortisone every other day. Thus, "alternate-day therapy" became a well-accepted method for treating asthma that did not respond to the conventional asthma drugs. Alternate-day therapy allowed many severe asthmatics to stay out of the hospital and lead relatively normal lives. Prednisone or prednisolone (Medrol) became the drugs of choice in alternate-day therapy, as they had a very short half-life. Even so, alternate-day therapy was not totally risk-free, as many patients developed serious side effects with long-term cortisone alternate-day therapy.

## The Cortisone Inhalers

The dangers posed by daily or alternate-day therapy prompted a search for safer cortisone drugs that could be delivered in relatively low doses with a metered dose inhaler. In 1951, inhaled cortisone was suspended in saline. This was followed in 1960 by release of the Decadron Respihaler, a potent adrenal-suppressive drug with severe cortisone side effects. Asthma specialists can thank their dermatology colleagues for the development of safer and more effective inhaled cortisone drugs. Beclomethasone, the first safe and effective inhaled cortisone drug used in asthma, was developed from a topical spray used in eczema sufferers. Changes in the structure of inhaled cortisone led to the development of compounds with a high degree of local activity and a low risk of side effects because of their reduced rate of absorption.

In the late 1970s two inhaled beclomethasone cortisone drugs, Vanceril and Beclovent, were introduced for asthma. In my opinion the development of this class of asthma drugs was and still remains the most important advance in asthma therapy in the twentieth century. Clinical experience with inhaled cortisone drugs over the past two decades has demonstrated their superiority in controlling chronic asthma in all age groups. Their ability to reduce and eliminate the need for oral cortisone drugs is unmatched by any other asthma medication.

Shortly after their introduction in the United States in the late 1970s cortisone inhalers were only recommended for patients with poorly controlled asthma. Clinical trials in European countries suggested that American dosing guidelines were too restrictive. Additional studies and experience with these drugs found that using higher doses in patients who did not respond well to conventional doses improved asthma and maximized the reduction in oral cortisone drugs. Early reports of the effectiveness of the cortisone inhalers have been amplified by long-term follow-up data in large numbers of patients. Oral cortisone doses can be reduced by 70 to 90 percent in children with severe asthma. Patients who have used inhaled cortisone for a number of years have fewer acute asthma episodes. Asthma specialists in Canada, Great Britain and the United States have expanded the indications for inhaled cortisone drugs in any patient with mild or moderate persistent asthma.

The five inhaled cortisone drugs currently available in the United States are beclomethasone (Vanceril, Beclovent), flunisolide (AeroBid), triamcinolone (Azmacort), fluticasone (Flovent) and budesonide (Pulmicort). Flunisolide and triamcinolone were approved for use in 1984, and the two more potent cortisone inhalers, fluticasone and budesonide, became available in the 1990s. Another inhaled cortisone preparation, mometasone (Asmanex), should become available sometime in 2001. The lack of a nebulized cortisone drug, a distinct disadvantage for infants and young children, was solved in September 2000 when budesonide (Pulmicort) became available in a nebulized solution called Pulmicort Respules.

A new and novel combination drug was approved by the FDA in 2000. This drug, called Advair Diskus, which is delivered by a breath-actuated powder device, combines a long-acting beta-agonist, salmeterol (Serevent), and the inhaled cortisone drug fluticasone (Flovent). This combination drug can be given as one puff once or twice a day to children and adults who need both a relieving and a controlling asthma drug on a daily basis. The convenience of having two medications in one and needing only two puffs per day will undoubtedly improve compliance.

The favorable results gained by more than 25 years of experience with these agents imply that their risk-benefit ratio favors the expanded use of these most potent of all anti-inflammatory or asthma controlling drugs. Before these drugs became available in the 1970s, I had at least two dozen or more patients in my practice with severe asthma that could only be controlled with alternate-day prednisone. Thanks to the availability of the inhaled cortisone drugs, I now treat very few patients who need long-term daily or alternate-day prednisone therapy.

## *Choosing an Inhaled Cortisone Drug*

Choosing one inhaled cortisone formulation over another is fraught with confusion. Health-care providers have a wide choice of several preparations with varying strengths and dosing schedules. The best way to compare different inhaled corticosteroids is to look at their therapeutic index. What is the therapeutic index? This is the ratio between desired and undesired clinical effects. The higher the therapeutic index, the better the risk-benefit ratio. Undesired effects are related to the amount of inhaled drug that is absorbed into the circulation and delivered to other body organs.

Older inhaled-cortisone drugs are more readily absorbed once the particles are swallowed, whereas the absorption from the newer inhaled cortisone drugs like fluticasone (Flovent) and budesonide (Pulmicort) comes from the inhaled fraction that enters the lung. The half-life or rate of elimination from the body also determines the systemic effect of any drug. Studies have concluded that all the inhaled cortisone drugs have side effects when given in high enough doses. No data exists to allow one to determine the superiority of one drug over another. Sometimes it is necessary to take the questions of cost, convenience, patient preference or HMO and insurance coverage into consideration.

In summary, inhaled cortisone drugs are the most effective long-term control medications for asthma. They carry less risk than other asthma drugs such as oral prednisone, theophylline or the long-acting beta-agonist drugs. When the inhaled corticosteroids are compared head to head to all other asthma drugs, such as cromolyn, long acting beta-agonists, theophylline and the newer leukotriene modifiers, the inhaled cortisone drugs always come out on top.

While serious side effects are uncommon, parents of asthmatic children and adults with asthma should be informed that these drugs are not completely risk-free, especially when used in higher doses. For those patients who require higher doses to control asthma, the potential for systemic effects is still less when compared to the complications in untreated asthma and the need for frequent bursts of prednisone. One must carefully weigh the risk-benefit ratio of the inhaled cortisone drugs and constantly try to "step-down" doses to achieve the lowest possible dose that maintains normal or near-normal lung function and quality of life. The 1997 NHLBI Guidelines identify inhaled cortisone drugs as the preferred treatment of asthma. To date no other asthma medication has been shown to be as effective as these inhaled cortisone drugs. I fully concur with the statement that inhaled cortisone drugs are the *"gold standard"* or cornerstone of asthma therapy. Over the past few years there has been an emerging trend in adults and children to aggressively use inhaled cortisone drugs early on, even in cases of mild persistent asthma. The pros and cons of this *"treat early and often"* approach will be discussed in chapter twenty-four, when I review the NHLBI treatment guidelines for asthma.

## *The Prednisone Pulse*

Most savvy health-care consumers are aware of the inherent dangers posed by the long-term use of daily or alternate-day oral cortisone or prednisone. However, many are not aware that the cortisone drugs used in asthma are vastly different from the anabolic steroids that athletes and weight lifters use to build up their muscle mass. These anabolic steroids are synthetic sex hormones that cause growth retardation, severe liver damage, psychological problems and other serious harm. Unfortunately, many patients (and some doctors) have "steroidphobia," which means that they are unduly apprehensive about using prednisone for short periods of time in unstable asthma.

Physicians like me who completed medical training in the 1970s, were taught that oral prednisone took a long time to exert its effect, and it should only be used in severe or life-threatening asthma attacks. Fortunately, these erroneous concepts have been recognized, and the pendulum has actually swung to the other extreme. Asthma specialists now mandate the administration of a short burst of cortisone or prednisone to any patient with moderate or severe asthma who is experiencing an acute asthma relapse.

The oral cortisone drug of choice in acute asthma is usually prednisone or prednisolone (Prelone or Orapred) in children. These drugs have a shorter half-life or length of duration of action than other oral cortisone preparations. Studies have shown the short-term use of oral prednisone is both safe and effective. A beneficial effect can sometimes be seen as early as three hours after the initial dose of oral prednisone. The prompt use of a well-timed pulse of prednisone reduces the need for acute emergency visits and hospitalization in both children and adults. It is the only drug that can prevent a near-fatal or fatal asthma attack. Emergency room studies have shown that prompt use of the prednisone pulse lowers the likelihood of an asthma relapse. Doctor Christopher Randolph followed 32 asthmatic children, aged three to 18 years, for 18 months. Randolph's patients were instructed to begin prednisone promptly, during the early signs of an asthma relapse. Their need for prednisone was based on clinical symptoms and peak flow readings. Patients were given a pulse of prednisone for five days, or until their peak flow rates returned to normal levels for 24 hours. None of these children required an emergency room visit or hospitalization during the study. Randolph appropriately concluded that aggressive use of prednisone minimized the need for emergency room care or asthma hospitalizations.

Patients who receive a prednisone pulse are more likely to have normal lung functions a week or two after taking prednisone. In my experience, many patients remain stable for weeks or months after just one short burst of prednisone. The prednisone doses used in acute asthma are strictly empirical, as there is little dose-response data dealing with cortisone and asthma. Since toxicity is directly related to duration of treatment, not dosage, most asthma specialists choose a high enough dose to be at or near the top of the dose-response curve. Most children and young adults respond to an initial dose of 30 to 60 milligrams of prednisone, followed by a seven to fourteen-day tapering dose. While some asthma specialists prefer to give full doses for four to five days and then abruptly stop prednisone, recent studies on the late-phase response of asthma favor a gradual tapering of the drug.

Patients with severe asthma may need two to three weeks of prednisone. Short-term prednisone therapy is a very safe and effective way to stabilize asthma that is out of control and not responding to the other asthma drugs. Recent studies in children have demonstrated that the prednisone pulse can be safely administered up to four to five times a year.

I usually prescribe a prednisone pulse to the following groups of relapsing asthmatics:

- Acutely ill patients with previous hospitalizations or a history of life-threatening asthma

- Relapsing patients who are overusing their cortisone aerosols or pocket inhalers

- Unstable asthmatics with poor breathing tests

- Unstable asthmatics who may be traveling or vacationing in remote areas where good medical care is unavailable

## Risks of the Prednisone Pulse

Potential side effects from the prednisone pulse include slight weight gain, increased appetite, menstrual irregularities, acne flare-ups, mood changes, muscle cramps and heartburn or indigestion. Muscle cramps, due to a loss of potassium, can often be prevented by drinking orange juice or eating bananas. Heartburn may be avoided by antacids, anti-ulcer drugs or taking prednisone after meals. Patients with tuberculosis, diabetes, high blood pressure, glaucoma, esophageal reflux, ulcers or psychosis will require closer observation when they take prednisone.

The long-term use of oral steroids has devastating side effects. Some of the more serious complications that will be discussed in the next chapter include adrenal gland failure, cataracts, decreased bone mass (osteoporosis), decreased growth rate in children, high blood pressure, elevated blood sugar and easy bruising. These more serious side effects are seen in those patients who take higher-than-normal alternate-day prednisone doses, usually over 30 milligrams every other day. Such side effects do not usually occur with the short-term use of prednisone or with conventional doses of the cortisone inhalers.

Patients who do require alternate-day steroids should take their dose in the morning every other day. This allows the adrenal gland time to work on its own on the off day. Prednisone is the least expensive of all asthma drugs, and comes in liquid and tablet forms in various dosing strengths. I prefer the five-milligram tablet strength, as it allows for more precise dosing schedules. Two liquid preparations, Prelone and Orapred, are very helpful for children and adults who cannot swallow tablets.

## Steroid-resistant Asthma

A small group of patients with asthma do not respond to high doses of inhaled or oral cortisone drugs. The term doctors apply to this group of patients is steroid-resistant asthma. Several factors that typify patients with steroid-resistant asthma include a longer duration of symptoms, low morning peak expiratory flow rates and increased bronchial hyperresponsiveness. The majority of patients with steroid-resistant asthma have an acquired form of steroid resistance induced by inflammation or immune activation. Steroid-resistant asthma poses a challenging problem for asthma specialists. Early identification of this form of asthma is important, not only to improve asthma control but also to avoid excessive and often debilitating cortisone side effects in patients who are not benefiting from cortisone.

Confounding factors such as GERD, aspiration syndrome, vocal cord dysfunction, sinus disease, environmental triggers, poor compliance with medications and psychosocial factors should be addressed prior to categorizing a patient as a steroid-resistant asthmatic. Patients with true steroid-resistant-asthma must be considered candidates for alternative anti-inflammatory asthma drugs such as cyclosporin, methotrexate, gold, dapsone, hydroxychloroquine and intravenous gammaglobulin or nebulized lidocaine.

# The **Side Effects**
## of the
## Cortisone Drugs

# 13

**W**hile the cortisone drugs are the most effective of all asthma medications, they also have the most potential to induce significant side effects. Adverse effects of cortisone therapy include adrenal suppression, osteoporosis or bone loss, increased appetite with weight gain, development of a moon-shaped face, a buffalo hump or swelling in the back of the neck, wasting of the extremities, atrophy of the skin, excess hair growth, eye cataracts, growth retardation in children and psychological disturbances.

Other less common complications include hypertension, peptic ulcer disease and diabetes. Most of the side effects listed above are seen with prolonged use of the oral forms of these drugs. However, the inhaled cortisone drugs may cause local and milder systemic side effects, especially when given in higher doses.

The most common problems encountered with the inhaled cortisone drugs are oral thrush, or white spots on the mouth or tongue, and a form of hoarseness called dysphonia. The incidence and severity of thrush and hoarseness, which is directly related to the daily dose of the inhaled drug, can be minimized by mouth-rinsing with water and using a spacer device to reduce particle deposition in the mouth and throat. Sometimes mouth rinsing with an antifungal agent like mycostatin will be required to control oral thrush.

## *Adrenal Suppression*

Our bodily functions are controlled by a group of glands in our body called the endocrine glands (Figure 13.1). These endocrine glands all secrete hormones into the blood stream that deliver messages to various organs and tissues. The production of these hormones is regulated by the brain's pituitary gland. This gland, the size of a hazelnut, is the most important of the endocrine glands as it serves as the control center for day-to-day function that regulates sexual features, breast milk production, growth, thyroid and adrenal gland function.

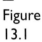

Figure
13.1

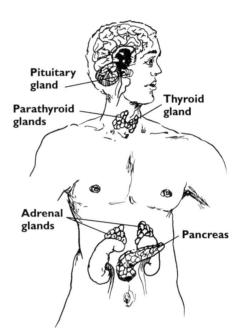

### *The Endocrine Glands*

Two of the more important parts of the endocrine system in asthma are the adrenal glands. These paired glands, small organs located in our abdomen behind our kidneys, produce several hormones including cortisone, androgens or sex hormones and adrenaline or epinephrine. These glands constantly exchange signals with the pituitary gland. When too much cortisone is circulating in our body, the pituitary gland sends out a signal to the adrenal glands that shuts down the production of cortisone.

Thus, when extra cortisone is introduced into our body, the adrenal glands stop cortisone production—this is called adrenal gland suppression. Any patient who takes an oral cortisone drug like prednisone on a daily basis for a long period of time will eventually experience adrenal gland suppression. This risk is somewhat minimized by giving the drugs on an alternate-day basis, which allows the pituitary and adrenal gland to overcome the effects of extra cortisone on the off day when cortisone is not administered.

Patients with adrenal gland suppression may experience acute adrenal insufficiency during times of acute stress brought on by surgery, acute illness or trauma. Acute adrenal insufficiency as a result of chronic cortisone therapy is a true medical emergency, and it requires prompt diagnosis and treatment with extra doses of cortisone. All patients on long-term oral cortisone should be considered to have adrenal suppression and wear a Medic-Alert bracelet that identifies them as being at risk for acute adrenal insufficiency. All adrenal-suppressed individuals should be given extra cortisone prior to any surgical procedure. Complete recovery from adrenal suppression may take six months to a year after cessation of long-term cortisone use. One of the major reasons for the enthusiasm for the inhaled cortisone drugs is that they minimize the risks of adrenal suppression, which is a rare complication of inhaled cortisone therapy. Nevertheless, the remote possibility of developing adrenal suppression posed by surgery, trauma, an acute illness or asthma relapse requires that patients who are taking inhaled cortisone drugs be given extra cortisone by mouth or injection prior to surgery or during an asthma relapse.

## Growth Retardation

The most recent controversy involving the inhaled cortisone drugs centers on the potential of growth retardation in children. Before getting into this debate, let us review the pattern of normal childhood growth. Normal childhood growth usually occurs in three stages. First, there is the rapid growth of infancy and early childhood. After age two this rapid growth slows down and is followed by more gradual increase in height—usually two to three inches per year. The rate of childhood growth normally dips to its lowest point during the two- to three-year period preceding puberty.

The third and final stage of growth that is controlled by growth and sex hormone output occurs in puberty. The timing of the growth spurt in puberty or adolescence is variable and may start as early as 10 years or as late as 16 years of age. Some children, often referred to as "late bloomers," have a pronounced delay in growth during this stage of life only to have a dramatic spurt later in adolescence.

How do cortisone drugs inhibit growth? Our adrenal glands make approximately 37 milligrams of cortisone each day, which is the equivalent of seven milligrams of prednisone. Cortisone is a vital hormone that fine-tunes all of our bodily functions, including growth. Growth is controlled by growth hormone, produced in the pituitary gland. Extra cortisone suppresses all functions of this pituitary gland, including the production of growth hormone. The result is a slowing of growth, as the large bones responsible for one's height are no longer stimulated to grow by growth hormone.

## Clinical Studies on Growth

The rising incidence of asthma leading to the widespread use of inhaled cortisone drugs in hundreds of thousands of children with asthma has created concerns about the possible effects of inhaled cortisone drugs on childhood growth. This circulating cortisone has the potential to shut down the output of growth hormone by the pituitary gland. Preliminary growth studies in children that were poorly controlled suggested that inhaled cortisone could impair childhood growth. Obviously if you look at childhood growth just before puberty you are going to see some sort of slowdown, even if the children are not taking inhaled cortisone medicines.

One study on the use of beclamethasone found a growth reduction of 1.4 to 1.5 centimeters, or one-third to one-half an inch per year. Another study found that there was no difference between final adult heights in those who took inhaled corticosteroids compared to controls not using inhaled cortisone drugs. It appeared that any growth rate reduction is limited to the first year of therapy. One other possibility is that adolescent growth could overcome any early effect of the inhaled cortisone on growth.

The debate generated by these findings prompted the FDA to address this issue, and in July 1998 the FDA recommended a labeling change for both nasal and inhaled cortisone drugs. This labeling change stated that nasal and inhaled corticosteroids have been shown to cause a reduction in growth velocity when administered to children and adolescents and that the long-term effects on growth were unknown. This FDA announcement created somewhat of a furor, leading to a formal statement from the national organizations of asthma specialists. The statement pointed out that the FDA labeling change did not imply that these products were unsafe, and warned against abrupt termination of these asthma drugs. Undue alarm would be an inappropriate response, and asthma experts stressed that inhaled cortisone drugs were still the most effective medications available for treating the millions of patients who suffer from asthma.

Fortunately, two studies published in the *New England Journal of Medicine* (NEJM) in October 2000 have put this growth issue to rest. The first study came from the CAMP or Childhood Asthma Management Program. The CAMP study tracked 1041 children, five to twelve years of age, for four to six years in eight asthma centers throughout the United States. Approximately one-third of the CAMP enrollees received the inhaled cortisone drug budesonide (Pulmicort), one-third got nedrocomil (Tilade), and another third took a placebo drug. The group treated with the inhaled cortisone drug fared best. They had fewer asthma relapses, less need for prednisone and fewer emergency visits or asthma hospitalizations. More importantly, no difference was noted in growth rates after one year of treatment with inhaled cortisone. In the second paper, Danish investigators tracked a group of children treated with inhaled cortisone budesonide for ten years. While they did find a small decrease in growth in the first year of therapy, at the end of 10 years, final adult height was not affected. Thus, it appears the FDA may have jumped the gun when they put out their warning about growth and inhaled corticosteroids in 1998.

These findings support my own observation about inhaled cortisone drugs and growth. In the days before we had the inhaled cortisone drugs, I frequently had to prescribe prednisone in order to control moderate to severe persistent asthma. It was well known at that time that asthma itself caused short stature and significant growth retardation. Major growth spurts were commonly observed after poorly controlled and very sick asthmatic children were placed on prednisone on an alternate-day basis.

My now 36-year-old son, who is 6 foot, 5 inches tall, has taken inhaled cortisone drugs since they first became available in the late 1970s. It is possible he may have been an inch or so taller if he had not used these inhaled cortisone drugs. But other than the fact he may have been a better rebounder in basketball, the improved quality of life offered to him by these drugs far outweighed the risk of a minimal reduction in his final adult height.

Any possible risks of inhaled cortisone drugs on growth need to be weighed against the effects of long-term under-treatment of the inflammatory process in asthma and poor lung growth that may lead to permanent scarring or lung remodeling. How can we lower the risk of growth suppression? I always attempt to use the lowest possible dose needed to control asthma. Using spacer devices with dose inhalers lowers the rate of systemic absorption. Their primary care provider or asthma specialist should closely follow children and young adults taking moderate to higher doses of inhaled cortisone drugs. The patient's height should be accurately monitored two to three times a year by a wall-mounted instrument called a stadiometer.

## Osteoporosis

Osteoporosis, the most common of all bone diseases, is estimated to affect 25 million individuals and result in 1.3 million fractures a year at a cost of $10 billion per year. The major risk factors for osteoporosis include gender (the rate is especially high in post-menopausal women) and race. Caucasians and Asians are more at risk for osteoporosis than blacks. Additional risk factors for osteoporosis include inadequate intake of calcium or vitamin D, lack of exercise, tobacco use, excess alcohol intake and the use of cortisone medicines. In osteoporosis the bones become very thin and fragile and are prone to break or fracture. Most common fracture sites are the wrist, back, hip and leg bones. Osteoporosis can be classified as primary—age or sex related, or secondary—due to other illnesses or drugs.

The most common cause of secondary osteoporosis is the use of oral cortisone drugs. When extra amounts of cortisone are introduced into our body, there is a significant disruption in the delicate balance between the hormones that control bone formation and bone density. Exogenous or extra cortisone inhibits the production of sex hormones like testosterone and estrogen and lowers the rate of calcium absorption. The end result is bone loss or osteoporosis. Between 30 and 50 percent of patients taking long-term oral corticosteroids will experience a bone fracture. Bone loss occurs rapidly (within six to twelve months) after beginning oral cortisone. The rate of bone loss is directly proportional to the cortisone dose.

What is the risk for osteoporosis for patients taking the inhaled cortisone drugs? Early studies on bone loss in patients taking inhaled cortisone were poorly done and inconsistent. Some placebo-controlled studies found that low to moderate doses of inhaled cortisone drugs have little effect on bone density. Pediatric studies have found no reduction in bone density in surveys of asthmatic children treated with low to intermediate doses of beclomethasone for several years. Remember—inhaled cortisone drugs are administered in microgram doses. A microgram is 1/1000 of a gram. Thus, in most cases not enough drug enters the blood stream to effect bone metabolism. Some people, especially postmenopausal women, who take inhaled cortisone drugs have a long-term risk for osteoporosis.

A study published in the *New England Journal of Medicine* in September 2001 implies that bone density should be monitored in young women taking higher doses of an inhaled cortisone drug. This study of 109 pre-menopausal women with asthma who inhaled higher doses (12 puffs per day) of triamcinolone (Azmacort), for three years found a loss of density of the hip bone, but not the long bones or spine. The decline in bone density was directly related to the number of puffs per year. It is believed that the decrease in bone density was the result of a decline in circulating estrogen. The drug used in this study, triamcinolone, is one of the older inhaled cortisone drugs which has been previously linked to bone problems. This study needs additional confirmation with the newer inhaled cortisone drugs such as fluticasone (Flovent) or budesonide (Pulmicort) that have less systemic absorption.

The best way to minimize any potential bone loss in this population is to use the lowest possible dose of inhaled cortisone drugs to control asthma and encourage weight-bearing exercises and adequate intake of calcium and vitamin D. In summary, the current thinking indicates that the daily dose of the inhaled cortisone drug, not the duration of therapy, adversely affects bone density. Supplemental estrogen therapy may offset this bone-depleting effect in postmenopausal women. The gold standard for diagnosing bone loss or osteoporosis is a bone scan or bone densiometer study. This screening test should be done on high-risk candidates for osteoporosis.

## Treatment of Osteoporosis

Once it has been determined that a patient on oral prednisone or a high-dose inhaled-cortisone drug has developed osteoporosis, early treatment is essential. Treatment programs include active exercise, especially gravity-dependent activities such as walking. Activities such as heavy lifting, high-impact aerobics and contact sports are not recommended, as they may cause fractures of the hip, spine or long bones. Medications should include supplemental calcium and vitamin D. The NIH recommends a daily dose of 1500 mg of calcium for women over age 50 not taking estrogen, and for all adults over age 65. A daily dose of 1000 mg of calcium is recommended for women age 50 to 64 who are taking estrogen, and for men age 25 to 64. An adequate dose of vitamin D (400 to 800 units) is recommended to help the body absorb calcium. Additional medications that may be indicated include some of the newer anti-osteoporosis medications like Evista, Fosamax and Didronel.

## Glaucoma and Cataract Risks

Cortisone drugs have been linked to glaucoma. The biggest risk for glaucoma occurs in patients using oral cortisone drugs or topical cortisone eye drugs. It is generally believed that cortisone raises the pressure in the eye by impeding the outflow of the watery fluid in front of the eye. A study done at McGill University in Montreal,

Canada assessed risk for increased eye pressure or glaucoma in nearly 50,000 adults over age sixty-five who used inhaled or nasal corticosteroids.

The study found that there was no risk for patients using low to medium doses of inhaled or nasal corticosteroids, but the risk for glaucoma was 44 percent higher in patients taking higher doses of inhaled cortisone, which was defined as 1500 to 1600 micrograms or more of daily inhaled cortisone.

The development of eye cataracts is another well-described complication of chronic cortisone use. The cataracts, while usually small, can at times significantly impair vision and require surgical removal. Although the mechanism involved in cortisone-induced cataracts is not clear, cortisone drugs may dehydrate the lens or alter carbohydrate metabolism in the lens. Small posterior cataracts have been observed to resolve in some asthmatic children after they changed from oral prednisone to inhaled cortisone drugs.

The risk for cataract formation in younger patients is negligible. Doctor Estelle Simons from Canada's University of Manitoba looked at the risk for cataracts in young children treated with inhaled cortisone and found no cortisone-induced cataracts in 95 patients who underwent eye examinations. The association between cataracts and inhaled or oral cortisone therapy in adult asthmatics is related to the daily dose and oral prednisone use, but not with dose or duration of inhaled cortisone therapy. In summary, the risk for cataract formation is minimal for patients taking low to moderate doses of inhaled cortisone drugs. The literature on this issue suggests that children and adults using oral cortisone drugs or higher doses of inhaled corticosteroids on a regular basis should have an annual eye exam to check for glaucoma or cataract formation.

## Psychiatric Side Effects

Psychiatric side effects to inhaled corticosteroids are rare, while such side effects to oral cortisone drugs are not uncommon. Frequent complaints include depression, irritability and mood disturbances. The risk of psychiatric side effects is usually dose-dependent. Such side effects cease to be a problem once the oral cortisone is tapered or discontinued. Those patients who require long-term oral cortico-steroids and experience significant psychological side effects may benefit from antidepresssive therapy.

## Cortisone Withdrawal

When asthmatics who were previously dependent on oral cortisone taper or stop oral cortisone, they can experience many unpleasant side effects from the cortisone withdrawal. Typical withdrawal symptoms include loss of energy, poor appetite, severe muscle aches, joint pains and a flare-up of co-existing problems like hay fever or eczema that were masked by the oral cortisone. Sometimes the symptoms of cortisone withdrawal are so severe that the drug must be tapered slowly over several weeks or months.

# The
# **Leukotriene**
# Modifiers

# **14**

## *A New Class of Asthma Drugs*

I n 1938, scientists discovered a new class of chemical mediators called slow-reacting substance of anaphylaxis, abbreviated SRS-A. Laboratory research over the next two decades, that culminated in a Nobel Prize, led to the discovery that SRS-A was composed of several chemicals called the leukotriene (pronounced lu-ko-try-een) mediators. High levels of leukotrienes were found in the sputum and urine of patients with asthma, leading to speculation that leukotrienes might be important triggers of bronchial asthma. These chemical mediators arise from a complicated metabolic pathway that induces smooth muscle constriction (bronchospasm), edema (swelling) and the influx of inflammatory cells like the all-important asthma-inducing mast cells and eosinophils.

This important discovery led to the search for compounds that could inhibit or suppress these mediators and relieve asthma. Intense research efforts at several of the world's leading pharmaceutical firms led to the development of four drugs which block or modify the actions of the leukotrienes. These drugs, known as anti-leukotriene drugs or the leukotriene modifiers, are the first new class of asthma drugs to be introduced in 25 years (Table 14.1).

These four leukotriene modifiers have been subjected to extensive clinical trials. They all have bronchodilating and anti-inflammatory activity. They block bronchospasm induced by aspirin in aspirin-sensitive asthmatics. Early clinical trials with the

**Table 14.1** Leukotriene Modifiers

| Generic Name | Brand Name | Dose |
|---|---|---|
| **montelukast** | Singulair | 10 mg adults<br>4 & 5 mg children*<br>*pediatric-chewable tablet |
| **zafirlukast** | Accolate | 20 mg twice a day<br>*must monitor liver<br>functions |
| **pranlukast** | Onon, Ultair | 225 mg twice a day<br>only available in Japan |
| **zileuton** | Zyflo | 600 mg four times a day<br>*must monitor liver<br>functions |

leukotriene modifiers in mild to moderate asthma showed improvement in symptom scores and a decreased need for beta-agonist rescue drugs. When leukotriene modifiers were compared to an inhaled cortisone drug, the patients on the inhaled cortisone drug had better pulmonary functions, but there was little difference in symptom scores or beta-agonist use. One distinct advantage of the leukotriene modifiers is that they come in pill form.

Most studies show that patients are more compliant or adherent when asked to take a pill once a day as opposed to using inhalers several times a day. One study found that patients on high doses of inhaled cortisone were able to cut their inhaled cortisone dose in half when a leukotriene modifier was added to their drug program. Thus, these drugs have a cortisone sparing effect, which means that they can lower the daily dose of inhaled cortisone needed to control asthma.

One leukotriene modifier, montelukast (Singulair), was studied in 336 children at private practices and medical centers throughout the United States. Singulair was found to be safe and effective, and to improve pulmonary functions in children from six to fourteen years of age. Once-a-day dosing with Singulair in adult volunteers protected against exercise-induced bronchoconstriction and reduced the need for breakthrough rescue therapy with beta-agonist inhalers. Singulair is now approved for use in adults and in younger children.

## First-Line Therapy?

Should the leukotriene modifiers be used as a first-line controller therapy or monotherapy (one drug only) in asthma? This important question is the subject of an ongoing debate between asthma specialists. Doctor Jeffrey Drazen from Partners Asthma Center in Boston, Massachusetts, believes that the leukotriene modifiers can be used in place of inhaled cortisone in mild persistent asthma. Drazen notes that these drugs are easier to take. They all come in pill form, and patients do not need extensive education techniques on inhalers and spacer use. Other asthma experts, such as Doctor Sally Wenzel from the National Jewish Asthma Center in Denver, Colorado, feel that leukotriene modifiers should not take the place of the inhaled cortisone drugs that are the cornerstone in the management of persistent asthma.

I tend to side with Doctor Wenzel on this issue. The inhaled cortisone drugs have a longer track record, and there are minimal risks for patients taking conventional doses. More importantly, inhaled cortisone drugs have been shown to have a greater anti-inflammatory effect that may prevent remodeling or long-term lung damage. At the present time the leukotriene modifiers can make no such claim, as they have only been around for a few years.

One in every four patients will not respond to a leukotriene modifier. The variable response to these drugs may be due to differences in genetic make-up. Some patients may not produce a particular mediator, and trying to block this mediator is a worthless endeavor. Therefore, you must administer a four-week trial to determine if leukotriene modifiers are effective, as it is impossible to determine which patients will not benefit from these drugs.

Thus, it is important to see a patient for a follow-up visit four to six weeks after starting a leukotriene modifier trial to determine if it is effective. I presently prefer montelukast (Singulair) as it has a once-a-day dosing schedule, pediatric dosing formulations and fewer reported side effects than the other agents.

## Leukotriene Modifier Side Effects

The leukotriene modifiers have been tested in thousands of patients and by and large have been found free of significant side effects in

197

clinical trials. While headaches and rashes were the most common side effects, the incidence was no more common than in the placebo group. The first leukotriene modifier released in the U.S., zileuton (Zyflo), can alter liver metabolism, as one to two percent of patients in clinical studies had elevated liver enzymes. Liver function studies are recommended in the first few months of therapy with zileuton.

In December 2000, a report in the *Annals of Internal Medicine* described three middle-aged women who developed a severe liver injury while taking zafirlukast (Accolate). One of these women required a liver transplant. These cases prompted the manufacturer of Accolate to revise its drug package insert to indicate that severe hepatitis and liver failure may occur in patients taking zafirlukast (Accolate). It is estimated that more than one million people have been treated with Accolate, so these toxic liver reactions are very rare.

Another noteworthy adverse effect of the leukotriene modifiers has been the rare development of an entity called the Churg-Strauss Syndrome. This is a syndrome characterized by vasculitis or inflammation of blood vessels throughout the entire body. The Churg-Strauss Syndrome usually occurs in patients who have tapered or stopped taking an oral cortisone drug like prednisone after starting a leukotriene modifier. It appears that the leukotriene modifiers do not directly cause the Churg-Strauss Syndrome. The vasculitis is probably due to an unmasking of this syndrome when oral steroids are tapered or discontinued. Most of the patients who develop the Churg-Strauss Syndrome have severe persistent asthma. The rate of this unusual complication appears to be very rare—about one in every 20,000 treatment-years.

## Summary

I feel the leukotriene modifiers can be used in the cases of mild persistent asthma—especially if exercise-induced asthma is a prominent feature or when there is a strong steroid phobia on the part of the patient or family. One distinct advantage of the leukotriene modifiers is that oral administration may relieve nasal symptoms in hay fever and control hives in asthmatics with chronic urticaria. When there is a risk of permanent lung damage or remodeling in more persistent and severe asthma, the leukotriene modifiers are at best add-on drugs. One unpublished study from

England by Doctor Peter Barnes found the leukotriene modifiers were of little value in sicker asthmatics dependent on oral cortisone drugs. The long-term effects of the leukotriene modifiers are still unknown. It sometimes takes several years before significant side effects surface with any new drug. Physicians should be aware that some leukotriene modifiers are potentially liver-toxic, and patients should be observed for signs and symptoms of hepatitis. Long-term experience with the leukotriene modifiers will ultimately lead to a better understanding of these drugs and define their proper place in asthma therapy.

# Additional and **Futuristic** Asthma Drugs

# 15

The previous chapters reviewed the major classes of asthma drugs. This chapter will discuss additional asthma drugs employed in asthma unresponsive to conventional therapy. I will also touch on some of the futuristic asthma treatments currently under development.

## Antihistamines in Asthma

Doctors have been traditionally taught to avoid using antihistamines in asthma because of their potential to dry up lung secretions and worsen asthma. Antihistamines contain a warning on their label or package insert that states that they should not be used in asthma. Many studies have shown this to be an unnecessary precaution, as most asthmatics can safely take antihistamines for sinus congestion, hives or hay fever without aggravating their asthma. Some patients with asthma actually stop wheezing when they take an antihistamine. People who do experience increased coughing or wheezing after taking an antihistamine should avoid antihistamines.

Previous efforts to treat asthma with older antihistamine drugs, like Benadryl, were unsuccessful because of their sedating tendency. Evidence now suggests that the new non-sedating antihistamines may play an expanded role in asthma. Today's newer drugs like Claritin, Allegra and Zyrtec have been a godsend to patients with allergic rhinitis or hay fever. These non-sedating antihistamines may prevent the early phase of the asthmatic response by blocking the release of histamine in the lung. One antihistamine, azelastine (Astelin), is a somewhat unique drug. While it has antihistaminic qualities, it also has an anti-allergic activity that relieves airway smooth muscle spasm and decreases inflammation in the bronchial tubes. Initial studies with azelastine in hay fever have shown it to be effective at a dose of one to two milligrams per day. Higher doses produced a marked decrease in symptom scores and less need for backup medications for patients with asthma. Azelastine's two most common adverse effects, sleepiness and altered taste, are dose-related and transient. This drug has not been evaluated under age 12, suggesting that FDA approval for children may be several years away.

## Expectorants and Asthma

One of the calling cards of asthma is an overproduction of thick sticky mucus that is difficult to cough up or expectorate. Thus, you might think that expectorants or drugs that thin out mucus would be useful in asthma. One of Sir William Osler's favorite asthma remedies was the expectorant potassium iodide. In theory this is a great concept, but too much iodide can cause thyroid problems. In real life most expectorant drugs are relatively useless in asthma. While some of the newer expectorants may be of some help, the best (and cheapest) of all expectorants is plain water.

## The Antibiotic TAO

Years ago asthma researchers discovered that an older erythromycin-like antibiotic, called troleandomycin or TAO, helped patients with severe cortisone-dependent-asthma. TAO interacts with cortisone by prolonging the half-life of cortisone in the body. This effect, called the steroid sparing effect, allows cortisone dependent patients to take less cortisone. Even though TAO reduces the total cortisone requirements, patients still have significant cortisone side effects despite a lowering of their total cortisone dose. In effect, TAO doubles or triples the dose of oral cortisone. Two reports of a fatal varicella (chicken pox) infection in patients taking TAO and the cortisone drug methylprednisolone (Medrol) have dampened my enthusiasm for TAO therapy. TAO may also cause significant liver problems. Only patients with severe cortisone-dependent-asthma should try TAO, and an asthma specialist should always monitor TAO therapy.

202

## Antibiotics in Asthma

I used to feel that most asthma doctors, including myself, were guilty of over-prescribing antibiotics in asthma relapses. While doctors know that most asthma relapses are triggered by viral, not bacterial, infections, it is difficult to withhold an antibiotic from a wheezing patient who is coughing up thick yellow-green-colored phlegm or sputum. A recent study that found secondary bacterial infections in patients coughing up yellow-green-colored sputum suggests that this approach is not totally wrong. Two situations where antibiotics are definitely indicated in asthma include acute or chronic sinus infection and mycoplasma pneumonia, a special type of lung infection.

## Vaccines in Asthma

You can prevent an asthma relapse caused by the influenza virus by taking an annual flu shot. Sometimes the flu vaccine induces a mild asthma flare-up, but studies show it is worth the risk as immunized patients have fewer flu-like illnesses and hospitalizations. I recommend flu vaccine for all my patients, including children, with persistent asthma. Even though bacterial infection is an infrequent cause of an asthma relapse, patients with chronic asthma, especially those over 50 years of age, should receive the pneumonia vaccine. Children with persistent asthma should receive the new pediatric pneumonia vaccine.

## Gold Therapy

The recognition that chronic inflammation plays a role in asthma suggests that drugs used to treat other inflammatory diseases, like rheumatoid arthritis, might be beneficial in asthma. Gold therapy, a favorite of Japanese physicians, has shown a favorable response in some patients with severe asthma. The drawbacks to gold therapy are twofold. It may require four to six months before any benefit is seen, and responders are limited to patients with allergic or IgE-mediated asthma. Side effects to gold therapy include skin rashes and stomatitis (inflammation of the mouth and tongue). Oral gold or Auronofin has been studied in America in a few oral cortisone-dependent patients with favorable results. Additional gold studies are needed to confirm these findings.

## Methotrexate Therapy

The safety and effectiveness of low doses of methotrexate, an older cancer drug, has been demonstrated in children and adults with rheumatoid arthritis. Seattle's Doctor Michael Mullarkey was the first to report the potential value of methotrexate in severe asthma. Long-term studies by Mullarkey have shown that methotrexate can be given over an 18- to 28-month period. Low-dose methotrexate may provide an alternative to the chronic use of high doses of daily or alternate-day prednisone. Two other methotrexate trials demonstrated improvement in asthma and a reduction in the need for oral prednisone. The most common side effects of methotrexate are gastritis, mouth irritation and low blood counts.

One word of caution before jumping on the methotrexate bandwagon. An 18-patient, placebo-controlled study at the National Jewish Hospital in Denver, Colorado, suggests that more aggressive management of asthma is necessary before entering into a methotrexate program, as 40 percent of the patients on the placebo drug in this study showed significant improvement. These patients were seen on a weekly basis, implying that close follow-up visits alone may improve severe asthma. Methotrexate is an experimental asthma drug. Patients and physicians should be fully aware of the potential risks and benefits of methotrexate therapy, as there are no guidelines for its use in asthma.

Another cancer-type drug being looked at in severe asthma is cyclosporin A. This compound was studied in 12 patients with severe cortisone-dependent asthma. Half of the cortisone-dependent patients were able to reduce their oral prednisone dose, from 30 milligrams a day to an average of 10 milligrams a day.

## Other Experimental Asthma Drugs

Hydroxychloroquine is an antimalarial agent used in rheumatoid arthritis and systemic lupus. A study of hydroxychloroquine in cortisone-dependent asthma found a reduction in the need for oral cortisone. Another placebo-controlled study in nine cortisone-dependent asthmatics showed no beneficial effect. Azathioprine is another antimetabolite shown to be a cortisone-sparing agent and immunosuppressant in a number of inflammatory diseases. In two studies in asthma, no benefit was seen with azathioprine. The popular anti-inflammatory gout medicine, colchicine, was administered to 10 asthmatics, who showed small improvements in symptom score and less need for beta-agonists, but no change in lung functions. No trials have been reported with colchicine in cortisone-dependent asthma.

## Intravenous Gammaglobulin

Gammaglobulin, the major antibody of our immune system that protects us from many major infectious diseases, has been successfully used in immune deficiency disorders. Monthly intravenous infusions of gammaglobulin increase antibody levels and protect against viral and bacterial infections. In higher doses, gammaglobulin acts as a modulator of the immune system by assisting the immune system in regulating the production of IgE antibody and the T-cells that cause chronic inflammation in asthma. Eight steroid-dependent asthmatics from the National Jewish Hospital, age eight to seventeen, received high-dose intravenous gamma globulin for six months. They had a three-fold reduction in their need for oral cortisone and increased pulmonary function tests, but no change in bronchial hyperreactivity. The positive findings in this small study suggest larger trials are needed with gammaglobulin, particularly in view of the fact that intravenous gammaglobulin costs approximately $25,000 per year.

## Lidocaine Therapy

Severe asthmatics who require oral cortisone are constantly being studied by asthma researchers, in a never-ending search to determine why their severe asthma requires daily or alternate-day prednisone. In one such study at the Mayo Clinic, doctors set out to analyze the mucus or sputum produced in the lung of patients with severe asthma. In this study, an instrument called a bronchoscope was passed down into the lung, and mucus or secretions were collected for laboratory analysis. In order to minimize discomfort from the procedure, the windpipe or trachea was sprayed with a local anesthetic prior to passing the bronchoscope. The local anesthetic used in this procedure was lidocaine or Xylocaine—the same drug used by your dentist during dental work.

Much to the surprise of the Mayo Clinic investigators, many of these cortisone-dependent asthmatics felt much better after the procedure. Several patients were able to cut back on their daily dose of prednisone. As the only variable in this study was the use of nebulized lidocaine, the Mayo Clinic doctors set up a pilot study to look at the effects of spraying lidocaine into the lungs of oral cortisone-dependent asthmatics. The results in a small group of adults with severe asthma were quite impressive. Many patients tapered or discontinued their oral prednisone. They then studied six children with severe asthma. Five of the six children given lidocaine were able to discontinue their oral cortisone three months after starting lidocaine.

The one advantage of lidocaine over other experimental asthma drugs like gammaglobulin, cyclosporin and methotrexate is its more favorable safety profile. These preliminary findings spawned additional investigations on local anesthetics in the treatment of severe asthma. Again a word of caution! This type of experimental asthma therapy should only be done in specialized clinics or asthma centers experienced in treating severe cortisone-dependent asthma.

## Antifungal Therapy

A possible link between adult-onset asthma and chronic fungal infection with *Trichophyton,* the fungus that causes athlete's foot, has been uncovered by investigators from the University of Virginia. The interest in this connection was triggered after a patient with severe asthma reported marked improvement in asthma after his chronic fungal infection was treated with an antifungal drug. This patient had severe asthma, chronic fungal infections of the hands and feet, and a positive skin test to the Trichophyton fungus. The Virginia group then administered an antifungal drug—fluconazole—to 11 patients with severe asthma, fungal infections and positive skin tests to *Trichophyton.* Treatment over several months led to a reduction in symptom scores and oral cortisone requirements, as well as improved pulmonary functions. These preliminary results imply that some forms of asthma might be triggered by chronic fungal infection of the skin and nails. Personally I feel this is a very rare entity. When these reports first came out several years ago, I added the *Trichophyton* test to my skin test panel. I find a positive skin test to this fungal antigen is rare and have yet to uncover a patient with severe asthma, positive skin tests and clinical fungal disease. However, in light of the beneficial response to antifungal therapy in the Virginia study, I intend to keep on looking.

## Magnesium Therapy

Magnesium, the fourth most abundant mineral in the body, regulates a series of enzymes systems critical to cellular metabolism. The exact mechanism by which magnesium exerts its effects is unknown, but studies suggest that it competes with calcium at the cellular level. Magnesium is a trace mineral found in leafy green vegetables, nuts, peas, beans and whole grain cereals.

The fact that magnesium had some bronchodilating properties was actually first discovered in 1912. In 1938, it was reported that magnesium reversed bronchoconstriction in guinea pig lungs, and shortly after, intravenous infusions of magnesium relieved bronchoconstriction in human subjects. Numerous follow-up studies have verified these early experiments, including some recent data showing that intravenous magnesium reverses severe asthma in adults and children who might have required mechanical ventilation.

In one study, researchers questioned 2633 adults about their diet and respiratory symptoms and tested their lung functions. Individuals who consumed the highest amounts of magnesium-containing foods had fewer bouts of wheezing from aeroallergens and better lung functions than those subjects who ate less magnesium-laden foods. Presently there is not enough scientific evidence to add a magnesium supplement to your diet, but eating liberal portions of leafy green vegetables, legumes and whole grain cereals makes good dietary sense.

One rather fascinating story on magnesium and asthma comes from the DMZ Rehabilitation Clinic located on the shores of the Dead Sea in Israel. The Dead Sea is a unique reservoir of minerals, and the content of its salt or brine is high in chlorides, bromides and minerals like magnesium. Apparently a microclimate is formed by high winds in this area that produce a mineral-rich haze that contains magnesium. It is believed that exposure to this microclimate is responsible for improvement in a variety of medical conditions. Researchers at this DMZ Clinic feel that patients with psoriasis, hypertension and asthma improve significantly when they are directly exposed to this climate. Such exposure includes topical application of the brine and mud from the Dead Sea.

In 1994, doctors at the DMZ Clinic observed that asthmatic patients attending the clinic for allergic skin diseases experienced less asthma and needed fewer asthma medications. This beneficial effect, that was documented by breathing tests and symptom scores, persisted for several months after their patients returned home. One possible explanation for their improvement was that they breathed air with a higher concentration of minerals, including magnesium. Ongoing research at this center and elsewhere may eventually shed more light on the role of magnesium therapy in asthma. At the present time there is not enough evidence to routinely recommend magnesium therapy in asthma.

## Futuristic Asthma Drugs

New asthma drugs have been slow in coming. Compared to the avalanche of new medications for heart disease, high blood pressure, gastrointestinal problems and migraine headaches, only one new class of asthma drugs, the leukotriene modifiers, has been approved for asthma in the past three decades. A variety of unique asthma drugs are under study. As there are approximately 150 million people in this world with asthma, the economic incentive for pharmaceutical companies to develop new asthma drugs is unlimited. Unfortunately, progress is painfully slow, as it takes several years and millions of dollars to bring a new drug to the marketplace.

Prior efforts to develop asthma drugs in the 1980s and 1990s focused on the endpoint of asthma—bronchial hyperreactivity and inflammation. Today, research is aimed at the beginning of the immune response, finding ways to block the immune system from traveling down the asthma-allergy highway. GlaxoSmithKline is developing a drug called Airflo to inhibit an asthma-inducing enzyme called phosphodiesterase. The mediators coming out of the T-cells are called interleukins. Immunex is studying an interleukin blocker called Nuance.

Other drugs in this class have entered early clinical trials. These drugs, called interleukin blockers, are probably several years away from FDA approval. As there may be 80 mediators involved in asthma, Doctor Peter Barnes thinks the next generation of asthma drugs will be one big anti-mediator pill that blocks several mediators. As I will discuss in the chapter dealing with immunotherapy, the final cure for asthma and other allergic disorders may lie in administering genetically derived vaccines to allergy-prone infants and young children.

## Anti-IgE Therapy

The IgE antibody is the immune protein that predisposes us to develop allergic diseases. The next new asthma-allergy drug that will be approved by the FDA is the IgE antibody-blocking drug, Xolair, which is expected on the market in 2002. Scientists have theorized that if you could shut down IgE production, you might cure asthma and other allergic disorders. Just a few years ago, this concept seemed to be nothing more than a dream. Now, thanks to enormous strides in immunology research, this dream has become reality.

Three major biotech drug companies, Novartis, Genentech and Tanox, are partnering to seek FDA approval for Xolair. This anti-IgE drug ties up circulating IgE antibody and prevents IgE from attaching itself to the mast cell. Preliminary studies in human volunteers at research centers in San Francisco and Denver found that IgE levels were reduced by 99 percent after receiving anti-IgE antibody intravenously or by injection. That's the good news. The bad news is that when the study subjects stopped taking the drug, IgE levels bounced back up to or above pretreatment levels. The rebound reaction is somewhat disturbing, as it looks like the drug will have to be taken at regular intervals on an indefinite basis for it to be effective.

This drug may help patients with allergic rhinitis. In one study Xolair and placebo injections were administered to 289 patients with allergic rhinitis once or twice a month for four months. Xolair-treated patients unresponsive to other therapies experienced a 45-percent reduction in symptoms. No adverse reactions occurred in the treated group. In two other asthma studies (1071 adolescents and adults and 334 children) the risk of hospitalization was reduced. Again no adverse reactions were noted. When approved, Xolair is most likely to be used in moderate to severe asthma. It may also find a niche in patients with severe allergic rhinitis. Another place for this drug might be to use it the first year patients are started on immunotherapy. Once immunotherapy injections start to take effect, the Xolair injections could be tapered or discontinued.

Are there any are potential drawbacks to this approach to the treatment of allergic disorders? First, as Xolair will be privately developed by biotech research companies (the drug will probably cost several hundred dollars per dose), managed care organizations will be very reluctant to approve it. Secondly, we must consider the following questions: Are we messing too much with Mother Nature? Remember that this IgE antibody once protected man from primitive parasitic diseases. Does IgE have any sort of a protective role in the twenty-first century?

One of the consequences of aging is that our immune system gets weaker as we get older. An aging immune system makes us more susceptible to all kinds of chronic and often fatal diseases. However, this winding down of the immune system is beneficial to many sufferers of asthma and hay fever, who become less allergic and less symptomatic with age. Yet, in my experience, many of my elderly patients do not always "outgrow" their hay fever or asthma, and they continue to have significant allergic-type symptoms well into their sixties and seventies. Over the past 30 years I have been very impressed by the overall good health of many of these "allergy-suffering senior citizens." They often look much younger than their stated age and frequently have no other medical problems other than hay fever or mild asthma. This observation, strictly a personal one, is not supported by scientific studies. Is it possible that IgE antibody may somehow protect some individuals from other non-allergic diseases by keeping their immune system in the high-speed lane? An overactive immune system may be fighting off other chronic diseases seen in the aging population, including cancer. One preliminary study found a lower incidence of lymphoma in individuals with higher IgE levels.

The other risk of shutting down the pro-allergic IgE-Th2 side of the immune system with an anti-IgE antibody is that you might push the immune system over to the non-allergic Th1 pathway. Excess stimulation of this Th1 pathway may lead to autoimmune diseases. This scenario has been observed in primates given other more advanced forms of an IgE suppressing antibody. Thus, before I endorse and prescribe a product that suppresses the allergic-IgE antibody, I would like to see studies that prove suppression of IgE antibody does not have any adverse effects on other parts of our protective immune system over the long term.

## Proceed with Caution

I prefer to take a yellow flag approach to all new drugs. In other words, I proceed with caution! Remember, most new drugs are tested on only 100 to 1,000 patients. More serious or rare side effects may not be seen until the drug has been used by thousands of patients. In the past, the FDA has been soundly criticized for taking too long to approve new drugs. Now the FDA may be acting too quickly. In 2000, the FDA review time for a new drug was down to 14 months, compared to 34 months in 1993. Paying a special FDA fee gets you a speedier process.

Since 1997, several new FDA-approved drugs have been removed from the market after they were found to cause serious injury and death. These drugs included the ulcer and reflux drug, Propulsid; the irritable bowel syndrome drug, Lotronex; and the diabetes drug Rezulin. The cholesterol-lowering drug, Baycol, was taken by 700,000 Americans before it was removed from the marketplace in 2001. Destruction of muscle cells resulted in kidney failure and 31 deaths in the United States and nine abroad. Baycol was the twelfth prescription drug to be removed since 1997. Remember that Seldane, one of the most popular antihistamines of all time, was available for several years and used in millions of patients before it was recognized that when it was taken with certain antibiotics or antifungal drugs it could trigger a serious and sometimes fatal cardiac heart rhythm.

# **Alternative**
## Therapy

**16**

The term alternative or complementary therapy refers to non-traditional medical treatments that have neither been approved nor shown to be effective in controlled studies by the established Western medical community. Alternative therapy includes treatments not subjected to the documentation of safety and efficacy through filing a New Drug Application (NDA) or an Abbreviated New Drug Application (ANDA) with the Food and Drug Administration (FDA).

Alternative or complementary products include, but are not limited to, phytopharmaceuticals (herbal agents), homeopathic remedies, nutraceuticals and anthroposophics. There is no financial incentive to test or study these products, as new drug applications are not needed. The 1994 United States Diet Supplement and Health Education Act (DSHEA) does not require proof of safety or efficacy by the FDA. The only way the FDA can remove an alternative medicine or herbal remedy is to prove that it is unsafe. This is in contrast to the United Kingdom, Germany and Canada, where these products are closely regulated by the government.

Over the past decade the popularity of alternative therapy has grown immensely. It is estimated that 40 percent of allergy and 10 to 20 percent of asthma sufferers in the United States now use some form of alternative medicine. In 1999, millions of American health-care consumers spent more than $12 billion on natural herbal supplements and $27 billion went to providers of alternative health care. The sales of alternative medicines increased 60 percent from 1990 to 1997. The number of homeopathic practitioners increased more than tenfold—from 200 in 1990 to 3,000 practitioners in 1998. More people now visit alternative medical practitioners than primary care physicians—600 million visits to alternative care providers versus 400 million encounters with primary care physicians. Nearly 2,000 global herbal products gross more than $20 billion a year.

When you look back on the history of pharmacological products in medicine, alternate drugs are not all that new. For example, the asthma drug cromolyn (Intal) was derived from Ammi visnaga, a Mediterranean plant used by Arabic physicians to treat intestinal colic 100 years ago. Theophylline was first extracted from tea leaves and coffee beans. The heart drug digitalis (digoxin) comes from the foxglove plant. Aspirin arose from the bark of the willow tree, and penicillin was discovered when a laboratory investigator accidentally found that penicillium-like molds were killing bacteria.

There are several reasons why alternative therapy is becoming more attractive. Alternative remedies offer a ray of hope for many patients confused by complicated drug programs. Patients justifiably fear traditional medicine and its outcome, as conventional prescription drugs cause 100,000 American deaths each year. Dissatisfied patients constantly surf the Internet to consult herbalists and seek alternative therapies. Up to 80 percent of patients who have undergone coronary artery bypass surgery use some form of alternative therapy. Courses in alternate therapy are now offered in medical schools and teaching hospitals. Most physicians, including me, have undoubtedly underestimated the potential benefits of alternative therapy. A United Kingdom study found that nearly six in every ten asthmatics were using alternative therapy, and the majority found it to be beneficial.

In 1991, the United States Congress responded to this explosion in alternative therapy by creating the Office of Alternative Medicine (OAM). In 1998, the NIH launched the National Center for Complementary and Alternative Therapy, which had a yearly budget of $100 million in 2000. Alternative therapies being investigated by the NIH include herbal remedies, nutritional supplements, acupuncture, hypnotherapy, relaxation techniques and chiropractic therapy. Some of the ongoing clinical trials are evaluating the use of St. John's Wort in depression, shark cartilage in lung cancer and the ginkgo herb in dementia. Of the 20,000 herbal supplements in the world, several recommended for additional study include Echinacea, Feverfew, Milk Thistle and Valerian. Echinacea, which is derived from the purple coneflower, is the most widely used product in Germany for prevention and treatment of the common cold. Its use is also increasing in the United States, where many believe that Echinacea is a mediator of immunity and benefits patients prone to frequent infections, fatigue or "low immunity."

The limited studies that have been done on alternative therapies have had mixed results. In one Yoga study, the combination of Yoga with cleansing techniques, vomiting, diarrhea and nasal throat irrigations increased lung functions and exercise capacity after two years of therapy. The results with acupuncture are mixed. In eight of thirteen trials the benefit was quite small. Buteyko Breathing Techniques showed no change in lung functions, but improved quality of life was noted. In 1998, 36 children who underwent massage therapy had a better attitude toward their asthma. When hypnosis was combined with relaxation exercises, study patients used fewer asthma drugs and had more symptom-free days.

## Herbalism

The development of modern-day herbal remedies is based on the philosophies and beliefs of ethnic groups derived from ancient Greek, Roman, Arabic and Chinese cultures. The basic components of herbal remedies are botanical products derived from natural plant life. Herbs are any part of a plant, including the leaf, flower, root, stem, fruit or bark, used to make a medicine, fragrance or food flavoring. Herbal medicines are touted as a safer and more natural approach to health care. Herbal supplements are packaged in teas, powders, tablets, liquids and capsules. Proponents of herbal medicine believe herbs contain naturally occurring chemicals with potent biologic and immunological activity.

The traditional Chinese medicine branch of herbalism relies on maintaining a balance between two forces, the yin and the yang, and the five major elements of fire, earth, water, metal and wood. Many Chinese asthma herbs are derived from *Ma huang,* the herb extracted from the *ephedra* bush. Chinese physicians or healers have used *Ma huang* for more than 4,000 years to treat asthma. The study of *Ma huang* led to the development of a western drug called ephedrine, a major ingredient of early asthma medicines in the twentieth century. Other popular herbal remedies include *Ginko biloba,* believed to improve memory and thinking ability. *Ginko* is the number-one herbal remedy used by older people. St. John's Wort is widely used by people with mood disorders. Glucosamine and chondroitin sulfate are popular alternative treatments for joint pain and arthritis. Some of the more common medical conditions for which people turn to alternative therapies include low back pain, allergies and asthma.

Commonly used herbs in asthma include *Ginko biloba* and *Atropa belladonna,* or deadly nightshade, where the primary ingredient is atropine, the basic ingredient of asthma cigars and cigarettes. *Licorice root* is a favorite of Chinese practitioners who recommend it as a cough suppressant to control coughing and wheezing. *Saikoku-to,* a popular herbal remedy in Japan, reportedly allows some asthmatic patients to reduce their doses of oral cortisone by prolonging the action of cortisone. *Tylorphorsa indica* has been used in India to treat asthma and bronchitis. Another Indian herb touted as a possible bronchodilator is *Coleus forskohli.*

Herbal research is in its infancy. Only 5,000 of the world's 500,000 plants have been studied. While the majority of herbal papers are written in Chinese or Japanese, millions of Americans with allergies and asthma utilize these unproven products. The typical herbal user is a well-educated, middle-aged Caucasian with a higher income. In other words, baby boomers are into herbal medicine big time. The effectiveness of some herbal products in asthma has been studied in China and Japan. Some of the more popular herbal preparations subjected to analysis include *Ma huang,* Minor Blue Dragon, Chai Ge Jie Ji Wan, Ginko biloba, ginseng and licorice root. Other asthma studies include the use of tea made with black pepper and cinnamon, doses of carbo-vegetables (vegetable charcoal), Ipecacuanha (ipecac) and juice therapy with onion and parsley juice.

Perhaps the most exciting study in herbal medicine and asthma to date was performed in mice. A recent article in the *Journal of Allergy and Clinical Immunology* reported on the use of a Chinese herbal formula used by traditional Chinese medicine practitioners to treat asthma. Using a mouse-asthma model, the investigators found very significant evidence for an anti-inflammatory and anti-asthma effect that was comparable to a cortisone drug. This herbal product, which contains 14 different herbal extracts, is currently under study. While a mouse is not a man, this promising study did show that herbal preparations may have potent anti-inflammatory properties.

## Herbal Side Effects

Presently there are no standards in the United States governing quality or strength of herbal products. The United States lags far behind European countries like Germany, where herbal products are classified as drugs. It has been suggested that the FDA classify herbal products as OTC medications. This would require manufacturers to provide proof of safety and effectiveness. There are several obstacles in the way of controlling herbal products. Isolation of the active ingredients in these plants is a very difficult and expensive process.

Many herbs will never be investigated, as the cost of bringing a new product to the marketplace approaches $500 million. Even if such a product were developed, it would not be protected by patent rights. The general public suffers under the misconception that all plant products are safe. Since they have a decided pharmacological action, it is wise to use herbal treatments only under the care of a qualified naturopath or herbalist, to avoid the common side effects listed below.

- Many herbs contain alkaloids that can damage the liver.

- *Ma huang* causes insomnia, tremors, urinary retention and irregular heartbeats.

- Lobeline can cause paralysis, coma and death.

- Sweet root contains oil of calamus, a potent carcinogen.

- Mandrake when misused can be a poisonous narcotic.

- Chamomile tea cross-reacts with ragweed and can cause allergic reactions in ragweed-sensitive patients.

- Overdoses of *Lobelia* have been linked to respiratory paralysis, fainting episodes and psychological problems.

- Sassafras, or "spring tonic," has been linked to cancer in lab animals.

- Many herbs contain the heavy metals, including arsenic, lead and mercury. Echinacea may cause allergic reactions in people sensitive to flowers of the daisy family, and aggravate diseases like lupus, tuberculosis and multiple sclerosis.

- St. John's Wort affects the action of the clotting drug Warfarin and the AIDS drug Crixivan.

- Licorice and grapefruit juice can interfere with steroids and cancer drugs.

- Valerian and kava kava interact with anesthetics during surgery.

- A higher risk of cancer has been reported with aloe, rhubarb (colon cancer) and capsaicin (gastric cancer).

- Ginko biloba may cause excessive bleeding during surgical procedures.

One disaster at a Belgian weight loss clinic involved the use of appetite suppressants and Chinese herbs. After the Belgian clinic made a switch to a toxic herb, nearly a hundred patients suffered kidney failure and several patients died. Fortunately, the FDA is becoming somewhat more proactive in regulating herbal products. They recently ordered an allergy-fighting compound called AllerRelief pulled off the shelves of health food stores. This herb contains the toxin aristolochic acid, the substance that triggered the outbreak of kidney problems and bladder cancer in the Belgian weight loss clinic. In the summer of 2000, the FDA seized cargo shipments from China suspected of carrying worrisome herbs. It also warned the herbal industry to police itself and sent a letter to practicing physicians urging a closer look at the use of herbal medicines by their patients.

Presently there are too many unanswered questions regarding the rate of absorption in the body, dosages and contaminants. All users of herbal products should buy reliable brands and monitor publications dealing with the potential side effects and drug interactions of herbal medicines. Reliable sources for such information include *Consumer Reports*, NIH publications, Medline, and *Prevention Magazine.* Patients and providers should report all significant adverse reactions to herbal products to the FDA at http://www.fda.gov/medwatch/report/consumer/consumer.htm

## Summary

Many health-care providers have been too bewildered to learn about alternative herbal products. There are nearly 2,000 herbal products currently available in the United States. Much of the care in this area is self-experimentation, where patients are more willing to rely on an unregulated herbal remedy than take an asthma drug. There is a growing need for educational efforts in the field of herbal medicine that will allow physicians to partner with their patients and make informed choices.

In the past I dismissed alternative care or complementary medicine as unproven and unscientific. I simply told my patients they were wasting their time and money. Now I have changed my approach to this issue. I try not to be judgmental, and work closely with alternative care practitioners. I warn patients about toxic or unsafe alternative medications or practices. A recent article in *Consumer Reports* noted that conventionally trained doctors were learning to be more sympathetic and less scornful. However, when one looks at the potential side effects of herbal products and assesses the fact that most studies of herbal remedies in asthma and allergic disorders are poorly controlled and done in only a few patients, at the present time I cannot endorse or recommend any herbal medicine as a form of alternative care in the treatment of asthma or allergic disorders.

For additional information and reading materials I recommend Natural Medicines Comprehensive Database, 3120 W. March Lane, PO Box 8190, Stockton, CA 95208; Tel: 209-472-2244; Fax: 209-472-2249; www.NaturalDatabase.com. This database, maintained by 21 full-time research staff, contains 1600 entries with literature reviews for effectiveness and safety as well as mechanisms of action. Additional Web sites can be accessed via the Internet. Directory Galaxy.com lists the top 10 places on the Internet for alternative health-care information.

## *Dietary and Vitamin Therapy*

Presently, there is no solid data on dietary therapy and asthma. In general, short-term dietary treatments have relatively little effect in chronic diseases like asthma. While many beverages and foodstuffs trigger asthma, few if any dietary substances appear to benefit asthma. Omega-3 fatty acids, found in fish such as salmon, tuna and mackerel, may help asthma sufferers by decreasing the production of leukotrienes. A few studies suggest that individuals who consume large quantities of fish oil have a lower threshold for developing chronic lung diseases like asthma, bronchitis and emphysema.

Additional studies are needed to look at the effects of maternal diet during pregnancy and in early infancy. Some researchers feel that exposure to antioxidants and omega-3 fatty acids in a developing fetus or newborn infant may reprogram the immune system and prevent the development of immune-mediated diseases like asthma.

The antioxidant vitamins, such as vitamin A (beta carotene), vitamin C (ascorbic acid), vitamin E (alpha-tocopherol) and vitamin B6 (pyridoxine) are our first line of defense against tissue injury and theoretically might benefit asthma sufferers. No specific studies have examined the role of vitamin A in asthma. Two studies with vitamin C examined the intake of fresh fruit and vegetables. In one study, children who never ate fresh fruit had a 25-percent greater chance of wheezing than those who ate one serving of fresh fruit a day. Similar results have been reported in adults. In another small study vitamin C was found to minimize exercise-induced asthma. vitamin E, found in vegetable oils, protects the lung against oxidant injury in animals.

One study in 77,866 nurses that examined vitamin E intake in adult-onset asthma found a 50-percent reduction in asthma in women with the highest vitamin E intake. Vitamin B6 is found in cereals, bread, whole grains, liver, spinach, bananas, fish, poultry, meats, nuts, potatoes, green leafy vegetables and avocadoes. A study utilizing a case-controlled design found that asthmatics had lower levels of vitamin B6 compared to normal controls. While there is no solid data to support the use of specific vitamins in asthma, taking a daily multivitamin can't hurt.

## Acupuncture

Ancient Chinese acupuncture involves inserting fine needles into various points on the body to restore the balance of energy flow throughout the body. While acupuncture has been widely used in China for asthma, the rise in popularity of acupuncture therapy for asthma in Western societies is not supported by clinical studies. One extensive review of acupuncture in asthma concluded that any possible benefit was mild at best. Anyone contemplating acupuncture should be sure their acupuncturist is certified by the National Certification Commission for Acupuncture and Oriental Medicine. Serious side effects are rare when acupuncture is performed by trained, certified professionals. Additional therapies from Eastern cultures that have been tried in asthma include massage therapy and shiatsu, a form of therapeutic practice also known as zone therapy or reflexology.

## Yoga

Exercise, meditation, and control of body functions have played important roles in medical practice and religion, especially in India. Breathing exercises and ritualistic chanting is often used as a means to aid meditative-self hypnotism, attain relaxation and decrease energy use. Such techniques are thought to benefit asthma, perhaps by reducing airway reactivity. Meditation may also lower oxygen consumption. Tantric yoga is a combination of cosmic or religious meditation and slow deep breathing to improve the distribution of energy flow through the body. Such practices are alleged to provide serenity and reduce fatigue. The Chinese have developed many forms of ritualized exercise, both for individual and group practice. The most popular of these practices is tai chi, where slow rhythmic body movements are associated with deliberate breathing.

## Homeopathy

Homeopathy is a 200-year-old system of medicine in which diseases are treated with diluted extracts of biological or plant extracts. Homeopathy is the most popular form of alternative therapy in France, where it is used by more than a third of the population.

Homeopathy is also increasing in popularity in Germany and the United Kingdom. It is estimated that more than a $1 billion a year is spent in Europe on homeopathic medications. In Britain, nearly one-third of general practitioners prescribe homeopathic remedies. The credibility of homeopathic medicine was given a boost by a report published in *Nature* in 1988. This paper from Paris demonstrated that homeopathic remedies lowered allergic or anti-IgE antibodies. A recent study randomized two groups of asthma patients. One group received an oral homeopathic preparation of a standard allergen and other patients received a placebo. All patients were allowed to take their usual medications. After four weeks symptom scores, pulmonary function tests and bronchial responses to histamine showed significant improvement in the treated group compared with the placebo. This is too small a study to hang your hat on, and additional data is needed before endorsing homeopathic therapy.

## Osteopathy

Andrew Still introduced osteopathy, a form of bone setting, in 1876. Still believed that most diseases could be improved by manipulating the joints and spinal column. Appropriate correction of immobilized joints allowed neuroendocrine function to be restored, thereby facilitating the improvement of physiologic disorders. In asthma, some osteopaths believe there may be an abnormality in the thoracic vertebrae and associated ribs. While manipulation of these joints can be of value in neuromuscular problems, there is no scientific evidence of direct benefit in asthma.

## Chiropractic Manipulation

In 1895, Daniel David Palmer introduced chiropractic care by claiming that many diseases could be managed by spinal manipulation. Classic chiropractic theory states that vigorous manipulation with the hands or mechanical devices readjusts the spinal column, removes nerve interference or spinal stress, and alleviates the symptoms of many chronic conditions including asthma. Current practice differs considerably from Palmer's original teachings. Chiropractic therapy has evolved into a holistic, nondrug-oriented form of care. Chiropractors often prescribe elaborate elimination diets with vitamin, mineral and antioxidant supplements to complement their use of massage and manipulation. Colon cleansing, heat and cold therapy, and other approaches alleged to remove toxins from the body are also popular. Specific chiropractic spinal manipulative therapy for asthma was recently reported to be no more effective than sham manipulation.

While there is no doubt that chiropractic therapy can help back pain, there is no evidence that spinal manipulation is of any benefit in asthma. In 1998, a study published in the *New England Journal of Medicine* compared active and simulated chiropractic manipulation in 91 children with active asthma. All children received four months of chiropractic treatment consisting of active or sham spinal manipulation. No difference in asthma symptoms or pulmonary functions was found in either group. The *New England Journal of Medicine* editorial on this article stated, "it is currently not appropriate to consider chiropractic therapy as a broad-based alternative to medical care for non-musculoskeletal conditions."

## Controversial Allergy Therapy

All new drugs and procedures should be well studied in animals and humans to determine if they are safe and effective before being approved for general use. During clinical trials, a new drug or experimental procedure is administered to patients who have given their informed consent. The FDA and national or local institutional review boards (IRBs) must approve these clinical trials. Unfortunately, these strict guidelines only apply to new drugs and medical procedures. Many older and outmoded controversial techniques have not been subjected to these stringent regulations. As a result, thousands of allergy and asthma sufferers are unknowingly victimized by unproven and controversial medical treatments.

Most medical and surgical specialists rely heavily on hospital support to practice medicine. When a doctor is judged to be incompetent or engages in unethical or questionable practices, the hospital can censure the offender or even suspend the doctor's hospital privileges. Regrettably, there are no such controls for some specialists or self-proclaimed allergists operating out of their private

223

offices or clinics. The FDA and most state medical societies do not regulate medical practice in a private office setting unless the doctor is negligent or prescribes dangerous drugs. The most common controversial techniques are cytotoxic testing, the provocation-neutralization technique, the Yeast Syndrome and clinical ecology.

## Cytotoxic Testing

In cytotoxic testing, a sample of your blood, specifically your white blood cells, is mixed with antigens to determine if you are sensitive to a specific allergen. Cytotoxic testing is quite different from the RAST test that is based on the presence of allergic IgE antibodies in your blood. Outstanding scientists have shown that there is no difference between the reactions seen in the white blood cells of allergic and non-allergic patients. There is no scientific basis to the cytotoxic test, branded as ineffective by the FDA. Federal Medicare and several states have permanently banned cytotoxic testing.

## Provocation-Neutralization Technique

This technique is supposed to provoke and thereby neutralize one's allergy. After the suspected allergen is ingested or injected, the doctor waits for symptoms to develop. If no symptoms occur, progressively stronger doses of the extract are given. When symptoms occur, a weaker dose is given to neutralize the reaction. If this dose is ineffective, stronger doses are injected until a full strength or a neutralizing dose is found. Patients are then given bottles containing the allergen and told to place drops under their tongue at regular intervals. This is called the sublingual method. Several controlled studies have concluded that this technique is ineffective. The United States Health Care Financing Administration (HCFA) has stated that the provocation-neutralization technique has no scientific evidence of effectiveness.

## The Yeast Syndrome

Another erroneous allergy school of thought that persists is the Yeast Syndrome. This syndrome, popularized by Doctors C. Truss and William Crook, preaches that an overabundance of the yeast germ

*Candida albicans* is responsible for many ailments, including fatigue, depression, hyperactivity, headache, skin problems and respiratory conditions. In his book, *The Yeast Connection,* Doctor Cook states that this is a common disorder which can only be verified by a favorable response to treatment over a period of time. "Yeast doctors" believe that high-carbohydrate diets, antibiotics, birth control pills and other drugs cause an overgrowth of yeast that weakens our immune system. Such a weakened immune system is more likely to react to foods, inhalants, odors and the chemicals in our environment.

Yeast treatment programs are designed to decrease the growth of yeast with special diets, anti-yeast drugs like Nystatin, yeast injections and placing yeast drops under the tongue. The American Academy of Allergy, Asthma & Immunology has stated, *"The concept is speculative and unproven...the basic elements of this syndrome would apply to almost all sick patients at some time. There is no published proof that yeast is responsible for this syndrome. Elements of the proposed treatment program are potentially dangerous."*

## The Clinical Ecologist

One group of doctors who use many of these controversial methods call themselves clinical ecologists. They practice clinical ecology, a school of thought that ascribes numerous ailments and symptoms to foods and chemicals in our environment. Patients are told that they are environmentally ill or hypersensitive to foods, odors, chemicals and pollutants in their environment. Clinical ecologists believe diverse conditions such as arthritis, alcoholism, depression, headaches, and learning disabilities are due to ecological allergies.

Clinical ecologists feel that traditional treatments are too restrictive. They impose strict diets and environmental controls that require major alterations in life-style. Home and working environments are altered to create safe rooms to avoid pollutants and common household chemicals. When avoidance is impossible, they utilize the neutralization-provocation and under-the-tongue techniques. The most incredible example of ecological treatment I have ever seen was in a young six-month-old infant whose mother was told to put diluted drops of kerosene under her child's tongue to control an allergy to automobile exhaust fumes. While the concept that our environment is responsible for a multitude of health problems is appealing, there is no scientific evidence to support the claims of the clinical ecologists. One of the benefits of the recent changes in the delivery of health care is that most insurers and managed care organizations no longer reimburse clinical ecologists for their controversial and unproven techniques.

# **Environmental**
## Controls

# **17**

O ne of the first doctors to associate environmental exposures with lung disease was the German doctor Georgius Agricola, who reported occupational pulmonary disease in miners caused by coal dust in the sixteenth century. The famous Italian physician, Gerolamo Cardano, went one step further when he inadvertently used environmental controls to treat John Hamilton, the Archbishop of St. Andrews.

In the seventeenth century Flemish physician Jan Baptista van Helmont, an asthma sufferer himself, realized that symptoms could be caused by inhalation of airborne dust. The most influential text on asthma from the nineteenth century was Henry Salter's book, *On Asthma: Its Pathology and Treatment,* in which Salter wrote that asthma attacks could be initiated by *"stroking a cat, sleeping on a feather pillow or passing a poultry shop."* In the nineteenth century Sir Charles Blackley, yet another allergy sufferer, stated, *"I have shown that the peculiar and distinctive action of pollen is seen in the oedema [swelling] which is produced in the cellular tissue of any part to which it is applied."*

In chapter seven I reviewed the common aeroallergens that trigger asthma. This chapter will review ways to control your environment and minimize or eliminate exposure to asthma-allergy triggers, including aeroallergens. In my opinion the most neglected area in asthma and allergy therapy is environmental control. When simple steps are taken to eliminate common irritants and allergens from one's environment, dramatic improvement and even clinical remission is a distinct possibility. Unlike medication programs, which are costly and may cause serious side effects, environmental controls can be put into place without risk, family disruption or major medical expense. Many of the more dramatic improvements in my patients with asthma are not due to drug therapy but are the result of employing effective environmental control programs.

## *Dust Mite Control*

Numerous studies have proved the value of creating a dust-mite-free bedroom. In a classic British study, nine dust-mite-allergic asthmatics moved into a hospital room where they carried on with their normal daily activities and took their usual asthma medicines. After sleeping in the hospital room for a few nights, all nine subjects were less symptomatic, took less asthma medications and showed improvement in their breathing tests. Doctor Andrew Murray studied two groups of children with allergic asthma in Vancouver, Canada. One group did not make any changes in their environment, while the second group instituted strict environmental dust mite controls. After one month, children who slept in the relatively dust-free bedrooms had far less wheezing and used less asthma medications than children who made no changes in their bedroom environment.

A study in schoolchildren in Los Alamos, New Mexico, a town located at high altitude in a dry climate, highlights the risk factors of cat and dog allergen. This Los Alamos study looked at the prevalence of asthma, allergy and exposure to indoor allergens. While the mite and cockroach allergen levels were very low in this dry climate, nearly four in every five homes housed a dog or cat. The strongest risk factor for asthma was cat allergen.

In temperate and subtropical climates there is a seasonal variation in dust mite levels, with some areas showing a substantial rise in mite populations in the autumn. In many areas this pattern of mite proliferation directly coincides with seasonal increases in asthma relapses and asthma hospitalizations. In 1985, I reviewed the patterns of emergency room visits and asthma admissions to the North Shore Children's Hospital in Salem, Massachusetts. There were two distinct peaks in asthma admissions. Following a period of few admissions (one to two a month) in July and August, admissions increased in September and October and peaked in November. In

December, admissions started to decline to another low point in the cold winter months of January and February. Admissions rose again in March and April, with a smaller secondary peak in May before they fell off again in June. This pattern of asthma relapses and hospital admissions coincides with the experiences of other hospitals and asthma specialists in the Midwest and northeastern United States.

Dust-mite-allergic asthmatics should focus on their bedroom and family room—the two most frequently inhabited areas of the home. A typical child spends 80 percent of his or her in-home time in the bedroom. An adult who averages eight hours sleep a night will spend one-third of their life in a bedroom environment. The illustration on the following page graphically depicts the ideal house-dust-mite-free bedroom that should be simply furnished and easy to clean. You should focus on two areas—the bedding and the carpeting. Pillows, mattresses, box springs and comforters should be enclosed in zippered airtight mite-proof covers. Avoid cheaper plastic covers, which are hot and sticky in the summer and cold and clammy in the winter. Comfortable, well-designed, durable, synthetic covers can be obtained from local department stores and allergy retail stores. The mail-order houses specializing in allergy-free products usually have the best prices and quality product lines. New products are lightweight and feel like linen. They are soft, easy to wash and come in several colors.

Down or feather pillows, a favorite breeding ground for mites, should be replaced with dacron or polyester pillows and covered with a mite-proof cover. The best blanket is a washable cotton or synthetic blanket. All bedding, including sheets, should be hot-cycled at 140 degrees F at least twice a month. Avoid electric blankets that keep the dust mites cozy and warm. The most important factor controlling dust mite growth is humidity.

Keep home humidity levels under 50 percent with dehumidifiers or air conditioners. Super-tight homes should be well ventilated, and kitchen exhaust fans should be installed. Whenever possible, homes in warmer humid climates should utilize central air conditioning to reduce dust mite and mold growth. Additional steps include covering heating or air conditioning vents with filters, keeping closet doors closed and avoiding heavy drapes in the windows.

# The Allergy-Free Bedroom

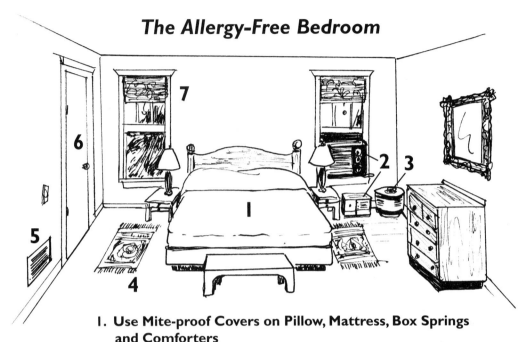

1. **Use Mite-proof Covers on Pillow, Mattress, Box Springs and Comforters**
2. **Air Condition and Dehumidify to 50% or Less Humidity**
3. **Use a HEPA Air Purifier**
4. **Remove Carpets, Use Washable Throw Rugs**
5. **Cover Vents with Filters**
6. **Keep Closet Door Closed**
7. **Avoid Heavy Window Drapes**

The second most mite-laden area of the home is in the rugs or carpets. The ideal bedroom or family room flooring is a wood or vinyl floor with washable area rugs. The next step is to consider replacing carpets with a wood or vinyl floor. When carpeting cannot be replaced, commercial carpet cleaners or mite-killing chemicals, called acaricides, can be applied to the carpets once or twice a year. One acaricide, called Acarosan, has been marketed in the United States. Another effective anti-mite spray is Allergy Control Solution, sold by Allergy Control Products. You cannot remove mites from a carpet by compulsive vacuuming, as mites burrow deep into the carpet and hold on fast with the little sucking pads on the ends of their legs. Normal steam cleaning is likewise an ineffective way to kill mites. One new method that combines active heat and steam treatments by delivering hot air and steam to mattresses, carpets and furniture reduced mite levels and bronchial hyperreactivity in asthmatic patients. In summary, I believe covering bedding and carpet removal to be the two most important steps in dust mite environmental control. Carpets in schools and public buildings may be another area for exposure to dust mites and animal allergens. Over the past 30 years, polished flooring has been replaced by carpets that are easier to maintain and reduce noise. Such carpets contain irritants and serve as host sites for allergens. Most schools do not have the money needed to clean carpets properly.

## Cockroach Allergen Control

Over the past three decades, asthma specialists have become aware that cockroaches play a very important role in asthma. Sensitization to cockroach allergen is common in older inner-city apartments and homes. Cockroaches have been reported to trigger asthma in many parts of the world, including Southeast Asia, Central America, India, South Africa and most recently Europe. Cockroach sensitization is not confined to inner-city populations. It occurs wherever substandard housing or older apartment buildings or homes sustain cockroach infestation.

Inner-city asthmatics have a much higher incidence of cockroach allergy. In some urban asthma clinics, one in every four asthmatics is allergic to cockroaches. There is also an increased risk for cockroach exposure in public buildings like supermarkets, grocery stores, restaurants, department stores and movie theaters. A cockroach allergy skin test is available, but telling people that they have an allergy to cockroaches can be a touchy situation. In my practice cockroach allergen is labeled "household insects" on our skin test panel. A positive cockroach test does not mean that you have cockroaches in your home. The skin test may remain positive years after exposure to cockroaches. I have seen several patients with a positive skin test due to past exposure to urban apartments in their student days or when they lived in semitropical or tropical climates. When the cockroach test is positive and there is no history of prior exposure, I tell the patient or family they may have a cockroach problem and to call their local exterminator, as cockroach removal often requires vigorous extermination procedures.

There is no sure-fire method for cockroach allergen control. Typical measures include removing food sources, setting bait traps and using insecticide sprays. Removing carpets from the bedroom may be helpful, as a study in Los Angeles found high skin-test reactivity to cockroach when a carpet was present in the bedroom. It is reasonable to assume that decreasing the population of living cockroaches will decrease the amount of cockroach allergen in the house. It is not known what length of time cockroach allergen persists, as a dead cockroach is still an allergenic cockroach.

In Baltimore, Maryland, infested dwellings underwent professional cleaning, vacuuming and cleaning of the kitchen plus application of the insecticide, ambacetin gel, to the kitchen and the rest of the home. Allergen was reduced by 80 to 90 percent in this eight-month study. Complete eradication was not achieved, as cockroach allergen levels still remained above the risk level in most homes. The difficulty of cockroach removal is probably due to the insect's ability to hide in difficult-to-reach places, like small cracks in walls or under appliances. Allergy injections with cockroach allergy is still in its infancy. No specific cockroach allergen has been proven to be effective in immunotherapy.

## *Mold Allergen Control*

In many damper climates it is virtually impossible to avoid outdoor molds. Many mold-allergic asthmatics do well in dry desert or high-altitude climates. When given a choice, I advise my mold-sensitive patients to vacation or retire in Arizona, not Florida. Mold likes it hot and sticky. Therefore, the key to indoor mold control is controlling temperature and humidity levels. Use a humidity gauge to monitor humidity levels throughout the home. Use air conditioners and dehumidifiers throughout the home where humidity levels are over 50 percent. Good ventilation with exhaust fans prevents mold buildup in books, bedding, kitchens, damp bathrooms, basements and laundry rooms. Avoid carpeting in bedrooms and damp basements. Keep bathroom tubs, tiles and shower curtains mold-free. Excess use of vaporizers or home humidifiers promotes mold growth within the home. Avid gardeners should avoid freshly cut grass, mulch piles, and raking leaves. Mold-inhibiting chemicals can

# *Mold Allergen Control*

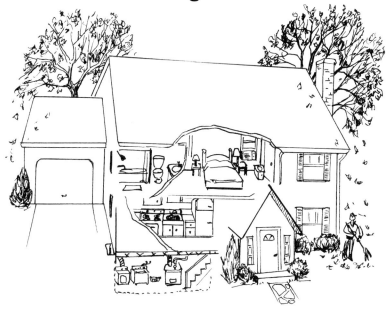

1. **Use a Humidity Gauge to Monitor Humidity Levels**
2. **Use Dehumidifers and Air Conditioners to Keep Humidity Under 50%**
3. **Use Exhaust Fans in Kitchen, Laundry Rooms and Basements**
4. **Avoid Carpets in Basements and Bedrooms**
5. **Keep Bathroom Tubs and Tiles Mold-Free**
6. **Avoid Excess Use of Humidifiers**
7. **Avoid Cut Grass, Raking Leaves or Mulch Piles**

be sprayed in areas where there is an excess build-up of molds, and mold-inhibiting paints can be applied to walls or ceilings. Molds are found in many foods. However, I feel the threat of mold reactions from foods is vastly overrated. Common foods that grow molds include cheese, particularly aged cheese; homemade wine; pickled foods; dried fruits; mushrooms and leftover bread. If these foods induce asthma symptoms, they should be avoided. Once you discover indoor mold growing in your home the following steps should be taken:

- Clean with a bleach or anti-mold solution.

- Repair leaky roofs and remove mold sources such as damp carpets and moldy shower curtains.

- Dry out damp areas with air conditioners, exhaust fans and dehumidifiers.

- Avoid carpeting on slab foundations or damp basement floors.

- Live and play above ground. Whenever possible, mold- (and house-dust-mite) sensitive patients should avoid sleeping in basement or cellar level family rooms or bedrooms.

- Ventilate damp rooms and crawl spaces under the house.

- HEPA air filters will help reduce the number of mold spores.

## Stachybotrys Mold

One newly rediscovered mold that bears watching is the *Stachybotrys* mold. This mold was first identified in 1931 in the Ukraine following an epidemic of a deadly immune disease in horses. This mold is found in water-damaged buildings with high humidity. *Stachybotrys* is a slow-growing black mold that flourishes on materials with high amounts of cellulose, like wood, dry walls, plaster board and ceiling tiles. It will not grow on bathroom tiles, concrete or food. What makes this mold especially dangerous is that it produces a toxin that can cause a fatal bleeding lung disorder in infants. An outbreak of *Stachybotrys* disease in Northern Ohio followed severe flooding in the spring of 1994. Dozens of cases of lung disease were reported in infants, a few of whom died.

In 1998, the American Academy of Pediatrics issued a policy statement that severe water damage and mold growth poses a risk for infants, and they recommended prompt cleaning (within 24 hours) of any water damage inside a home. This policy statement recommended removing any saturated cardboard, dry wall or paper products, which could serve as a food source for the deadly *Stachybotrys* mold.

## Animal Allergens

One of the more frustrating aspects in educating patients and their families about environmental control revolves around animals and household pets. All-too-familiar statements from my pet-allergic patients and families are, "Our children would rather get rid of me than our family dog, and our cat is part of the family." Such responses is understandable when you consider the strong relationship of love and companionship that develops between man and animals. Animals, like dogs, may be needed for security purposes. The emotional benefits of owning a pet may have to be weighed against their capability to induce asthma or allergic rhinitis. Dogs and cats are the most frequent offenders, but any furry or feathered animal, including gerbils, guinea pigs, hamsters, birds, rats and rabbits, can trigger asthma. Once you become allergic to any one species of animal, you are quite likely to develop an allergy to other furry or feathered animals when given the proper exposure.

Many allergists insist on animal removal. Some hard-liners refuse to treat patients who do not comply with their orders to remove offending pets from the home. When allergic animal owners are unwilling to give up their pets, a compromise may be necessary. Limited exposure may be an acceptable approach, and avoidance of the animal should be considered.

- Keep the animal outside the home or out of bedrooms.

- Routine grooming is essential.

- Treat a pet's skin conditions aggressively.

- Maintain wood floors and leather or vinyl furnishings.

- Wash your hands immediately after touching an animal.

- Reduce carpeted surfaces in the home by using hardwood or vinyl floors with washable scatter rugs.

## Dog Allergen Control

Dog allergen behaves much like cat allergen in that it is easily airborne without disturbing the indoor air. This is in contrast to exposure to dust mite or cockroach allergens, that only become airborne after vigorous air disturbance and exposure predominantly occurs overnight during sleep. Many mite or cockroach-allergic patients cannot identify allergen exposure and tie it to their symptoms, although many are worse in the morning. Dog and cat-allergic individuals, on the other hand, begin to sneeze and wheeze immediately after entering a home where these animals reside.

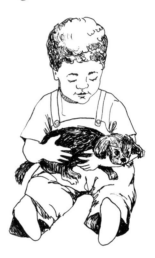

There is some encouraging news for dog lovers and families unwilling to part with their dogs. No one covets their dogs as much as the British people, who reside in a country with an estimated seven million dogs. I have had the opportunity to golf in England on several occasions, and some days there are more well-behaved dogs than golfers on the links. In 1999, a study in England measured dog allergen levels in homes before and after dogs were washed and shampooed twice weekly. Significant reductions in airborne allergen and reduced amounts of allergen in the dog's clippings were found. No effect was noted when the dogs were vacuumed. This survey concluded that you should wash your dog at least twice a week, as allergen levels increased just three days after washing.

Another way to minimize exposure to dog allergen is to confine the dog and keep it out of the bedroom and family room. Factors that increase dander production or cause excess shedding of hair or skin should be controlled. Dogs with common skin conditions like fleas and seborrhea that lead to excess dander production and dry skin will require special attention from their owner or veterinarian.

Routine grooming procedures should be performed outdoors, preferably by a non-allergic family member. Commercial hypoallergenic cleansers and dog shampoos have not been shown to reduce allergen levels.

## Cat Allergen Control

Cat ownership is associated with a high incidence of asthma. Cat allergy is more common than dog allergy, even though more homes house dogs than cats. This may be due to the fact that cat allergen is more widely dispersed in our society. Cat allergen is a very small, sticky, invisible particle that is carried about on the clothing of cat owners to all kinds of places, including churches, schools and other public buildings. The difference in the asthma prevalence rate between New Zealand and Sweden is interesting. New Zealand has one of the world's highest rates of asthma—16 out of every 100 citizens have asthma. Sweden has one of the lowest rates of asthma—only four in every 100 people. Sixty-three percent of all New Zealand homes have cats, while only 23 percent of Swedish homes house cats.

Reducing cat allergen in a home where cats reside is a daunting task. It has been estimated that an average cat that carries 60 to 130 milligrams of cat allergen on its coat can spread 100 milligrams of allergen on a carpet every day. This explains why you may not see any reduction in cat allergen levels months after a cat has been removed from a home if carpets are left in place. Therefore, whenever possible, carpet removal or extensive carpet cleaning is essential when a cat is removed from the home or a cat-allergic asthmatic moves into a dwelling previously occupied by a cat.

In contrast to mite allergens, high efficiency particulate air filters (HEPA) reduce levels of cat and dog allergen by 70 percent in rooms with polished flooring. In contrast, only a 30 percent reduction is achieved in carpeted rooms. Frequent vacuuming is somewhat helpful as long as the vacuum is equipped with a HEPA exhaust filter or double-thickness bag. The efficacy of treating carpets with tannic acid solutions is questionable at low allergen levels, and almost certainly useless at high allergen levels.

Controlling the source of cat allergen remains difficult. Cat allergen is produced in the salivary and sebaceous glands and is also found in the voided urine of cats. Studies from Johns Hopkins University Asthma Center and the University of Virginia have produced both good and bad news for cat lovers. The bad news is that when a cat is removed from the home, it may take weeks or several months to rid the home of cat allergen. Homes with carpeted floors accumulate cat allergen 100 times faster than homes with polished floors. The good news is that weekly washing of the cat with soap and water or plain water dramatically reduces levels of cat allergen in the home. Studies at the University of Virginia show that washing the cat on a weekly basis, removing carpets and upholstered furniture, using HEPA air purifying devices, vacuuming and regular cleaning significantly lowers cat allergen levels. Surprisingly, one recent study found that the color of cats may be important. People with dark-colored cats were two to four times more likely to have cat allergy symptoms.

One other common type of animal sensitivity is horse allergy. Avoidance is the easiest solution for most horsehair-allergic patients, but this may be impossible for jockeys, horse groomers or avid riders. Many horse-allergic patients can tolerate exposure to horses if they take medications before riding and avoid barns and grooming procedures. Undisturbed insulation in old houses with horsehair-plastered walls does not pose a problem unless the home undergoes remodeling.

## *Pollen Control*

The major pollens that trigger asthma are reviewed in chapter seven. While there are no sure-fire ways to completely avoid outdoor pollens, the following steps help reduce symptoms:

- Do not pick or sniff allergenic plants.

- Close home windows and use air conditioners.

- Use HEPA-type air filters in bedrooms or family rooms.

- Keep car windows closed during pollen seasons.

- Watch weather forecasts. Dry, warm, windy days promote high pollen counts, while rainy, colder days will lower the pollen load. Daily pollen counts in your area are available through the National Allergy Bureau at 1-800-9Pollen.

- If possible, plan outdoor activities later in the day, as pollen counts are higher in the early morning hours.

- When outdoors, wear a visor or cap and sunglasses to keep the pollen out of your eyes.

- Keep your lawn cut short, as longer, more mature grass generates more pollen.

- Shower and shampoo before going to sleep to keep pollen off your pillow and bed.

- If you live near a vacant lot that becomes a ragweed garden, cut the ragweed down in late July or early August before it pollinates. There is no need to cut down nearby pollinating trees, as tree pollen can travel many miles and such an action is not likely to reduce exposure to tree pollen.

- Do not dry clothes or bedding outdoors where it can collect pollen.

## Home Humidifiers

The amount of moisture in the air, called relative humidity, is the amount of water vapor the air can actually hold. Ideal indoor air should neither be too dry nor too moist. Death Valley, the driest area in the United States, has a relative humidity of 20 percent. Many northern homes become drier than Death Valley in the winter months, when indoor humidity levels may fall as low as 10 percent.

Dry indoor air acts like a giant sponge, soaking up moisture from your respiratory tract and dehydrating your skin, mouth, nose and lungs. Low humidity causes dry skin and nosebleeds, and it accelerates the transmission of respiratory infections between household members. The hazards posed by dry indoor air can be partially overcome by proper use of machines called humidifiers that add water vapor to the air.

Ideal in-home humidity, which varies with the local climate, is usually between 40 and 50 percent. An inexpensive instrument called a hygrometer can measure indoor humidity. When humidity levels fall below 40 percent during the heating season in the northern climates, it is time to use humidifiers in bedrooms or family rooms, especially in homes heated with fireplaces, coal or wood stoves. To avoid mold build-up in the humidifier, frequent cleaning is a must. Rinsing with a bleach solution (one tablespoon per pint of water) usually does the trick. Do not add cleaning agents (other than bleach) or mold-inhibiting tablets to your humidifier, as they can produce toxic emissions. Overusing a humidifier during the non-heating season promotes mold and dust mite growth within the home. Humidifiers that directly attach to hot air heating systems are ideal breeding grounds for all kinds of organisms. Such units should be replaced, drained or cleaned on a monthly basis. Ultrasonic cool mist humidifiers are safer, quieter and more efficient than the older cool-mist vaporizers and are less likely to grow molds.

A *Consumer Reports* article on humidifiers warns people who live in homes that lack a vapor barrier to avoid excessive use of humidifiers. A vapor barrier prevents moisture condensation in house walls. Older homes that do not have vapor barriers are prone to wood rot and paint peeling if the indoor air becomes too moist. A word of caution is indicated. My bias for humidifiers is colored by the fact that my winters are spent in a cold, dry New England climate where indoor humidity often reach intolerably low levels. In warmer, moist climates, humidifiers are hazardous as they accelerate the growth of dust mites, molds and bacteria. Do not use home humidifiers unless you live in a cold, dry winter climate where the humidity levels routinely fall below 40 percent.

## Air Purifiers

Some indoor allergens and air pollutants can be removed from your home or office with air purifier devices. Many types of air purifiers are available, and their effectiveness is usually directly proportional to their cost. Some air purifiers are effective and some are not. Air purifiers work in two ways—by mechanical filtration or by putting an electrical charge on particles of allergen in the air that are then deposited on a screen or grid. This latter method is called electro-static precipitation.

Air filters are classified by their efficiency, or ability to remove particles of various sizes. When you are filtering air, you want to remove the small, lung-damaging particles that are invisible to the naked eye. Most of the less expensive filters do not remove particles less than 10 microns in size. The best and most expensive filters are the HEPA, or high-efficiency particulate air filters. HEPA filtration, first developed by atomic scientists at the Manhattan Atomic Bomb Project, is the air purifying method employed in operating rooms, microchip manufacturing, space research and "boy in the bubble" isolation chambers. True HEPA filters are 99.97% effective at removing particles as small as three microns. A typical strand of hair is 75 microns wide. This means that if 10,000 particles were passed through a true HEPA filter, 9,997 particles down to three microns in size will be trapped by the filter! This three-micron-sized particle is critical, as it is the particle size most likely to be inhaled deep into the lung.

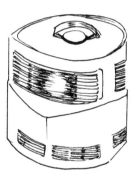

HEPA Air Purifier

The cost of HEPA filters varies depending on the size of the area or room where they are used. Smaller HEPA filters for a typical small eight by ten foot bedroom cost around $100. Larger HEPA filters cost $300-$500. The cost for a full HEPA system in a central air system approximates several thousand dollars. Shop wisely—beware of less efficient filters not labeled as true HEPA filters. HEPA filters are very quiet and energy efficient, consuming no more electricity than a 40-watt bulb. Widely advertised portable table or desktop air purifiers are ineffective. Most medical insurance companies will not cover the cost of air purifiers.

Doctor Robert Reisman of Buffalo, New York, tested the Enviracaire HEPA Air Cleaner in the homes of 40 patients with nasal allergies and asthma. Some of the machines had real HEPA filters in them, while others had sham or blank filters. The study subjects then recorded symptoms and their need for medications for two months. The patients who had the real filters in their homes had fewer symptoms and needed less medication than those with the dummy or blank filters.

Studies have shown that air cleaners are not effective in controlling dust mites unless their use is combined with mite-proof mattress encasements. This observation is probably due to the fact that the larger-sized dust mite particles only become airborne when the surrounding air is disturbed. On the other hand, smaller-sized dog and cat allergens are more likely to be airborne and are easily captured by air cleaners. The first study to prove that HEPA air purifiers helped control the environment of pet-allergic asthmatics who maintained pets in their home looked at asthmatic Dutch children who were allergic to cats or dogs. Twenty children participated in a placebo-controlled study where air cleaners were placed in their living rooms and bedrooms. The placebo group had inactive or sham air cleaners placed in their homes, while the active treatment group used real HEPA filters. Substantial amounts of pet allergen were captured in the homes with the active filters. Children in the homes with the active filters had less airway responsiveness and better peak flow scores than the placebo group. Surprisingly, higher amounts of pet allergen were captured in the living or family room than the bedroom. As a result of this study, I now advise pet-allergic asthmatics to install HEPA air purifiers in both their bedroom and family room.

## Air Conditioners

The most useful appliance for patients with mold or pollen allergy is a room or automobile air conditioner. Bedroom air conditioning protects the sleeping asthmatic during the early morning hours, when trees, grasses and weeds begin to release their pollen. They also indirectly lower dust mite and mold counts by acting as a dehumidifier. You must use an air conditioner that circulates indoor room air as most air conditioners do not filter pollen from outdoor air. Air conditioners must be cleaned frequently to prevent buildup of dust, mold and pollen. Automobile air conditioning is a must for any pollen-sensitive asthmatic that spends a lot of time traveling by car. Patients who do not sleep in an air-conditioned bedroom should install adjustable fiberglass filters in their bedroom windows.

## Dehumidifiers

Indoor relative humidity is the key factor determining the growth and survival of dust mites and molds within the home. A dehumidifier is just the opposite of a humidifier. It removes water vapor or moisture from the air, which in turn reduces the growth potential of molds and dust mites. In order to do this successfully, relative humidity must be maintained below 50 percent for at least 22 hours per day in areas when outdoor humidity levels are high. Dust mite populations usually peak in the summer months. Thus, removal of water vapor from the air is critical at this time of year. Dehumidifiers

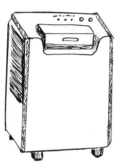

should be used in moist areas of the home, especially damp cellars or basements. In temperate climates, humidifiers are most helpful in the warmer, humid months of the year, but they can be used year-round in semitropical or tropical climates.

## Summary of Environmental Controls

Proper environmental controls may cost several hundred dollars. This expense is justified, and more than offset by the savings in prescription drugs and medical care at the doctor's office or hospital. Although most medical health plans do not cover these costs, any expense directly related to improving your home environment, from buying mite-proof covers for your bedding to an expensive overhaul of your heating system, is a legitimate income tax medical deduction. Table 17.3 summarizes the 10 basic steps in environmental control.

**Table 17.3.** Ten Basic Steps in
Environmental Control

**1.** Add dust-mite-proofing to the bedding.

**2.** Remove carpets from the bedroom.

**3.** Relocate, confine or wash pets.

**4.** Do not allow smoking in the home.

**5.** Avoid strong odors and chemicals.

**6.** Install kitchen exhaust fans.

**7.** Use humidifiers with caution.

**8.** Use bedroom air conditioners.

**9.** Install HEPA air filters.

**10.** Install a dehumidifier in your damp cellar.

## Traveling and Asthma

People with asthma should take special precautions when traveling. Avoid flying if you have a sinus or ear infection. Always carry a second set of medications in your carry-on bag in case your luggage is lost or stolen. If you have to fly on a foreign airline that allows smoking, request a seat as far away from the smoking section as possible. Many airlines allow passengers to carry caged pets on board their aircraft. The major airlines vary in their allowance for pets in airline cabins. American Airlines allows a maximum of five pets per cabin. Several other airlines limit the number of pets to one or two per cabin. Southwest Airlines prohibits pets completely. The animals have to be small enough to fit into a carrier that goes under the seat in front of you. This makes it quite likely that the caged pet is a cat as most dogs are too big to fit into the carrying device. If you are allergic to pets and encounter this situation, ask the flight attendant to change your seat. Pet-allergic asthmatics should contact their airline in advance and carry their medications, including a battery-powered nebulizer, to deal with an allergy or asthma attack.

Try to take an early flight and sit in the front of the plane or in a window seat where the air is fresher. There are anecdotal reports that passengers in first or business class get more fresh air as there are fewer passengers sharing the same space. Most of the time bad air triggers headaches and dry noses and throats, even in non-allergic individuals. Another common problem for air travelers with asthma is dehydration resulting from exposure to the dry, poorly humidified air in aircraft cabins. Use a salt-water nasal spray and drink plenty of liquids to avoid dehydration. Avoid consumption of alcohol or caffeine beverages that promote dehydration. Dry airline cabin air also promotes the dissemination of respiratory infections. Frequent hand washing is the best way to reduce your chances of picking up a cold or viral infection from fellow passengers.

Peanut- and tree-nut-sensitive asthmatics are at risk when they fly, as small particles of aerosolized peanuts or tree nuts can trigger a severe allergic reaction (anaphylaxis) or an asthma attack. Peanut particles are released into the air when a bag of peanuts is opened. High levels of airborne peanut allergen occur when a hundred or more people on an airplane open bags of peanuts at the same time. Peanut protein has also been found in the filtering devices onboard commercial aircraft. There are reports of fatalities in airplanes at high altitudes in peanut-allergic fliers. In response to this risk, many commercial airlines no longer serve peanut snacks. Many carriers will exclude peanuts from a flight when so requested well in advance of the flight.

Hotels and motels are notoriously bad environments for dust-mite and mold-sensitive asthmatics. Carry your own pillowcase covers. Ask if your hotel offers a dust-mite-free or so-called "green room" with mite-proof bedding and air purifiers. Avoid sleeping in musty rooms with antiquated air conditioners or stuffed furniture. If mold-sensitive, request a room in a dry, sunny area away from indoor swimming pools. Avoid rustic cabins that have been shut up for long periods. Ask the owner to air out such cabins hours before arrival. Camping equipment also provides an ideal site for dust mite and mold infestation. Air out tents and sleeping bags before camping trips. Allow damp camping equipment to dry out before repacking.

When traveling by car, bus or train, potential irritants include dust mites, mold, pollens, perfumes and air pollutants. If possible, travel in the early morning when traffic is lighter and air pollutant levels are lower. Asthmatics should carry a portable nebulizer that is battery powered, or one that can be plugged into the car cigarette lighter. Before entering a car, turn on the air conditioner to clear out pollen or mold spores.

In some remote areas or foreign countries, you may be the "best asthma doctor" within hundreds of miles. When traveling overseas for prolonged periods or on a frequent basis, consider joining organizations designed to help travelers with medical needs. The International Association for Medical Assistance to Travelers (IAMIT) is a nonprofit organization that provides a physician directory of English-speaking physicians who have trained in a western country. IAMIT also provides a Traveler Clinic Record for your doctor to complete prior to travel. While there is no charge for an IAMIT membership, a donation is appreciated. For information call 716-754-4883 or visit their Web site at www.sentex.net/iamit

The Travelers Emergency Network (TEN) offers members 24-hour access to a worldwide network of physicians and provides contact information for doctors where you are traveling. The annual membership fee is $99. For information call 1-800-ASK-TEN or visit their Web site at www.tenweb.com

## A Glimpse of the Future

Innovative discoveries in the arena of aeroallergens and their role in asthma are very exciting. Clinical studies assessing the risk factors posed by outdoor and indoor allergens have proven that scores of allergens play a major role in asthma. Most doctors have been converted by these studies and have turned away from the old dogma that allergens are not important asthma triggers. Laboratory techniques that allow health-care providers to measure the amount of allergen in the patient's environment make it easier to determine if their patients are complying with environmental care instructions. Researchers can scientifically assess the effectiveness of air filters, vacuum systems, air conditioners and anti-mite chemicals.

Just as the 1980s and 1990s gave us new drugs and asthma education programs, the twenty-first century may become known for advances in environmental controls. It has been suggested that maternal exposure to allergens after the twenty-second week of pregnancy may play an important role in the development of asthma and allergy. There is an increasing body of evidence showing that the priming of our immune system before birth or in early infancy may send the immune system down the allergy pathway. Thus, reducing exposure to allergens during pregnancy, early infancy- and childhood may prevent the development of asthma and allergic diseases. A study in the Isle of Wight in England found that modest reductions in dust mite allergen in the home reduced the prevalence of mite allergy and bouts of wheezing in the first four years of life.

An ongoing study in Manchester, England, is following a group of infants with a high-risk profile for developing allergy and asthma. The Manchester study selected a group of unborn children with two allergic parents. In the control group, nothing special was done within the home. In the active or treatment group, strict dust mite avoidance measures were implemented in the parents' bedroom. Dust mite levels were measured throughout pregnancy, immediately after birth and again at age six months and one year. Dust mite levels were reduced by nearly 98 percent in the treated group. The control or untreated group had 29 times more dust mite allergen in their homes than the treated group. Long-term follow-up of these children will determine if strict environmental control measures during pregnancy and early infancy reduce the risk of developing asthma. One area that needs additional study is the day care setting. Analysis of dust mite allergen in day care settings in the warm and humid setting of the southeastern United States found high levels of dust mite allergen. Scandinavian day care centers and schools house large amounts of dog and cat allergen. As 50 percent of all children now attend a day care center, these sites may be as important as in-home exposure in the allergic sensitization of a young, immature immune system.

## Is Animal Exposure Protective?

There is solid evidence that exposure to dust mite allergen plays an important role in asthma. In contrast, recent population studies have suggested that having pets in the home, especially cats, may decrease the risks of allergic sensitization and asthma. Doctor Thomas Platts-Mills and co-workers have investigated the immune response to cat and dust mite allergen among 226 seventh- and eighth-graders, including 47 children with asthma who had a wide range of allergen exposures in New Mexico and Virginia. In this study Platts-Mills found that, in contrast to dust mite exposure, cat allergen exposure produced certain antibodies, called IgG or IgG4 antibodies, in children who did not develop allergies or asthma. This may explain why some children exposed to higher levels of cat allergen appeared to be protected from allergies and asthma. Thus, in some patients exposure to animal allergens in infancy or early childhood may induce an state of immune *"tolerance"* to allergens.

These IgG antibodies are the same protective antibodies produced after the administration of allergy injections or immunotherapy. There may be two distinct groups of children. One group develops asthma or allergy when exposed to cat allergen. The other group is protected by exposure to high levels of cat allergen. At the present time, there is no way to pick out those children who will be protected by cat allergen exposure. More studies are needed to unravel this issue. Thus, I still recommend that infants and children at risk for asthma and allergic disorders (positive family history, eczema, hay fever or food allergy) avoid exposure to animal allergens.

Clinical studies in this area are confusing. Some, such as the Tucson, Arizona, study that tracked 1,246 babies since 1980 suggests that early exposure to cats and dogs may be protective and pet avoidance in early life may not be useful. However, it may be inappropriate to tell non-allergic families who wish to prevent allergies in their children to rid their home of pets. These studies raise the intriguing possibility that early exposure to an allergen, like cat allergen, either through allergy injections (immunotherapy) or natural exposure, may signal the all-important T-cells and B-cells to produce mediators and protective antibodies that prevent asthma and allergic rhinitis.

# Immunotherapy
## in Asthma

# 18

n 1911, two ingenious pioneers in allergy research, Drs. L. Noon and J. Freeman, discovered that hay fever victims who were injected with an extract of grass pollen before the grass pollen season suffered fewer symptoms once the grass pollinated in early summer. Modern research has documented their observations, and allergy injections, or immunotherapy, is an accepted treatment for many allergic conditions including asthma, allergic rhinitis and sensitivity to stinging insects.

In immunotherapy, a very dilute dose of an allergen is injected once or twice a week for three to four months. Each succeeding dose delivers a higher concentration of the allergen. These weekly injections build up to a maintenance dose that is usually the highest dose the patient can tolerate without risking an allergic reaction. Once this maintenance dose is reached, injections are given every two to four weeks and continued for at least three to five years on a year-round or perennial basis.

The much older practice of giving injections for several weeks prior to a specific pollen season, called pre-seasonal or co-seasonal therapy, has given way to the more effective year-round method. When allergy injections are deemed to be successful, they are continued for three to five years. When it is clear that allergy injections are not helping or are causing adverse reactions, they should be discontinued. Patients who are relatively symptom-free for two consecutive years or pollen seasons deserve a trial vacation from allergy shots. Highly allergic individuals or those with continued allergen exposure (cats in the home) often require more than five years of allergy injections.

## How Do Allergy Injections Work?

Allergy injections work by directly stimulating your immune system as shown in Figure 18.1. When an antigen or allergen is injected into your body, the immune system handles this allergen in two ways. The T-cells release chemical mediators that signal the immune system's B-cells to stop making allergic or IgE antibody to the injected substance. The T-cells also stimulate the B-cells to produce a gammaglobulin or IgG antibody called a blocking antibody. Later on, when an allergen is confronted by the blocking antibody, it neutralizes or blocks the allergen before it can get to the mast cell and trigger an allergic antigen-antibody reaction.

The net result of all this immune interplay is a lowered level of IgE antibodies, a higher level of blocking antibodies and a decreased capacity to mount an allergic reaction. In essence, allergy injections may push the immune system in the direction of the non-allergic Th1 pathway and away from the Th2 allergy response. When allergy shots are successful, patients have fewer symptom days and require less medication to control their hay fever or asthma.

■
Figure
18.1

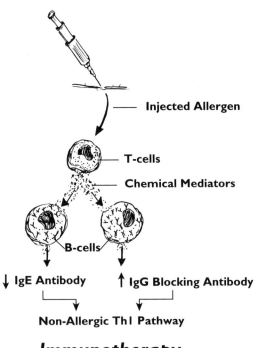

**Immunotherapy**

Immunotherapy has not always been a well-accepted mode of asthma therapy. There are several reasons why doctors have questioned the value of immunotherapy in asthma. First, immuno-therapy for asthma is a difficult treatment to study. There are relatively few well-designed, double-blind, placebo-controlled studies dealing with immunotherapy and asthma. In a double-blind study, some patients get an active drug (in this case an injection with the actual allergen), while others receive a placebo or inactive drug. Neither the patient nor the doctor knows who is getting what until the study ends. Few patients are willing to take the chance of receiving placebo injections (salt water) for several years.

The second reason for the poor acceptance of allergy shots in asthma is that many patients with asthma do not have allergies. Scores of unscrupulous "shot doctors" fail to prescribe correct medications or implement proper environmental controls before they sentence their patients to years of worthless allergy injections. Such poor and inappropriate treatment has given immunotherapy a bad reputation. Bad press is another reason for skepticism regarding immunotherapy. Doctor N. Franklin Adkinson from Johns Hopkins Asthma Center in Baltimore, Maryland, argues that immunotherapy should be more effective and less toxic than other therapies.

Adkinson correctly points out that most allergy injections are given by non-allergy specialists and dosing errors are common. Adkinson was the lead investigator in a 30-month immunotherapy trial in 121 children with moderate to severe asthma. When children who received immunotherapy were compared to children who did not get allergy injections, there was no difference in the clinical outcome. This study, published in the *New England Journal of Medicine* in 1997, was widely circulated in the lay press and media. Proponents of immunotherapy argued that many children in this Baltimore study had more severe asthma and resided in inner-city, cockroach-infested dwellings.

In my earlier teaching days, I believed that allergy shots were effective in asthma when administered to carefully selected patients, but at that time there was no concrete proof to present to skeptical medical students or house staff. Fortunately, advances and dis-coveries in the field of immunology, combined with well-designed clinical studies, have conclusively shown immunotherapy to be effective in hay fever, stinging insect allergy and allergic asthma.

Immunotherapy with dust mites, pollens and cat allergen significantly lowers the overall reactivity of the asthmatic lung. Immunotherapy reduces both the early- and late-phase response and skin reactivity to allergens. One proponent of immunotherapy, Doctor Jean Bousquet from Montpellier, France, notes that despite the best efforts in environmental control and optimal medical management, the rate of adequate symptom control may only approach 50 percent. Bousquet has published several papers showing that immunotherapy is effective with dust mites and pollen allergens. Unlike many American allergists, Bousquet stresses the need to use single allergens which means that each allergen is injected separately and not mixed together as one shot. This approach allows one to administer more precise doses of each allergen. Bousquet adds that the safety of immunotherapy has vastly improved with the availability of standardized allergy extracts.

One review of 62 immunotherapy studies published between 1966 and 1998 found that immunotherapy significantly reduced asthma symptoms, medication requirements and bronchial reactivity. Another review of 20 well-controlled studies concluded that immunotherapy consistently improved asthma symptoms, reduced airway reactivity, improved pulmonary function tests and lowered the need for asthma medications. This review suggested that immunotherapy is cost effective by reducing the need for expensive asthma medications, emergency care and hospitalizations.

Recently, an exciting study on grass immunotherapy in England found that low symptom scores continued for several years after immunotherapy was stopped. A report from Sweden and Denmark is of special interest to cat lovers. Doctor Gunilla Hedlin investigated the effects of three years of placebo-controlled cat and dust mite immunotherapy in 29 children with moderate asthma. Hedlin found a general reduction in asthma symptoms and bronchial reactivity after three years of treatment. She also noted an improvement in the tolerance to cat allergen exposure. This study is important due to the increasing prevalence of cats in our society. A Swedish study found that 53 percent of asthmatic schoolchildren were cat allergic. As cats are so abundant and cat allergen can be found anywhere, cat allergen immunotherapy may be the only way to control cat-induced asthma in some patients.

## Indications for Immunotherapy

I generally employ one or more of the following guidelines to determine when immunotherapy is indicated:

- Allergic or IgE mediated asthma for more than two years
- Excess loss of school and workdays or repeated hospital visits
- Allergic asthma that is not responding well to medications or environmental controls
- Inability to tolerate asthma medications
- Co-existing diseases such as allergic rhinitis or eczema
- Positive skin tests that correlate well with the clinical history
- Persistent asthma and exposure to cats in the home

## Risks of Allergy Injections

Allergy injections are not entirely risk-free. They should always be given under the supervision of a physician. After receiving your injections, you should remain in the clinic or doctor's office for 30 minutes, as most injection reactions occur within this time frame. Allergy injections should not be self-administered at home or by well-meaning relatives, neighborhood nurses or others who lack experience in administering allergy shots or treating systemic reactions induced by allergy injections. The most common injection reaction is a local swelling at the site of the injection. The size and intensity of this local reaction often determines the strength of the next dose. Sometimes patients experience what is called a systemic reaction, in that they develop symptoms of an acute allergic reaction.

Mild systemic reactions cause itching and sneezing, while more severe reactions may induce asthma symptoms. Most injection reactions respond promptly to an antihistamine like Benadryl or an injection of epinephrine. Whenever a patient experiences a significant reaction to an allergy shot, the doctor should make a careful dosing adjustment prior to the next injection visit to prevent a recurrence of the systemic reaction.

In rare instances, a severe anaphylactic or allergic reaction may occur, blocking a patient's airway or causing a drop in blood pressure. Deaths from allergy injections and skin testing have been reported. Fortunately, they are extremely rare. Doctor Richard Lockey compiled data on 46 fatalities associated with skin testing or allergy injections. These deaths took place between 1954 and 1985—a rate of about one a year. Persons at risk included those experiencing seasonal symptoms and patients on beta-blocking drugs. Additional data in Lockey's study suggest that patients with the greatest risk are women with unstable severe asthma and low lung function tests. I have stopped giving injections to patients who fit this profile. In my opinion, allergy shots usually do not work very well in this group of patients.

## Treatment Failures

As with any form of medical treatment, immunotherapy treatment failures are bound to occur. The five most common causes of treatment failures in immunotherapy are the following:

- Allergy "shot doctors" treating people with non-allergic asthma

- Poor control of the environment such as keeping pets in the home

- Failure to keep appointments and follow a regular injection schedule

- Development of new allergies not covered by the present injection program

- Inability to give an effective dose because of severe sensitivity to the injected allergen

## New Frontiers in Immunotherapy

Over the past two decades I have been quite conservative, perhaps too conservative, in my approach to immunotherapy. When confronted with allergic patients, especially young children with developing allergies and allergic rhinitis or asthma, I usually relied on medications and environmental controls before starting allergy injections. In my experience, younger atopic children first become sensitized to tree pollen. These youngsters come into the office in April or May with severe nasal and eye allergies and wheezing. As the peak period for tree pollen levels in Greater Boston occurs in early to mid-May, allergy specialists often call this "Mother's Day Asthma." When I treated this typical pre-school child with tree pollen allergy, I held off recommending allergy injections until later childhood as most of these children would develop additional allergies to grass and ragweed pollen over the next several years. Otherwise I would be adding a new allergen to their injection treatment program every year or so, which would require endless office visits and allergy injections. If these children developed a full-blown spectrum of allergies and were still having symptoms later on in childhood, I would recommend immunotherapy. I told these patients and parents that it took a long time—several months to a year or two—before immunotherapy took effect. There are several evolving reasons why this may be the wrong approach to immunotherapy.

Asthma and allergy drug therapy is aimed at reducing symptoms—the end result of the immune reaction that triggers the sneeze, wheeze and itch response. Environmental controls attempt to prevent the immune reaction by removing offending allergens. Neither of these treatments alter the basic cause of the asthma-allergy immune response. The only form of therapy that down-regulates the inflammatory response of the immune system in allergic disease and asthma is immunotherapy.

Thanks to advances in the immunology lab, we now know there are four effects from immunotherapy: an early effect, a persisting effect, a long-term effect and a preventive effect. The early effect may be seen as early as eight to twelve weeks after starting allergy injections. The persisting effect is achieved during the next three to five years of therapy. New data has revealed that a long-term and preventive effect may last up to six years and perhaps indefinitely after stopping immunotherapy. Emerging evidence implies that there is a strong link between hay fever and asthma, as nasal allergies often precede the onset of asthma. It may all be part of one evolving disease process. Perhaps allergists should be starting young toddlers on allergy injections when they show their first signs of an allergic reaction to an aeroallergen like tree pollen.

Fascinating studies from France led by Doctor Bousquet have shown that administration of dust mite immunotherapy to young children prevented the development of new allergies later on in childhood. This observation supports Doctor Platts-Mills's theory that early natural exposure to an allergen like cat allergen may induce a state of immune tolerance and prevent allergy and asthma for a lifetime. French investigators are now starting pre-school children on allergy injections, an uncommon practice in the United States. Most American allergists wait until later childhood before recommending immunotherapy as I do. An ongoing study in six European allergy centers, called the PAT or Preventative Allergy Treatment Study, found that non-asthmatic children with nasal and eye allergy who were started on immunotherapy to birch and grass pollen had a lowered incidence of asthma five years later than allergic children who did not receive allergy injections.

Large multi-center trials in Europe will determine if early administration of immunotherapy to young patients with allergic rhinitis prevents the onset of asthma. I am very tempted to jump on this early-immunotherapy bandwagon. If these studies confirm that the early use of immunotherapy prevents the onset of additional allergies and asthma later on in childhood, I will radically change my indications for recommending allergy injections in children.

Allergy specialists have relied on natural products for the diagnosis and treatment of allergic diseases for a hundred years. One of the reasons for my conservative approach to immunotherapy was that many allergy extracts were not standardized and varied in quality and potency. While the quality and purity of allergy extracts have vastly improved over the past 20 years, the development of natural allergy extracts may have peaked. Tremendous progress in molecular biology now allows researchers to develop "super allergens" that will be more immunogenic and less allergenic.

One promising approach to immunotherapy is the development of antigens derived from proteins, called peptides. A peptide is actually a small fragment of a whole allergen that is altered by gene vaccination. Peptides directly affect the T-cells or lymphocytes that program the allergic-inflammatory reaction. Their advantage is that peptides have little risk of causing systemic reactions and can be given in higher doses. The development of other types of new allergens offers exciting prospects for allergen-specific therapy.

Traditional immunotherapy requires that the allergen be injected on a regular basis for several years. New allergens may be administered by mouth or inhaled into the nose or lungs.

Another important breakthrough will be the development of antigen-selective DNA vaccines capable of triggering a powerful protective immune response. One DNA-derived peanut vaccine has been shown to block sensitization and severe allergic reactions or anaphylaxis in peanut-allergic mice. Such therapy holds great promise for those patients prone to severe life-threatening reactions to peanuts or tree nuts. Human clinical trials with such a product are now underway. Someday it may be possible to use a single allergen as a vaccination in infancy or early childhood and thereby prevent the development of asthma or allergy for a lifetime. While these are only some of the possible scenarios for the refinement in immunotherapy, they are enough to suggest that immunotherapy may be the asthma therapy of the future.

# Special Types
of Asthma

# 19

everal forms of asthma deserve separate discussion. In this chapter I will review four special types of asthma, including hidden or cough-variant asthma, nocturnal asthma, aspirin-sensitive asthma and occupational asthma. Subsequent chapters will cover the special features of exercise-induced asthma, childhood asthma, asthma in women and adult asthma.

## Cough-Variant Asthma

Coughing, wheezing, shortness of breath and chest tightness are the most common symptoms of asthma. Yet not everyone with asthma has all these telltale symptoms. In some patients the only asthma symptom is a persistent cough. This form of asthma is called hidden or cough-variant asthma. Although cough has been recognized as a clinical feature of asthma for centuries, the recognition that cough may be the only asthma symptom was not appreciated until 1975, when Doctor Regis McFadden described a group of adult asthmatics whose only complaint was a chronic cough.

In 1982, I described a group of 26 children with cough-variant asthma. On long-term follow-up, three-fourths of these children with cough-variant asthma eventually developed more obvious signs of asthma. This suggests that cough-variant asthma may represent the early stages of persistent asthma. Doctor Peter Konig found that patients with hidden asthma were often misdiagnosed and mistreated. Doctors failed to consider asthma as a possibility because the cough was not accompanied by wheezing, and they prescribed all sorts of ineffective medications, such as antihistamines, cough medicines, decongestants and antibiotics. This is most unfortunate, as patients with hidden asthma have a mild form of asthma that usually responds quite nicely to asthma medications.

The quality of cough may help determine the cause of a cough. The cough due to a postnasal drip or a chronic sinus problem is usually a dry, nonproductive "tickle in the back of the throat" cough. The cough in tracheobronchitis or childhood croup is a barking-type cough. A goose-like honk or seal-like cough suggests a tic or habit-type cough. The cough from gastroesophageal reflux disease (GERD) is often worse at night or after eating, and is aggravated by stooping, reclining or lifting.

The cough in hidden asthma is quite different. This cough has a bronchial quality, interrupts sleep and is frequently triggered by cold air or exercise. The cough is often nonproductive (no mucus or sputum) and may persist for several years before the diagnosis of asthma is made. Risk factors that trigger cough-variant asthma include indoor and outdoor air pollution, tobacco smoking, domestic pets and respiratory infections. Asthmatic children attending day care centers are more likely to report cough than those not attending day care, possibly as a result of more frequent respiratory tract infections.

In summary, cough is a very common symptom among adults and children, as up to 30 percent of the general population have recurrent episodes of coughing that prompt a visit to the doctor's office. Medical studies have shown that 30 to 50 percent of people with a chronic cough may have unrecognized asthma. The take-home lesson here is an obvious one. Not all asthmatics wheeze, and if you, or someone you know, repeatedly coughs during sleep or exercise, cough-variant asthma is a distinct possibility. One way savvy parents, teachers, coaches and gym instructors can uncover cough-variant asthma is to recommend an asthma evaluation for anyone who repeatedly coughs during sports, gymnastics or outdoor exercise programs.

## *Nocturnal Asthma*

Nighttime or early morning asthma, commonly called nocturnal asthma, was first described by Sir John Floyer. In 1698, Floyer wrote,

*"I have often observed the Fit always to happen after Sleep in the Night when Nerves are filled with windy Spirits and Heat of the Bed has rarefied the spirits and Humours."* Numerous surveys have shown that nearly 90 percent of asthmatics wake up coughing or wheezing some time during the night—most commonly between 3:00 and 5:00 A.M. Many patients are unable to return to sleep without specific asthma treatment. The major consequence of nocturnal asthma is sleep loss, resulting in deterioration of daytime performance at school or in the workplace. Nocturnal asthma in children obviously affects all members of the household.

Doctor Margaret Turner-Warwick, from Brompton Hospital in London, England, collected data on more than 7,000 asthma patients who reported nocturnal wheezing. Sixty-four percent of these patients wheezed three out of seven nights a week, and more than one-third wheezed every night. The surprising finding of Turner's study was that nearly 25 percent of subjects who considered their asthma to be mild wheezed every night, and nearly half were awakened three times a week. Doctor Turner-Warwick concluded that being awakened at night by asthma symptoms was very common, and patients frequently overlooked nocturnal asthma.

Health-care providers should instruct their patients to use peak expiratory flow meters to record the severity of nighttime asthma and response to treatment. Patients whose peak flow readings drop in the morning, called "morning dippers," are more prone to nocturnal asthma. Additional studies have found that nocturnal asthma attacks are more severe than episodes in the evening or early morning hours. Nocturnal asthma attacks are far more dangerous than daytime episodes, as most near-fatal and fatal asthma attacks occur suddenly and unexpectedly between midnight and 8:00 A.M.

The causes of nocturnal asthma are not fully understood. Plausible explanations include a fall in circulating cortisone and epinephrine levels, gastric reflux (regurgitating food or acid from the stomach), high allergen exposure to animal dander or dust mites in the bedroom, and nighttime changes in the tone of the nervous system's control of the airway. Recent studies found airway inflammation to be more severe in the prone versus the upright position, suggesting that the recumbency may be the main trigger of nocturnal asthma. It is quite likely that some or possibly all of these factors lead to an increase in airway reactivity severe enough to awaken a sleeping patient.

What is the best drug for the control of nocturnal asthma? The treatment of nocturnal asthma should follow the stepwise approach of the asthma guidelines outlined in chapter twenty-four. First, anyone who awakens more than two to three times a month should take an inhaled anti-inflammatory or asthma-controlling drug daily. When this approach does not relieve nocturnal asthma, your health-care provider has several options, including the addition of long-acting beta-agonists, leukotriene modifiers or theophylline drugs. I used to use theophylline drugs in all my patients with persistent nocturnal asthma, as studies from the 1970s and 1980s clearly showed that, at that time, theophylline was the best drug for nighttime asthma. However, many patients cannot tolerate a bedtime dose of theophylline due its insomnia-inducing caffeine-like side effect.

I now prefer a long-acting beta agonist drug such as salmeterol (Serevent) in nocturnal asthma. Patients who take a long-acting beta-agonist drug must be warned that they should not be used to relieve an acute attack of asthma. If one wakes up wheezing in the middle of the night, one should only use a short-acting bronchodilator like albuterol. When nighttime asthma does not respond to an inhaled cortisone drug, a long-acting bronchodilator or a leukotriene modifier, I will prescribe a long-acting theophylline drug. Sometimes changing the timing of the daily dose of asthma medications by taking your drugs later in the day—about 3:00 to 4:00 P.M.—successfully blocks nocturnal asthma.

## Aspirin-Sensitive Asthma

First manufactured in Germany in 1899, aspirin remains the most widely used drug in the world. American drug firms produce nearly 20 tons of aspirin each year, and the American public consumes 100 to 150 million aspirin tablets a day. The average adult takes 60 aspirin tablets a year. For most of these millions of consumers, aspirin is a safe and effective drug. Not so for people with asthma, especially adults with asthma, who are 10 times more likely to develop an allergic reaction to aspirin. A small subset of asthmatics experience adverse reactions to aspirin and any drug that acts like aspirin. Symptoms of aspirin sensitivity include nasal congestion, hives, swelling and wheezing. Asthmatics who react to aspirin are classified as aspirin-sensitive or aspirin-intolerant. Aspirin allergy is more common in patients with chronic rhinitis, sinusitis and nasal polyps. Patients are identified as being aspirin-sensitive only after they have experienced hives, swelling or wheezing following ingestion of aspirin or other non-steroidal anti-inflammatory drugs (NSAIDs). Common NSAID medications that act like aspirin include ibuprofen (Advil or Motrin) and naproxen (Aleve, Naprosyn or Anaprox).

Aspirin-sensitive asthma usually starts in adulthood and does not favor either sex or any ethnic group. After having been in good health, or having hay fever or mild asthma during childhood, the typical patient with aspirin-sensitive asthma experiences a cold or bronchial infection which does not resolve in 10 to 14 days. Nasal congestion and discharge persists for weeks. This is not your typical runny nose—it produces copious amounts of watery nasal discharge that requires several handkerchiefs a day. These patients eventually lose their sense of smell or taste and develop grape-like growths in the nose called nasal polyps. Eventually, they develop asthma or experience an asthma attack after taking aspirin.

This triple-threat combination of sinus disease—nasal polyps, asthma and aspirin allergy is known as Aspirin-Sensitive Asthma or Samter's Syndrome. This syndrome is named after Doctor Max Samter, who first described this entity. I might mention that I had the opportunity to train under this wonderful physician at his Asthma Institute in Chicago in the late 1960s. While aspirin asthma is rare in children, it is estimated that two million adults have this potentially severe form of asthma. Patients with nasal polyps and asthma should not wait to have a reaction to aspirin before taking steps to avoid aspirin or NSAID medications. The only effective painkillers or anti-inflammatory drugs that do not usually cross-react with aspirin are codeine and acetaminophen or Tylenol. Some of the commonly used NSAID drugs that cross-react with aspirin are listed in Table 19.1.

Hundreds of non-prescription OTC (over-the-counter) medications contain aspirin or an NSAID drug, including Bufferin, Alka-Seltzer, Anacin, Pepto-Bismol and many cough or cold preparations.

**Table 19.1.** NSAID Drugs that Cross-React with Aspirin

| Generic Name | Brand Name |
| --- | --- |
| indomethacin | Indocin |
| fenoprofen | Nalfon |
| naproxen | Aleve, Naprosyn, Anaprox |
| tolmetin | Tolectin |
| ibuprofen | Motrin, Advil, Nuprin |
| mefenamic acid | Ponstel |
| sulindac | Clinoril |
| meclofenamate | Meclomen |
| piroxicam | Feldene |
| phenylbutazone | Butazolidin |
| flurbiprofen | Ansaid |
| ketoprofen | Orudis |
| diclofenac | Voltaren |
| diflunisal | Dolobid |

Aspirin-sensitive asthmatics should compulsively read all drug labels in order to avoid hidden sources of aspirin or NSAIDs. Researchers from La Jolla, California, have shown that it is possible to desensitize patients with aspirin or NSAID allergy. During this desensitization procedure, the aspirin-sensitive patient is given a tiny amount of aspirin that is progressively increased over a period of several hours or days. Once desensitized, the patient must take aspirin every day or the sensitivity to aspirin rapidly reappears.

In the late 1990s a new class of NSAIDs was marketed for victims of arthritic diseases. This class of drugs, known as the COX-2 inhibitors, blocks only one form of the enzyme cyclooxygenase, unlike aspirin which blocks both COX-1 and COX-2. While these new COX-2 drugs may not be that much more potent than aspirin, they have less of a tendency to cause gastritis and ulcers when taken on a long-term basis. Some preliminary reports suggest that COX-2 drugs can be used in patients with a history of aspirin or NSAID sensitivity. Our practice has carefully tested and successfully challenged several patients with a history of aspirin allergy or NSAID reactions with Vioxx, the new COX-2 inhibitor. The majority of our patients have tolerated these challenges without any adverse reactions. It should be emphasized that oral challenges with aspirin or any NSAID drug may induce severe bronchospasm and nasal reactions. Physicians conducting such challenges should be experienced in the proper techniques of challenge procedures and prepared to aggressively treat allergic reactions or asthma attacks.

Doctors have always thought that NSAID-allergic patients could safely take acetaminophen or Tylenol, but this may not be true. Doctor Guy Settipane has challenged 50 aspirin-sensitive asthmatics with 1,000 and 1,500 milligram doses of acetaminophen, and found that one-third reacted to higher doses of acetaminophen. Thus, it may be wise to avoid higher doses of Tylenol in aspirin-sensitive asthmatics.

Also, certain chemicals may cross-react with aspirin and the NSAID drugs. The most commonly cited chemical is the FD&C Yellow Dye No. 5, or tartrazine, that is widely used to color foodstuffs yellow. Many asthma specialists warned their aspirin-sensitive asthmatics to avoid this yellow dye. Doctor Ronald Stevenson put this myth to rest when none of 150 aspirin-sensitive asthmatics he challenged with tartrazine experienced any broncho-spasm or nasal reactions. I no longer tell my aspirin-allergic or NSAID-sensitive asthmatics to avoid tartrazine.

## Occupational Asthma

In his *Affections*, Hippocrates wrote, *"When you come to a patient's house you should ask what sort of pains he has, what causes them, how many days he has been sick, whether the bowels are working and what sort of food he eats."* In 1713, Bernadino Ramazzi, the father of occupational medicine, added an important question to Hippocratic medical history when he asked, *"What occupation does he follow?"* As early as the sixteenth century, researchers described asthmatic symptoms in grain handlers. Many centuries later, non-organic agents were identified as triggers of asthma in the workplace. Occupational asthma can be defined as asthma due to causes and conditions attributable to a particular occupational environment and not to stimuli encountered outside the workplace. It is important to differentiate true occupational asthma from pre-existing asthma aggravated by an irritating or chemical exposure in the workplace. There are two types of occupational asthma. The first and most common type occurs after prolonged exposure and allergic sensitization to the offending substance. The second form of occupational asthma occurs shortly after exposure to toxic levels of irritants, gases and compounds not considered to be allergens. This form of occupational asthma is often called RAD, or "reactive airways disease."

It is estimated that more than two million Americans have occupational asthma. The exact number is difficult to pinpoint, as mandatory reporting guidelines vary from state to state. In many cases a wheezing worker is unwilling to report symptoms for fear of job loss. Job-related asthma is increasing in frequency and severity. More than 300 different chemicals used in the workplace have been linked to asthma. Sometimes asthma occurs immediately after starting work, whereas in other cases it may take months or years before the asthma symptoms surface. Both allergic and non-allergic substances trigger occupational asthma. In some cases allergic asthma occurs when the worker is exposed to aeroallergens like plants, enzymes or other biological agents.

The diagnosis of occupational asthma, while difficult to establish, is usually based on clinical history and appropriate lab and skin tests. Serial monitoring of lung functions in the workplace or direct bronchial challenges may be necessary to nail down the diagnosis. Occupational asthma has many disguises. A factory or office worker may report to work on Monday morning feeling well, only to suddenly develop a fever, chills, wheezing or a flu-like illness which workers call the *"Monday morning miseries."* Other workers may have a delayed onset of symptoms, and they do not get sick until later in the week. Most people with occupational asthma improve on long holiday weekends or vacations. The triggers of occupational asthma include both the allergic and non-allergic materials. A typical non-allergic example of occupational asthma is the housewife who wheezes in her poorly ventilated laundry room when she inhales irritating ammonia or bleach fumes. An allergic example of occupational asthma would be the veterinary worker who wheezes when exposed to dogs or cats.

Compounds that induce occupational asthma can be broken down into two different groups based on their size or molecular weight. The high-molecular-weight group includes sensitizing proteins capable of eliciting a true allergic or IgE-mediated reaction. Such compounds include proteins like latex, enzymes and plant products. One of the best examples of this form of occupational asthma is Baker's Asthma, where chefs and restaurant workers become allergic to wheat flour. In some forms of occupational asthma, workers are sensitized to minute amounts of chemicals used in the workplace. The two most common examples of this type of occupational asthma are TDI-induced and TMA-induced asthma. TDI (toluene di-isocyanate) is a chemical widely used in the electronic and foam manufacturing industries. When released into the factory air in high enough concentrations, TDI is a potent irritant to the skin, nose and lungs of normal individuals. Some workers have become sensitized to TDI when exposed to an air concentration as small as one part per billion.

The cause of TDI-induced asthma is poorly understood, as it is neither a simple irritant nor an allergic reaction. Heavy smokers and workers with a past history of asthma are more prone to TDI asthma that may evolve into a very debilitating illness. A more lethal form of occupational asthma was uncovered by Doctor Roy Patterson and co-workers of Northwestern University. Patterson's group reported that TMA (trimetallic anhydride), a widely used epoxy resin, caused all types of reactions including the Monday morning miseries, allergic asthma and a severe sensitivity reaction which induced respiratory failure and even death.

The treatment of occupational asthma is avoidance and environmental control. Employers must take appropriate steps to minimize or eliminate a worker's exposure to offending chemicals. One of the more successful models of industrial environmental control took place in the detergent industry. Doctor I. Leonard Bernstein and his co-workers from the University of Cincinnati discovered that detergent factory workers were developing asthma at an alarming rate. Bernstein's detective work revealed the asthma-inducer was an enzyme, *Bacilis subtilis,* which was added to the detergent to improve its stain-removing qualities. The detergent industry quickly responded to this threat and installed industrial environmental controls in their factories to minimize exposure to this enzyme. In 1970, it was estimated that 1,000 of 4,000 workers exposed to the detergent enzyme had developed sensitization to the chemical. By 1985, the number of cases had decreased to only one percent of exposed detergent workers. Detergent Worker's Asthma was virtually eliminated as an occupational health hazard. The possibility of disability from chronic occupational asthma can be reduced significantly once an early diagnosis is made. Drug treatment of asthma should not be considered as an alternative to avoidance. However, when avoidance is impossible, pretreatment with asthma drugs may minimize the response to inhaled chemicals in the workplace.

# **Exercise** and Asthma

# 20

Exercise-induced asthma has intrigued physicians for more than 2,000 years. In A.D. 200, Aretaeus stated, *"If from running or gymnastic exercise or any other work, the breathing becomes difficult, it is called asthma."* Sir John Floyer, himself an asthmatic, wrote that violent exercise-induced shortness of breathing and dancing was more asthmagenic than walking. Floyer suggested that exercise was related to *"putting the Spirits to a great expansion or making the Blood boyl."* In 1864, H. A. Salter, who recognized that cold air triggered asthma, speculated that the passage of fresh and cold air over the bronchial mucosa triggered asthma by irritating the nervous system.

These accurate descriptions have stood the test of time. The occurrence of wheezing during or after exercise is now called exercise-induced asthma. Asthmatics born in the nineteenth century and the first five decades of the twentieth century were often confined to their home as there were no effective medicines for exercise-induced asthma that would allow them to participate in sports and outdoor activities. Jim Davis, the creator of the cartoon cat, Garfield, attributes his talent to having to spend most of his childhood drawing indoors because of his asthma. Other creative artists whose success may have been due to their asthma that did not allow active outdoor play include Ludwig Van Beethoven, Charles Dickens and Robert Louis Stevenson.

## *Incidence of Exercise-induced Asthma*

Surveys in Georgia, Connecticut and Alabama that evaluated young athletes with questionnaires, physical exams and exercise challenges found that exercise-induced asthma is a widely under-diagnosed condition. Doctor Margaret Guill found that 13 percent of surveyed athletes in Georgia had exercise-induced asthma, a much higher rate than previously reported in college and Olympic athletes. Doctor Christopher Randolph reported similar numbers in Connecticut schoolchildren. Doctor J. Wyler of the University of Iowa evaluated players on this Big Ten football team with an asthma questionnaire and an inhalation challenge with methacholine, an asthma-provoking chemical. Twelve percent of the Iowa football players had a history consistent with the diagnosis of asthma and, somewhat to the surprise of the investigators, nearly 50 percent had a positive methacholine challenge.

Doctor William Busse evaluated 304 collegiate athletes from the University of Wisconsin over a three-year period. These Wisconsin athletes completed a medical history, physical exam, skin testing and methacholine challenge. Fifty of the 295 athletes reacted to methacholine inhalations. Sixteen had symptoms consistent with asthma. In a study at the Air Force Academy, undiagnosed exercise-induced asthma was found in 94 out of 224 Air Force Academy recruits. High school football players in urban Philadelphia were found to have a high incidence of unrecognized exercise-induced asthma.

Most, if not all, patients with asthma cough or wheeze when they exercise, especially when they exercise in cold, dry air. This syndrome has various names, including exercise-induced asthma, exercise-induced bronchospasm and sports-induced asthma. The duration and intensity of any exercise activity is governed by one's physical conditioning and endurance level. During exercise, the bronchial tubes normally open up or dilate to improve the exchange of oxygen and carbon dioxide. This dilation of the bronchial tubes is due to release of adrenaline from the adrenal gland. Just the opposite occurs when an asthmatic exercises. The bronchial tubes tighten and, within five to ten minutes after starting exercise, the exercising asthmatic starts to cough or wheeze (Figure 20.1).

While some individuals are able to continue exercising or "run through their attack," others must stop exercising altogether. Sometimes the asthma symptoms do not begin until after exercise is completed. A few patients do not cough or wheeze until several hours after exercising. This is called delayed exercise-induced asthma. Most attacks of exercise-induced asthma subside within 30 to 60 minutes,

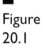
Figure
20.1

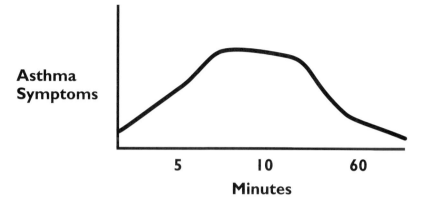

even when untreated. Several factors, including climate and the type of exercise, influence the severity of exercise-induced asthma. Exercising in cold, dry air is much more likely to trigger asthma than exercising in warm, humid air. Running is more asthmagenic than swimming or cycling. The duration of exercise is also important. A longer exercise period increases the likelihood of exercise-induced asthma. Many patients with exercise-induced asthma only wheeze during the allergy season or during periods of high temperatures and humidity when air pollution levels are high.

Exercise-induced asthma is essentially a mini-asthma attack, and for some patients it may be their only form of asthma. Exercise-induced asthma occurs only in asthmatics, and most asthmatics have exercise-induced asthma. A negative history for exercise-induced asthma may be due to the fact that many patients with asthma never exercise strenuously enough to develop symptoms. They either cannot exercise or have been advised not to exercise by their family physician.

Whenever I confront a patient with asthma who does not cough or wheeze with exercise, I will closely question the diagnosis of asthma. When exercise is the only asthma trigger, I use the medical term exercise-induced bronchospasm, not exercise-induced asthma. Putting the buzzword asthma into a medical report or insurance form may result in being declared ineligible for entrance into the armed forces, flight schools or service academies, or raise the premiums of your health or life insurance coverage.

## *Mechanisms of Exercise-induced Asthma*

The basic mechanism of exercise-induced asthma has been a mystery to researchers for decades. Australian doctors were the first to unravel the puzzle of exercise-induced asthma when they recognized the advantages of swimming over free running. Young asthmatic Aussies were encouraged to take up swimming at an early age. As a result of their swimming programs, several Australians with asthma have won Olympic medals in swimming, the most famous being Shane Gould, who won several gold medals in the 1972 Summer Olympic Games. In retrospect, this Australian experience hinted at the basic cause of exercise-induced asthma.

Another study that helped uncover the cause of exercise-induced asthma was performed in Israel, where physicians noted that children from dry, arid areas of Israel had more problems with exercise-induced asthma than children who lived in the more coastal humid areas. These observations suggested that exercising in cold or dry air was more asthmagenic than exercising in humidified swimming pools or coastal climates.

Inhaled air is normally humidified and warmed to body temperature by the time it reaches the lung. By testing people with asthma in laboratory settings, researchers have learned that when asthmatics hyperventilate during exercise, they do not warm or humidify their inspired air as well as non-asthmatics. Thus, they inhale dry, colder air that acts as a potent bronchoconstricter. This explains why exercise-induced asthma is more likely to occur while jogging outdoors on a cold winter morning, versus swimming indoors in a well-humidified pool. The exact location of this temperature and humidity defect is unknown.

The swelling of the nasal passages and increased secretions in exercise, especially in cold air, also limit airflow and warming of the lower airways. These important observations have led to very simple advice for athletes who have asthma, especially wintertime joggers. Wear a protective mask or scarf over your mouth and nose when exercising in cold dry weather! Such a mouth covering allows you to rebreathe warmer, more humid expired air.

## Diagnosis of Exercise-induced Asthma

The diagnosis of exercise-induced asthma is usually quite easy. The basic question I ask my patients is, "Do you cough or wheeze when you exert yourself, especially in colder, dry weather?" When the answer is yes, the diagnosis of exercise-induced asthma is almost a certainty. Sometimes physiologic shortness of breath or simply being out of shape may be confused with exercise-induced asthma, and an exercise challenge may be necessary.

I sometimes conduct an informal exercise challenge where a patient is seen in the office, and a baseline breathing test and a chest exam are performed. The patient then runs outdoors (weather permitting) for a period of five to ten minutes and returns to the office for a reexamination and breathing test. The presence of wheezing or a drop of 15 to 20 percent or more in one-second vital capacity (FEV1) or peak expiratory flow rate usually confirms the diagnosis of exercise-induced asthma. Such a free-run challenge may be more asthmagenic than a laboratory treadmill test, as it can be conducted in the real-life outdoor setting of cool, dry air. Patients and parents can often help make the diagnosis of exercise-induced asthma at home or on the athletic field by measuring their peak flow rates before and after exercise. Exercise challenges in adults with known or suspected cardiovascular disease should only be performed in laboratory facilities with the capability of monitoring heart rate and blood pressure.

One condition that may be confused with exercise-induced asthma is exercise-induced laryngeal stridor. This condition is more common among top trained, young female athletes who develop stridor or a croupy-like breathing pattern during maximal exercise. Unlike those athletes with true exercise-induced asthma, they do not cough or wheeze during or after exercise. Exercise-induced laryngeal stridor is essentially the same as vocal cord dysfunction which was discussed in chapter five.

## Elite Athletes with Asthma

Exercise-induced asthma is more common in world-class athletes who compete in endurance events such as cycling, swimming or long-distance running. Even though swimming is less asthmagenic than free running, the incidence of exercise-induced asthma is very high in competitive swimmers, especially if they have hay fever. Doctors William Pierson and Robert Voy evaluated athletes at the 1984 Olympic Games in Los Angeles. They found that 67 of the U.S.A. team members, or 11 percent, had exercise-induced asthma. These 67 Olympians with exercise-induced asthma won 41 medals in all. Fifteen athletes won gold medals, including women track stars Jackie Joyner-Kersee and Jeanette Bolden. Jeanette Bolden developed asthma in infancy. Her asthma was so severe that she had to be placed in a home for children with asthma in her native Los Angeles. Bolden credits her Olympic triumphs to the fact that this home taught her to accept and control her asthma.

Medal winner Jenny Gilder's asthma was so severe that while enrolled at Yale University she was put on athletic disability. When Gilder started using the correct asthma medications, her life changed completely. She was able to compete in running and cross country skiing and win a silver medal in rowing.

Cross country gold medal winner Bill Koch may be the most remarkable of all asthmatic athletes, as he won his gold medal while competing in very cold, dry, winter air. In 1982, Koch became the first American skier to capture the world cup, a difficult competition involving 10 races held at various places all over the world. Koch admits that in 1984, he raced without taking his asthma medicines. He tried other approaches to managing his asthma, including a special warm-up program. Koch feels that his disregard for medications brought his 1984 Olympic hopes to an abrupt halt. Amy Van Dyken from Colorado was diagnosed with asthma at age 18 months. When she first started swimming, it took her six years to swim a single length of the swimming pool. Van Dyken's perseverance obviously paid off, as she became the first American woman to win four gold medals in the 1996 Summer Olympic Games in Atlanta. Many well-known professional athletes have asthma but have kept it quiet. One reason they keep their asthma in the closet is that any public acknowledgment that they have asthma might weaken their position during contract negotiations.

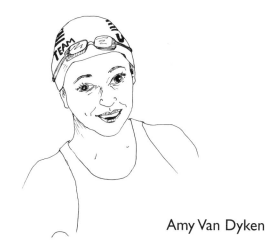

Amy Van Dyken

## *Yet Another Epidemic*

The incidence of exercise-induced asthma has paralleled the rise in allergies and asthma, especially in elite athletes. A team of researchers from the University of Iowa analyzed questionnaires filled out by 699 athletes who participated in the 1996 Summer Olympic Games. The purpose of this study was to determine if the prevalence of asthma had increased in highly competitive athletes just as it had in the general population. Indeed, asthma did increase in frequency in these athletes. Olympic athletes with the highest incidence of asthma were the cyclists and mountain bikers, who had a prevalence rate of 45 percent, and swimmers, who reported a 25-percent incidence of asthma. Approximately 17 percent of these 699 elite athletes used asthma medicines, and 10 percent took asthma drugs on a regular basis. This compares with an 11-percent asthma incidence in Olympic athletes who participated in the 1984 Summer Games. Thus, the prevalence of asthma in Olympic athletes in the 1996 Summer Games increased more than threefold compared to the 1984 Games.

A survey of 738 competitive swimmers found that 21 percent had asthma and 19 percent had allergic rhinitis. When the risk factors for allergy were combined with competitive swimming, the risk for having asthma was 97 percent greater than that for the non-allergic swimmers. Competitive swimmers who swim up to 30 hours per week inhale and aspirate all kinds of chemicals, including chlorine, chloroform, formaldehyde and acetaldehyde. In a two-hour training period, a competitive swimmer may be exposed to an amount of chlorine that exceeds the recommendation of a worker with an eight-hour exposure. It is thought that airway inflammation in swimmers is an irritant response from inhalation of these pool chemicals. A survey of 103 runners from the Finnish national teams found that 15 percent had exercise-induced asthma. When Finnish runners had other allergies, they were six times more likely to have asthma.

## Sports-induced Asthma

Is exercise-induced asthma being over-diagnosed in the general population, especially in children and adolescents? In my opinion the answer is definitely yes. Most individuals, except highly conditioned athletes, become short of breath during vigorous aerobic exercise. The degree of shortness of breath is directly related to one's endurance or physical conditioning. Over the past decade I have seen a growing number of patients, usually children or young adults, referred for evaluation of exercise or "sports-induced asthma." These children and young adults often have no other signs of asthma, such as coughing or wheezing when exposed to allergens or during respiratory infections.

The typical patient with sports-induced asthma is usually an active junior high or high school athlete—more often a soccer player.

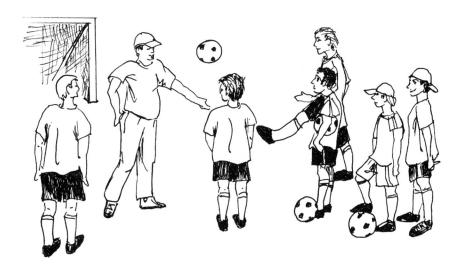

These patients are frequently accompanied to the office by their father who, as luck may have it, is also the kid's coach. Dad relates that his child, who has been active in a sport such as soccer for several years, can no longer run as fast or as long as his or her teammates. After competing in vigorous activities for eight to ten minutes, this youngster develops a shortness of breath that limits his or her performance level. The under-performing athlete has usually seen his or her primary care provider, who without the benefit of an exercise challenge or a lung function test, makes a snap diagnosis of "sports-induced asthma" and prescribes an asthma inhaler. When these student-athletes did not respond to the inhaler and athletic performance did not improve, they were then referred to my office for further evaluation.

On close questioning it becomes apparent that these individuals with "sports-induced asthma" rarely cough or wheeze, and they have no other history of allergy problems like hay fever or eczema. The proper approach to these patients is to take a careful history, perform a breathing test before and after inhaling a bronchodilator and do an exercise challenge. Sometimes it may be necessary to perform a methacholine challenge test. Between visits the patient is told to record peak flow reading before, during and after exercise. The diagnosis of sports-induced asthma should be discarded when the evaluation fails to show any evidence of exercise-induced asthma or cardiovascular problems.

Most children experience a growth spurt in late childhood and adolescence. This growth spurt is accompanied by a substantial increase in height and weight that means that it takes more endurance and physical conditioning to perform at a higher level of competition. Soccer is a particularly strenuous sport, as it involves free running outdoors, often in cold, dry air. It also is a sport with no time-outs or rest periods. Over the past decade, soccer has grown in popularity. In many cities and towns hundreds of young children start playing soccer at an early age. As children grow older and enter high school, the level of competition intensifies and team selection becomes more competitive. Only the very best and fastest players are chosen for the "select teams." This pyramid effect leads to significant fallout, and disappointed parents begin looking for medical reasons why their child can no longer run as fast and as long as the better players. In my opinion this is a major reason for the over-diagnosis of sports-induced asthma.

Is exercise-induced asthma also being over-diagnosed in elite athletes? This question was raised by Doctor Sandra Anderson from Australia, who noted that high-endurance athletes move more air in and out of their lungs per minute when they exercise, especially during long periods of exercise like long distance running or cycling. It stands to reason that these elite athletes breathe in more allergens, air pollutants or cold air during competition than the casual week-end jogger. Track and field athletes are obviously at greater risk for outdoor pollen exposure. This may explain why elite athletes have more exercise-induced asthma, especially when they exercise outdoors. One must ask the question: Is exercise-induced airway narrowing in elite athletes the same as true exercise-induced asthma? Exercise-induced asthma may not be the right diagnosis in these athletes, as their lungs are exposed to more cold air, allergens and air pollutants and are more likely to lose water. Doctor Anderson suggests that the wheezing seen in elite athletes may not be true exercise-induced asthma, but simply a defense mechanism to water loss combined with high exposure to inhaled allergens, cold air and air pollutants.

## *Treatment of Exercise-induced Asthma*

Exercise-induced asthma can usually be effectively treated. Warming up before exercise will reduce the intensity of exercise-induced asthma. This is based on the observation that exercise challenges performed 60 minutes after exercise produce less bronchoconstriction than the first exercise period. A warm-down exercise may also decrease the degree of delayed exercise induced asthma. Individuals with exercise-induced asthma who are engaged in intensive competition should perform light exercises every 30 to 40 minutes when there are long intervals between events. Avoiding too quick a return to a cold environment after exercising in warm air (or vice versa) also lowers the degree of exercise-induced asthma. In my college days in New Hampshire, I always wheezed after I left the gymnasium and went out into the cold New Hampshire winter air.

Patients should try to exercise indoors when air pollutant levels are high. Wear a mask or scarf when exercising in colder air. Nasal breathing is not recommended during intense exercise, as most athletes do not move enough air through their nose to meet the high oxygen requirements of aerobic exercise. Doctor Robert Strunk evaluated the fitness of children with asthma at the National Jewish Hospital in Denver and found that most asthmatic children at this institution were very much out of shape. Strunk found that patients with asthma could improve their performance in activities such as bicycling, running and swimming by improving their physical fitness.

The most effective medicine in relieving and preventing exercise-induced asthma is the beta-agonist drug albuterol. Albuterol will prevent or reduce bronchospasm for up to two hours when taken 10 to 15 minutes before exercise. When albuterol does not work, I add cromolyn sodium (Intal) 30 to 60 minutes before exercise to block or minimize exercise-induced asthma. Inhaled cortisone drugs do not reduce exercise-induced asthma if administered as a single dose before exercise, but they may minimize exercise-induced asthma when administered over an extended period.

In July 1998, two articles in the *New England Journal of Medicine* described a new approach to exercise-induced asthma. Doctor Regis MacFadden reported that the long-acting bronchodilator salmeterol (Serevent) provided protection against exercise-induced bronchoconstriction for up to nine hours when patients cycled on a stationary bike and breathed frigid air for 30 minutes. The second article noted that the leukotriene modifier, montelukast (Singulair), reduced exercise-induced asthma by an average of 47 percent after 12 weeks of study. However, this protection was only seen in three of every four patients. Thus, patients taking montelukast for exercise-induced asthma should be told there is a one chance in four that the drug may not work.

Another approach in patients who do not respond to albuterol or Intal is to use both Serevent and Singulair. While this two-pronged approach may help asthmatics who vigorously exercise more than once a day or for longer periods of time, due to the potential risks of using a long-acting, beta-agonist drug as monotherapy, I only recommend this combination in patients who are taking inhaled cortisone on a daily basis.

## Rich Dumont and Marax

Years ago Olympians who took asthma drugs during competition were severely penalized. In 1972, USA swimmer Rich Dumont forfeited his 400-meter gold medal when it was discovered that he had taken an older asthma medication (Marax) before his race. Unfortunately, Marax contained ephedrine, a known nervous system stimulant that is banned from Olympic competition. Dumont's misfortune forced the Olympic Committee to change its rules. Dumont should be awarded a much larger medal by society for alerting the world to the plight of the asthmatic athlete and showing just what an athlete who had asthma could accomplish. Olympic athletes used to be able to take asthma medicines prior to competition as long as they notify the Olympic Committee well in advance. In August 2001 these rules were changed.

Asthma medications' use in the 1998 Winter Olympics ranged from a high of 60 percent in cross-country skiers to a low of three percent for bobsledders. The International Olympic Committee (IOC) now feels that it is quite possible that some athletes are using asthma medicines as performance-enhancing drugs, especially the beta-agonist drugs, which are classified as stimulants. In August 2000, the IOC toughened up its requirements for the use of asthma medications. Athletes must now provide clinical and laboratory evidence that they have asthma, including lung function tests, before competing. These tests will be reviewed and approved by a panel of medical experts. Hopefully, such stricter requirements will not discriminate against athletes with true asthma. The Medical Commission of the IOC has approved and banned certain drugs which are listed in Table 20.1.

Readers who wish to learn more about exercise-induced asthma should read *Asthma and Exercise* (Henry Holt and Co. 1990). Written by Nancy Hogshead and Gerald Cousens, this fine book details the asthma experiences of Nancy Hogshead, an asthmatic who won four Olympic medals in swimming at the 1984 Summer Olympics. Hogshead vividly explains that she had undiagnosed asthma up until the 1984 Olympics. It was not uncommon for her to develop shortness of breath and coughing after a race. She simply thought she had small lungs. After finishing fourth in the 200-meter butterfly, Hogshead was short of breath and began to cough. A nearby doctor

## **Table 20.1.** IOC Asthma and Allergy Medications, 1999

*Allowed to use*

- Sodium cromolyn (Intal) or nedocromil (Tilade)
- Leukotriene modifiers
- Ipratropium bromide (Atrovent)
- Theophylline
- Antihistamines

*Permitted by notification*

- Inhaled albuterol (Proventil, Ventolin), salmeterol (Serevent)
- Inhaled cortisone drugs

*Strictly prohibited*

- Systemic or oral corticosteroids
- Other inhaled beta-agonists than those noted above
- Systemic or oral beta-agonists
- Inhaled or systemic epi

asked her if she always coughed like that after a race and suggested that she possibly had asthma. After she returned to Duke University, lung function tests determined that she did have exercise-induced asthma. Hogshead's book convincingly demonstrates how essential it is for a patient or family to take control of exercise-induced asthma and not be controlled by it. The authors present clear and detailed advice on how adults and children with asthma can cope with exercise and sports. Hogshead and Cousens describe the asthma experiences of several famous athletes who took control of their asthma and went on to high achievement, including Jackie Joyner-Kersee, Mike Gminski, Danny Manning, Jim Ryan, Cheryl Durstin-Decker and Sam Perkins. *Asthma and Exercise,* an important edition to anyone's asthma library, contains many resources and outlines a number of safe exercise programs.

## *Scuba Diving and Asthma*

The term scuba, which is the abbreviation for self-contained underwater breathing apparatus, describes the diving apparatus that allows divers to carry their own air supply. Scuba diving became a worldwide recreational activity after modern Scuba gear was developed by Jacques Cousteau and Emile Gagnon in 1943. Now there are nearly six million certified divers in the United States.

The most common reason for a death during scuba diving is drowning. The second most common cause of death is arterial gas embolism. When divers ascend to the surface, the volume of air in their lung expands. If the diver ascends too quickly, air cannot be exhaled fast enough and it is forced into the arteries supplying blood to the lung. When air bubbles enter the blood stream, they cause an air embolism to other organs of the body, including the brain. Air may also leak into tissues surrounding the lung and cause a pneumothorax or collapse of the lung. This condition occurs because increased pressure causes more nitrogen to be dissolved in the blood. When the diver comes up too quickly, the increased nitrogen reverts to its gaseous state, causing nitrogen bubbles. The end result is called decompression sickness or "the bends." In milder cases, symptoms consist of localized joint pain and skin rashes, whereas in more serious cases air embolism to the brain and spinal cord can lead to paralysis and death.

What is the risk of diving if you have asthma? It is commonly agreed that symptomatic asthma is a contraindication to diving due to exercise limitations and mucus plugging. Air trapped in the lungs may predispose the asthmatic to an air embolism when he or she ascends to the surface. The bottom line is that asthmatics who are coughing or wheezing should not dive.

What about asthmatics who are not having symptoms? Several surveys by popular diving magazines have found hundreds of divers with asthma who reported that they dove on a regular basis with little or no problems. Older recommendations cautioned that asthmatics with a history of active asthma within the past five years should not dive. More recent publications reported that patients with normal lung functions and little airway reactivity in response to exercise or cold air have no greater risk for barotrauma than normal subjects. Thus, the recommendations regarding the risks of scuba diving in asthmatics is sketchy and conflicting. Recently published ACAAI (American College of Allergy, Asthma & Immunology) guidelines for scuba diving state

- Any individual with active asthma should refrain from diving even if their lung functions are normal.

- Persons with a remote history of asthma who are completely without asthma symptoms and have normal lung functions can probably safely engage in diving.

- Persons with a vague history of asthma should be examined and studied before being allowed to dive.

Doctor Arthur Torre, an asthma specialist and avid diver, is a member of PADI or the Professional Association of Diving Instructors. PADI and other diving organizations had formerly stated that asthma was an absolute contradiction to diving. In 1995, Doctor Torre and his fellow diving physicians reviewed the data on this issue and came up with the new recommendation that asthma was a relative contraindication to diving. This meant that if your asthma was not well controlled, you should not dive. Under current guidelines most diving organizations, including the Underseas Hyperbaric Medical Society, state that to dive safely, an asthmatic should have normal lung functions before and after exercise. Those individuals who maintain normal lung functions, even with medication, should be able to dive.

The data collected by the Divers Alert Network found that divers with asthma have no greater risk for air embolism than non-asthmatics. Doctor Torre recommends measuring lung functions before and after exercise and monitoring lung functions with a peak flow meter twice a day a few weeks before diving and during a diving trip. When lung functions are normal and the patient has no asthma symptoms, Doctor Torre feels the chances of having asthma problems while diving are relatively small.

I agree with Doctor Torre. If you have active, persistent, uncontrolled asthma, you should not dive. Individuals with controlled asthma should be evaluated by lung function tests and seek authorization from qualified physicians before diving. If you have mild intermittent asthma with normal lung function tests, diving is probably safe. Pre-dive administration of a short-acting bronchodilator will minimize the risk of bronchospasm during a dive. Asthmatics who dive should also be checked and treated for ear and nasal-sinus problems, as barotrauma of the middle ear and sinus cavities is the most common medical complication in divers.

For further information on diving and asthma, contact the Divers Alert Network at Duke University in North Carolina (1-800-445-2671 www.diversalertnetwork.org.). This network maintains a list of health professionals familiar with the health issues related to scuba diving.

# Childhood
## and
# Young Adult Asthma

# 21

**A**sthma is a common childhood illness. Studies from England, Australia, Canada and the United States suggest that one child in ten has asthma. Pediatric asthma is the most frequent reason for missed school days and emergency room visits in pediatric centers. Asthma accounts for one in every four pediatric asthma admissions to inner-city hospitals, and produces more in-hospital days than any other childhood disease.

One-third of children who develop asthma do so before their third birthday, and nearly 80 percent of all asthmatic children start to wheeze before they enter the first grade. The sex distribution changes with age. Asthmatic boys outnumber girls in early childhood. In middle childhood the sex ratio evens out, whereas in adolescence and young adulthood females outnumber males by a three to two margin.

## The Wheezing Infant

Asthma specialists now know that asthma is a common disease of infancy and early childhood. Doctors at the Mayo Clinic studied the medical records of the residents of Homestead County, Minnesota. They found that 60 percent of all asthmatics of any age had been diagnosed by age three, and almost 90 percent had developed asthma by age six. It is easy to both over-diagnose and under-diagnose asthma in infancy and early childhood. The first one or two episodes of a wheezing illness in infancy are usually called wheezy bronchitis or bronchiolitis by the family doctor or pediatrician. Nearly 50 percent of infants experience a transient wheezing illness from time to time because of the small size of their airways. When children grow, their airways enlarge and many outgrow the tendency to wheeze when they have a respiratory infection. Doctors have to be careful not to over-treat infants who have two or three bouts of transient wheezing, as many do not develop full-blown asthma. Only one-third of wheezy infants go on to develop persistent wheezing or true asthma. One of the more blatant examples of over-treatment occurs when an infant or toddler has his or her first episode of wheezing. Many family physicians and pediatricians jump the gun and prescribe a nebulizer for home administration of bronchodilators. Not only is this overkill from a treatment standpoint, it is economically unsound as many of these children never experience another bout of wheezing, and unused and expensive nebulizers simply gather dust in the closet.

Sometimes the diagnostic pendulum swings the other way. When an infant or young child experiences three or more episodes of a wheezy-type illness, the likelihood of asthma increases. The correct diagnosis of asthma is often delayed, as many doctors are unwilling to put the word "asthma" into play. Doctors call it persistent wheezing, bronchitis or bronchiolitis, as using the word asthma implies that the child may have a chronic disease that might last several years or even a lifetime.

The hesitancy of doctors to label a wheezing youngster as having asthma is not unique to America. Doctor L. Hey of Tyneside, England, found that 11 percent of all the children in his town had asthma symptoms, yet only one in three was prescribed appropriate asthma medicines and only one in ten families knew their child had asthma. The salient point here is that reluctance by doctors to use the term asthma can lead to delayed, inappropriate and poor care.

I fully concur with Hey's observations. I have evaluated scores of children who have been coughing and wheezing for many years, yet the diagnosis of asthma has never been entertained. Parents are totally shocked when the diagnosis of asthma is brought up. Doctors have told the parents that their child is "bronchial," a misnomer that leads to under-treatment of a very treatable condition. In summary, any infant or child who experiences three or more episodes of wheezy bronchitis may have asthma. The diagnosis of asthma is almost a certainty when a child persistently coughs or wheezes between respiratory infections, during exercise or while sleeping.

## Natural History of Childhood Asthma

The potential for developing asthma and other allergic diseases at a young age depends upon one's genetic make-up combined with environmental exposures that send the immune system down the allergy-prone Th2 pathway. What is the natural history for the unfortunate infant born with the asthma-allergy genetic coding? The earliest sign of difficulty is often an allergic reaction to milk or eggs. Typical symptoms of food allergy in infancy include colic, vomiting, diarrhea or hives. These infants often develop a scaly, itchy skin rash called eczema or atopic dermatitis.

The presence of food allergy or eczema before three months of age places the infant into a higher risk group for developing asthma. The first hint of asthma is wheezing or chest congestion during a respiratory infection. Most milk and egg food allergies are outgrown by age four or five, only to be replaced by the development of allergies to inhaled allergens such as dust mites, molds, household pets and pollens. The exception to this food allergy scenario is the young child with peanut or tree nut allergy, which can persist for years or a lifetime.

A United Kingdom study in Wales followed 440 infants from birth to age seven. Infants destined to become allergic asthmatics were different in several ways. They had more egg allergy, eczema and high serum IgE levels in infancy. The onset of egg allergy before six months of age was a very sensitive marker for the future development of asthma and other allergic problems. Whether allergy to eggs influences the development of future allergies or is simply a signal of things to come is not known. Additional risk factors for asthma in these young infants included maternal smoking and exposures to high levels of dust mites. Animal allergen exposure is widespread throughout the world.

One Swedish study that looked at the association between dog and cat allergy in young children with asthma found that exposure to cats, especially in children under age four, greatly increased the chances of developing asthma. Another study found this risk was highest in damper homes where cats resided. The risk of asthma from exposure to cat allergen appears to be augmented by exposure to cigarette smoke. Preliminary results of the CAMP or National

Childhood Asthma Management Program have shown that skin test sensitivity to dog or cat allergen increases the likelihood of asthma. When confronted with an infant or young child with food allergy, eczema or asthma, I strongly advise the parents not to introduce pets, especially cats, into the home even if the child is not yet allergic to animals.

Do environmental controls and dietary precautions by the mother during pregnancy or while breastfeeding prevent the development of asthma or asthma in their offspring? Several investigators have attempted to answer this difficult question. Doctor Robert Zeiger of San Diego divided high-risk families and their mothers into a prevention and a control group. The mothers in the prevention group avoided allergenic foods during pregnancy and while breastfeeding. They were asked to eliminate pets and institute strict dust mite controls within their home. The control group made no changes in their diet or lifestyle. While the incidence of food allergy and eczema was much lower in the prevention group in infancy and early childhood, the rate of allergy and asthma was the same in both groups by age four. While maternal environmental precautions and avoidance of allergenic foods lowered the incidence of food allergy and eczema in early childhood, these measures did not prevent children from eventually developing allergies or asthma later on in childhood.

It is fairly easy to identify those infants who may develop true asthma later on in childhood. The high-risk children have food (egg or milk) allergy or eczema at an early age (before age three), a family history of asthma or allergy, smoking mothers and high levels of IgE antibody or eosinophils. Is allergy skin testing of any value in early infancy in these children? One myth perpetuated by pediatricians and family physicians is that infants and young children with eczema or food allergy are too young to undergo skin tests, as skin tests are not very reliable at this age group. Nothing could be further from the truth.

Skin testing is an easy and reliable way to pick out those youngsters at risk to develop additional allergies or asthma. Why do allergy skin tests in an infant or a young child who has had an obvious reaction to milk or eggs? When the clinical history is consistent with a food reaction, I may not test for that specific food. The main reason to do limited skin tests to other foods and allergens in this age group is that you may uncover unidentified allergies and implement preventive dietary and environmental precautions. The other reason for skin tests in this age group is to rule out allergy and minimize unnecessary and sometimes expensive environmental precautions. I frequently encounter young children with negative skin tests whose parents have already removed family pets and have spent hundreds of dollars on unnecessary environmental precautions within the home.

## Late-childhood Asthma

Sometimes asthma may not begin until late childhood. Australian investigators found that asthma that starts in the early school years which they labeled, infrequent episodic asthma or transient wheezing, had an excellent prognosis. Wheezing episodes during viral infections that began after age three were rarely troublesome. Nearly 50 percent of Australian children in this study stopped wheezing by the age of 10, and very few had persistent asthma in adulthood.

A study in Aberdeen, Scotland, looked at three groups of adults who had asthma and wheezing as schoolchildren: those who had doctor-diagnosed asthma in childhood, those whose parents reported wheezing only in the presence of a cold and those who had no respiratory symptoms whatsoever. Subjects with doctor-diagnosed asthma in childhood were 14 times more likely to wheeze, and seven times more likely to be using asthma medication and have decreased lung function as adults. The outlook for children who only wheezed with colds was much better than for those who had allergen-induced asthma. As adults their symptoms were mild and did not usually interfere with normal life, and their lung functions were normal.

This Scottish study suggests that the transient wheezing syndrome during the early school years is quite different from that in children with persistent asthma. The transient wheezers do not wheeze between respiratory infections; they have negative skin tests, low IgE levels, and no eczema or food allergy. Only one in three of these children will be wheezing by age 11. On the other hand, over 80 percent of children with eczema, food allergies, positive skin tests and a maternal history of asthma were still wheezing at age 11.

The preceding discussion illustrates the complexity of the variations of asthma at different ages. It is now clear that persistent asthma is associated with a well-defined set of risk factors. Older children (aged eight to eleven years) with persistent wheezing have more severe symptoms, increased daily variability and more allergy problems. In the Australian study, early-onset asthma often predicted chronic asthma that persisted into adult life. In these patients, the most troublesome period was between the ages of eight and fourteen, when asthma symptoms persisted for months at a time. Many of these children were seldom wheeze-free. The majority were males who were highly reactive to airway challenges. Only five percent of these children were wheeze-free as adults, although boys seemed to improve more during puberty than girls. Lung function levels were significantly lower in this group when compared with those with infrequent episodic asthma or with asymptomatic controls.

More importantly, there is mounting evidence that most of the deterioration in lung function seen in older children and adults with asthma occurs in early school years. Most children who develop persistent wheezing start life with normal lung functions. By the age of six, the persistent wheezers have significant deterioration in lung function as compared with children who are wheeze-free. It appears that the persistent bronchial reactivity characteristic of chronic asthma may alter lung development during the period of fastest lung growth—between birth and age seven. Whether the poor lung function observed in these children is associated with severe asthma or is only a marker of severe asthma is unknown. It is imperative that children who fall into this high-risk group be promptly diagnosed and aggressively treated at an early age. Proper asthma treatment in the high-risk preschool child may prevent permanent remodeling or lung scarring and a lifetime of asthma.

## Adolescent-onset Asthma

When asthma begins in adolescence, the outlook is not so rosy. Adolescent-onset asthma is more common in girls and is likely to be a non-allergic form of asthma with less chance of a remission, especially in females. A survey in the Mississippi River Valley looking at junior high and high school students found that 16 percent had asthma. Girls had more asthma than boys, and their asthma was more severe than that found in the male students. The risk of developing Samter's Triad (asthma, nasal polyps and aspirin allergy) is also higher in this age group. Young adults with asthma pose a special challenge to asthma care providers. Adolescent-onset asthma is often quite severe and can be difficult to control. The teenage years can be a bumpy road on the path to adulthood. Peer pressures and a desire not to be different lead to non-compliance and disease denial on the part of young adults with asthma. Near-fatal and fatal asthma attacks are more common in young adults than children. Many of the errors in care by these patients include overuse of rescue inhalers, failure to take anti-inflammatory medicine on a regular basis, smoking and disregard of environmental controls. Special educational efforts are needed to ensure compliance with medication programs and identification and avoidance of asthma triggers. Adolescents should be encouraged to take charge of their asthma action plans.

## Will My Child Outgrow Asthma?

One of the more commonly asked questions by parents of asthmatic children is, "Will my child outgrow asthma?" I used to tell parents that it was a coin toss—one-third outgrew their disease, one-third got better and one-third did not improve. New epidemiological studies offer a more promising outlook for childhood asthma. The majority of children below three years of age who only wheeze with respiratory infections stop wheezing by mid-childhood. Among 2,345 children in the United Kingdom who wheezed before five years of age, 80 percent were wheeze-free by age 10. The more wheezing episodes before age five, the less chance the child had of outgrowing asthma. Ninety-two percent of children with one wheezing episode by age five were symptom-free at age 10. In contrast, only 60 percent of children with more than 10 episodes of wheezing were symptom-free at age 10.

Long-term follow-up studies suggest that most children with asthma improve during adolescence, and up to 50 percent are wheeze-free in adulthood. Nevertheless, about 80 percent of symptom-free young adults still have evidence of a twitchy lung or bronchial reactivity and may redevelop asthma at any time in adulthood. Thus, having childhood asthma significantly increases one's risk of redeveloping asthma as an adult, especially if the first attack occurred after age two or if there were more than 10 attacks during childhood. Additional factors that predict adult asthma are being female, a history of eczema or food allergy, low lung functions, smoking mothers, and a parental history of asthma.

## Recurrent Croup and General Anesthesia

Two additional conditions that are risk factors for childhood asthma are repeated bouts of croup and exposure to general anesthesia. Many children experience recurrent croup throughout childhood. Some of these children are seven to eight years of age, well beyond the classic age for croup. I have had some personal experience with this problem, as my oldest daughter, whose twin brother has asthma, had numerous episodes of croup up until age twelve. I never really associated croup with asthma, but it appears that some croupy children have a different form of asthma that only affects their large airways. A study in Belgium found that a high percentage of children with asthma had recurrent croup. The Belgian investigators found a strong association between a positive family history of asthma and croup. If recurrent croup is indeed a unique form of asthma, the good news is that most children will outgrow it as my daughter did. Doctor Douglas Johnestone of Rochester, N.Y., reported that children subjected to general anesthesia at a young age had a much greater chance of developing asthma. This paper was of particular interest to me. My oldest son, who developed asthma at age four, underwent a rather difficult hernia repair at age two that required nearly two hours of general anesthesia.

## Role of Parents and Caretakers

In the days before sophisticated asthma therapy became a reality, parents and caretakers of children with asthma simply administered a quick-relief inhaler or an oral asthma medication and hoped for the best. When the child did not improve, they would seek additional help from their primary care doctor, asthma specialist or local emergency room. The availability of more complex asthma-care programs mandates that parents and all caretakers of children assume a more responsible role in managing asthma. The fundamental role of parents and caretakers is education and time. Parents and all caretakers of children with asthma must avail themselves of the wide range of educational materials available for asthma care, and they must devote the time it takes to care for a child with asthma. This concept becomes more problematic when children are being raised in alternative family structures, including the divorced or single parents, the commuter parent and stepparents.

Doctor Mary I. Enzman-Hagedorn has found that parental responsibilities are more burdensome in alternative family structures versus the traditional two-parent family. In divorce situations where the parents are maintaining two homes, the division of the child's time may lead to significant stress. It becomes necessary to institute environmental controls in two households instead of one. A lonely single parent often seeks companionship from a dog or cat, which poses an obvious problem for the pet-allergic child. Financial problems, coupled with the need to maintain a full-time job and care for a child with a chronic illness, may overwhelm single or working parents.

Asthma can be a time-consuming and exhaustive illness, especially for working parents who have to commute long distances to work or who travel a great deal. The unpredictable nature of asthma leads to a buildup of fear, guilt and anxiety. Disrupted family structures often lack a comprehensive plan for asthma control. At-risk families must learn as much as possible about controlling asthma. This includes being able to identify warning symptoms, understanding asthma triggers and asthma medications, and having a sound asthma action plan to put into place when asthma relapses occur. Clinic and office-based nurses play a key role in presenting educational programs to patients and their families.

Many families with asthmatic children become housebound because of their inability to transfer the care of a child with asthma to responsible babysitters. Everyone needs a break in their daily activities, and a housebound approach is detrimental to the overall psyche and well-being of the entire family. Asthma education programs should involve all caretakers of the child. The following set of guidelines was developed by the American Lung Association to help responsible parents be comfortable leaving the care of an asthmatic child to caretakers or babysitters:

- Use babysitters who will follow directions and comply with a simple asthma action plan.
- The babysitter does not have to be an expert in asthma care.
- Do not employ smoking babysitters.
- Provide proper training and education, including a list of asthma medications and asthma triggers to avoid.
- Babysitters must know how to administer medications, especially when younger children require nebulizers.
- Encourage the babysitter to treat your child no differently than other children.
- Provide a written asthma action plan that includes where parents can be contacted and emergency phone numbers of your doctor and local hospital.

## The School and Asthma

Asthma is the chronic illness that is the leading cause for school absenteeism. Nearly six million schoolchildren have asthma, and lost school days number over five hundred thousand each year. The following section provides a guide for school personnel to develop and maintain an asthma management program in their school. Any school asthma program should

- Provide an equal opportunity for a normal learning experience.
- Not allow students to feel sickly or different.
- Allow participation in all physical activities up to the student's physical capacity.
- Reduce school absences and disruption in the classroom.
- Guarantee medical support during acute attacks of asthma.

Effective school asthma management programs require a partnership between the student, parents or guardians, health-care providers and all members of the school staff. Any successful program must coordinate school procedures for administering medication and follow an asthma action plan for each child with asthma that contains a complete list of asthma medications, their doses and a course of action to be followed during an acute attack including emergency procedures and key telephone numbers. The specific roles of the school staff are outlined below.

## The School Nurse

The school nurse is the team captain and plays the leading role in developing a health-care plan for students with asthma which coordinates between the student, parents, teachers, coaches and gym instructors. The school nurse should

- Meet with parents to assess asthma triggers in the home environment. If students have not been tested for allergies or the family has a poor concept of environmental controls, parents should be advised to see their health-care provider or consult an allergy specialist.

- Review the student's asthma treatment program and action plan and be sure the student uses inhalers properly. Students who appear fatigued during the school day should be checked for nocturnal asthma symptoms that may be interfering with sleep.

- Monitor early warning signs of unstable asthma and follow these patients with peak flow meters.

- Assume responsibility for educating teachers and physical education instructors about allergy and asthma.

- Take responsibility to minimize the exposure to allergens or irritants in the students' classroom and ensure they follow specially prescribed diets in the school cafeteria. Students with peanut or tree nut allergy require extra supervision, as most near-fatal or fatal allergic reactions to peanuts and nuts occur in asthmatic patients outside the home.

- Allow students to use asthma medicines, and permit students to self-medicate when fully authorized by parents and the physician.

- Stay in close contact with physical education instructors to ensure fair grading for students with allergies and exercise-induced asthma.

## The Classroom Teacher

The classroom teacher who spends most of the day with students is in the best position to observe the student's daily progress from a health and educational standpoint. The classroom teacher should

- Be provided with information and educated about asthma and the side effects of asthma medications.

- Inform the school nurse and parents if the student has a significant deterioration in school performance or develops behavioral problems.

- Keep the classroom relatively dust-free and not allow furry or feathered animals in the students' environment.

- Be prepared to handle an acute asthma attack.

- Allow the student extra time to make up missed work or exams due to absences.

- Treat the student as a normal human being and provide a normal learning experience.

- Minimize chalk dust exposure by using a wet cloth or sponge, not an eraser, to clean blackboards.

- Be aware that asthma is a very treatable condition.

One role of the classroom teacher may involve environmental control. Emerging evidence implies that exposure to animals, especially cat allergen, in the classroom can trigger asthma in students who do not have cats in their home. Segregating cat owners from non-cat owners may lower the exposure to cat-allergic asthmatics and decrease asthma symptoms. Simply seating the cat-allergic child away from students who have cats at home may prevent cat-induced wheezing in the school classroom. In day care or nursery settings where children spend a lot of time playing on the floor or in traditional classroom settings, removing or limiting allergen-laden carpeting may be helpful.

## *The Coach and Physical Education Instructors*

Physical education instructors and coaches have a unique opportunity to impact the life of a student with asthma by encouraging active participation in gym and sports activities. All too often I have encountered well-intentioned, but poorly informed, physical education instructors and coaches who turn promising athletes with asthma into couch potatoes by limiting their participation in strenuous activities. Physical education instructors and coaches should

- Be provided with education detailing the telltale signs and symptoms of asthma and allergic conditions.

- Permit and encourage the student to participate in regular physical activities.

- Notify parents if the student cannot fully participate in gym. Do not allow the student to stop taking gym classes unless so directed by a doctor.

- Allow for a reduction in outdoor activities during cold weather or periods of air pollution. Excuse the student from classes if he or she has significant asthma symptoms.

- Attempt to determine the child's physical limitations. Encourage the child to function within those limits.

- Do not force the student to exceed his or her limitations, such as running laps outdoors on a cold day, when such activity is likely to trigger asthma. Encourage warm-up activities and exercises.

- Become familiar with exercises that are best tolerated by the student with asthma.

- Allow the student to set his or her pace on a daily basis.

- Permit the student to take the prescribed asthma drugs before or during exercise, including after-school activities like games or practices, with no inconvenience.

## The School Administrator

The school administrator must ensure that the school has an ongoing asthma management program. Responsible school administrators should

- Ensure that the student has a safe environment, free of allergens or air pollutants. Whenever possible, new school construction and maintenance projects should be done during vacation periods or after school hours. The new studies on animal allergens in the school setting suggest that classroom carpeting should be avoided.

- Require the school nurse to keep up-to-date medical records and provide education classes for all other school personnel.

- Allow the asthmatic student to be bused, especially on colder winter days when walking to and from school may trigger an asthma attack.

- Prevent discrimination by coaches, phys-ed instructors or classroom teachers which would interfere with the student's learning experience.

- Develop a concise policy on the use of medications during school hours in gymnasiums and after school hours on playing fields.

As children and young adults spend a large part of their lives in a classroom, school personnel have a dramatic impact on the treatment of asthma. The Asthma and Allergy Foundation of America (AAFA) has developed an Asthma Action Card for asthma. These AAFA cards allow the physician and the family to provide clear concise information on triggers, prevention and emergency treatment. This card outlines the patient's basic allergies and common asthma triggers, and lists a medication plan that utilizes peak flow readings. In the opinion of many school nurses in the National Association of School Nurses, the size of the asthma and allergy population in schools is increasing.

In a survey in Los Alamos, California, nearly 20 percent of students were thought to have health problems related to asthma or allergic diseases. A school nurse survey by the Asthma and Allergy Network (AAN-MA) uncovered a significant need for improving the health and educational process of children with asthma and allergies. Responders indicated that children experienced some degree of embarrassment surrounding the use of asthma medications. Many schools lacked full-time nurses, and only a few schools had a peak flow monitoring program. The AAN-MA report pointed out that schools should allow children with asthma to have access to medications, receive appropriate medical assistance during a relapse and have freedom from the embarrassment generated by the need to take asthma medications.

## Inhalers in the School

One of the major problems encountered by a student with asthma is that many schools do not allow them to carry their own asthma medicines or inhalers and assume responsibility for their own care. The most frequent indication for an asthma medicine in the school setting will be exercise-induced asthma. When a school prohibits the student with asthma from self-medicating with an asthma inhaler, the student must then go to the school office or nursing station before or after a gym class or exercise period to get the inhaler to prevent or relieve exercise-induced asthma. This is both an embarrassment and a great inconvenience for the student. In large schools, the gym class may be completed by the time the student returns from the nursing office. Under such circumstances, most asthmatic students will only go to the school office or the nursing station in an emergency situation. Not only is this unfair, it is a violation of one's rights, as the student is being deprived of his or her basic rights to fully participate in everyday school activities.

The Drug Committee of the American Academy of Allergy, Asthma & Immunology studied this problem and published a position statement that encourages schools to allow responsible students of any age to keep inhalers in their possession and assume responsibility for self-management with asthma inhalers.

## *Preparing the Student for the School Year*

A report by The Allergy and Asthma Network-Mothers of Asthmatics nicely outlines the appropriate steps to take to approach asthma in the school setting. Proper communication and information sharing is the best way to minimize parental concerns, and teacher and student apprehension and fear. Parents should meet with the school nurse, teachers or administrators before the school year begins. If the child has food allergies, the cafeteria manager should be included. The important topics to discuss in such a meeting include

- The student's allergy and asthma medical history.
- The goal of any treatment plan.
- How to identify and handle emergencies.
- How to use allergy and asthma medications.
- How to use spacers, peak flow meters and EpiPen.
- Who to contact during the school day.
- The student's ability to self-medicate.
- A list of food allergies and asthma triggers.
- A plan to make up missed school work.

Every once in a while I confront parents who are having problems with school personnel who usually through ignorance discriminate against their asthmatic children by keeping pets in the classroom, not allowing them to make up missed work or examinations, excluding them from athletic or gym activities or prohibiting self-medication by responsible students. These problems are usually solved when administrators, teachers or gym instructors are reminded that students with asthma are protected by federal law under section 504 of the Rehabilitation Act of 1973, the Individuals with Disabilities Education Act.

Parents whose children do not receive proper support from school authorities should inform them that they plan to file a formal complaint with the state department of education or the regional office of the United States Department of Education-Office for Civil Rights. In my experience this approach solves most, if not all, discriminatory problems in the school setting.

## *When the Student Leaves Home*

When the asthmatic student leaves home for the first time to attend school or college or to travel, special steps need to be taken to build a solid foundation for asthma self-management. The departing student, who will be independent for the first time in his or her life, should have a sound grasp of the fundamentals of asthma therapy. He or she should know how to use medications and when to seek additional care for acute asthma.

The student's physician or asthma doctor should prepare a summary of the student's medical history and a current list of medications that allows school health-care providers unfamiliar with the student's medical background to follow an asthma treatment program. The student's doctor should also write a letter to school housing authorities requesting non-allergenic bedding, non-smoking roommates and air-conditioned dormitories. Many boarding schools and colleges are situated in remote, rural areas where competent asthma care may not be readily available. The student should be encouraged to communicate by phone with parents or doctors during an asthma flare-up.

As many students tend to neglect their medications and environmental controls during their first semester, I usually schedule a brief follow-up visit during a vacation period to make sure they are following their treatment program. Many parents, including me, have noted that school dorms or apartments are potential dust bins. Fortunately, they often have less carpeting and upholstered furniture and no exposure to dogs or cats. Therefore, many dust-mite and pet-allergic students experience dramatic improvement during their first few months away from home. Some students are able to stop daily asthma medications once they move from their dust-mite- and pet-allergen-infested home. A severe relapse is not uncommon when they return home for the Thanksgiving or Christmas holidays. Re-exposure to a homestead with high levels of dust mites, dog or cat allergen is usually the cause of such holiday asthma relapses.

## *Key Steps for Savvy College Students*

- Whenever possible, choose an air-conditioned dormitory.
- Keep room furniture to a minimum.
- Bring your own pillow.
- Avoid dusty upholstered furniture and old rugs.
- Use dust-mite-proof covers on your mattress.
- Hot wash your bedding weekly.
- Use HEPA Air Purifiers.
- Prohibit smoking in your room.
- Keep pets out of your room.
- Keep a list of your asthma medications.
- Do not stop taking your asthma medications.
- Continue allergy shots at the school health facility.
- Get an annual flu shot.
- If needed, know where to find an asthma specialist.

# Asthma
## in
# **Women**

# **22**

here is a gathering body of evidence that age and sex strongly influence the risk for developing asthma. In early puberty the sex ratio of asthma gradually evens out with the incidence of asthma increasing among girls and catching up with the rate of asthma in boys. In later adolescence or in young adulthood the pendulum dramatically shifts with asthma becoming more common and more severe in women—a pattern that persists throughout adulthood. In a Tucson, Arizona, study, the incidence of adult-onset asthma was twice as common in females versus males. This sexual trend is most pronounced in women over 40. There is a wide gender disparity in the severity of asthma at various ages. Young boys (under age 10) are twice as likely as girls of that age to require hospitalizations, whereas adult women are three times more likely than men to be hospitalized. Adult women are hospitalized for longer periods of time, and are more prone to near-fatal and fatal asthma episodes. The reasons for this striking difference in the incidence and severity of asthma in adolescent and adult women are poorly understood. The possibilities include genetic factors, hormonal imbalances and increased exposure to indoor allergens.

## *Premenstrual Asthma*

Hormonal factors undoubtedly play a key role in asthma. Up to 40 percent of asthmatic women experience an increase in their asthma symptoms prior to and during their menstrual period. One emergency room survey found that four times as many women sought emergency room care before or during their menstrual cycle. The authors of this paper speculated that a rapid decline in circulating estrogen prior to menses predisposed women to an asthma relapse. Conflicting reports have found that hormonal replacement both improves and worsens asthma. Thus, at this time it is impossible to make any recommendations on the use or nonuse of hormone replacement therapy in postmenopausal women with asthma. Until clinical trials prove that premenstrual asthma is a significant problem, conventional therapy is recommended in the premenstrual state. On the other hand, if a woman has frequent asthma relapses in the premenstrual cycle, asthma medications could be started or stepped up during this period.

## *Asthma and Pregnancy*

Asthma may be the most common medical problem that occurs during pregnancy. One in every 10 pregnancies is complicated by asthma. What happens to women with asthma when they become pregnant? The standard answer to this question was one-third get worse, one-third are unchanged and one-third improve. It is rare or unheard of for labor and delivery to be complicated by acute asthma. Furthermore, most women revert to their pre-pregnancy asthma status within three months after their delivery.

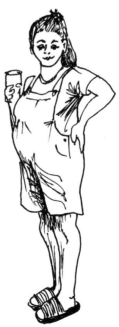

Women with mild asthma usually remain stable during pregnancy, whereas women with more moderate to severe asthma are likely to worsen. Such patients will need closer observation during pregnancy than those women with mild asthma. As asthma may increase the risk of complications for both the mother and the baby, we must determine the reasons for asthma complications during pregnancy. Poorly controlled asthma may lead to low oxygen levels, elevated blood pressure and dehydration, all of which adversely affect the mother and developing fetus. Mothers with lower lung function tests have more intrauterine growth retardation, implying that poor asthma control leads to adverse outcomes. Studies that compared asthma in pregnancy managed by asthma specialists versus non-specialists found a lower rate of mortality and low birth weight infants in patients who received specialty care.

## Risks in Pregnancy

Some of the older medical literature on pregnancy and asthma downplayed the risk asthma poses to the fetus and mother. I no longer tell my pregnant mothers not to worry. Several studies comparing outcomes in mothers with asthma to outcomes in non-asthmatic mothers reported an increase in infant mortality, premature or low birth weight, toxemia of pregnancy and high blood pressure. The risk of these complications is much higher in asthmatic mothers who smoke, especially African-American women who smoke.

Doctor Kitaw Demissie studied nearly 500,000 births in several New Jersey hospitals between 1989 and 1992. Demissie identified 2,289 asthmatic mothers and compared their pregnancy outcomes to non-asthmatic mothers. The mothers with asthma had more than three-fold greater risk of delivering a premature or low-birth-weight infant. Asthmatic mothers were more likely to have preeclampsia or high blood pressure in pregnancy, require a longer hospital stay and need a Caesarian section. The risk for congenital defects was only slightly higher in the mothers with asthma. Asthma control in these New Jersey mothers may have been less than ideal, as most mothers did not receive specialty care during pregnancy.

Asthma specialists believe that when asthma is well controlled in pregnancy, the risk for complications is minimal. This concept is supported by a report from Kaiser-Permanente's Prospective Study of Asthma During Pregnancy. In this study of 486 pregnant asthmatic women actively managed by asthma specialists, there was no increase in the incidence of preeclampsia, perinatal mortality, prematurity or congenital defects. Upper respiratory tract infections are the most common triggers of severe asthma in pregnancy. The peak incidence of asthma relapses in pregnancy occurs between the 24th and 36th week of pregnancy. Asthma usually improves during the last four weeks of pregnancy. One study that needs to be confirmed is a recent survey in Finland that found that infants delivered by Caesarian section were at more risk to develop asthma.

## Birth Defects and Asthma

Fortunately for mankind, birth defects are relatively rare. Approximately three to five percent of all children born in the United States have a developmental defect, ranging from mild deformity to severe heart defects or mental retardation. Two-thirds of all birth defects have no known cause. Only two to three percent of all birth defects are classified as teratogenic, or malformations resulting from the mother's environmental exposures.

A teratogen is any plant, food, drug or physical agent that interferes with a developing fetus and causes a congenital defect. The science of teratology started in the 1930s after pregnant pigs fed a diet high in vitamin A produced a large number of offspring with congenital malformations. The human counterpart to this pig experiment occurred in the 1950s, when the pregnancy-terminating drug, aminopterin, produced several malformed children after the drug failed to abort pregnancy. The thalidomide experience of the 1960s demonstrated that a drug that had little or no effect on the mother could produce devastating malformations in the developing fetus. This led the FDA and other regulatory agencies to institute stricter requirements for research and animal testing in new drugs before they were released for general use. It is estimated that there are three million persons living in the United States with developmental defects due to in-utero exposure to a teratogenic compound. Not all fetuses exposed to potential teratogens develop congenital defects. Genetic factors may put some infants at risk. For example, only 10 percent of the infants exposed to thalidomide developed a congenital defect. The time of exposure to a teratogen is critical. Exposure during the first trimester of fetal development is much more dangerous than exposure in later stages of pregnancy. Although relatively few asthma drugs have been proven to be harmful in pregnancy, and less than one percent of congenital malformations are attributed to drugs, ethical considerations make it unlikely that any drug will ever be declared totally safe during pregnancy.

## *Drug Therapy in Pregnancy*

The principles of asthma therapy during pregnancy differ very little from the treatment in non-pregnant patients. The proper approach combines drug therapy, environmental controls and, when indicated, allergy injections or immunotherapy. There should be no holding back of drugs considered to be safe in pregnancy. The benefits of taking asthma drugs in pregnancy far outweigh the risks of uncontrolled asthma that could endanger the life of the fetus and mother.

What then are the best asthma medicines for the pregnant asthmatic? The Food and Drug Administration has divided all drugs into categories A, B and C, based on their relative level of safety during pregnancy. No asthma medication licensed by the FDA falls in the safest category A. Several drugs are listed in categories B and C. The National Asthma Education Working Group on Asthma and Pregnancy has published recommendations for preferred medications in pregnancy. The tendency is to use older, more proven medications that have a longer track record than the newer asthma drugs. The Asthma Education Working Group recommended that pregnant and breastfeeding mothers avoid the following drugs:

- Alpha-adrenergic compounds (except pseudoephedrine)
- Epinephrine (except in anaphylaxis)
- Iodides
- Sulfonamides

- Tetracyclines
- Quinolones

Asthma medications preferred for use during pregnancy are the following:

- Inhaled beta-agonists (no specific one was endorsed)
- Terbutaline when systemic beta-agonist therapy is required
- Theophylline
- Cromolyn sodium (Intal)
- Vanceril, Beclovent, Q-VAR, Pulmicort
- Prednisone or prednisolone

Several new asthma medications, including salmeterol (Serevent), nedocromil (Tilade), the leukotriene modifiers and many potent inhaled cortisone drugs have become available since the Working Group completed its report. Animal studies with nedocromil have been reassuring (FDA Category B), while those with salmeterol have not (FDA Category C). There is no solid data in pregnancy on the leukotriene modifiers. Most asthma specialists prefer the shorter-acting, beta-agonist drugs like terbutaline (Brethine), or albuterol during pregnancy. Terbutaline is commonly used to control premature labor, and the doses used in premature labor have not increased the incidence of congenital malformations.

When an inhaled cortisone drug is needed during pregnancy the drug of choice is now budesonide (Pulmicort Turbuhaler). In January 2002, data from Sweden prompted the FDA to upgrade the pregnancy rating for budesonide (Pulmicort Turbuhaler) to Category B—making it the first and only inhaled cortisone drug to receive this rating. The FDA based this labeling change on data that looked at more than 2,000 pregnancies in Sweden from 1995–1997 that found no increased risk for congenital malformations when budesonide was administered during early pregnancy—the period when most major organ malformations can occur. This drug is also the only inhaled cortisone drug with a once-a-day dosing indication for children and adults with mild to moderate asthma.

The data on oral cortisone use in pregnancy is not encouraging. Pregnant women who took oral cortisone drugs had more pregnancy complications. Again, it is believed that the complications in pregnancy were due to the severity of the asthma and not the oral cortisone. In cases of severe asthma, the benefit of oral cortisone for the mother and baby far outweighs the risks of severe asthma. While theophylline has generally been considered to be safe in pregnancy, a recent report on asthmatic women who took theophylline throughout pregnancy raises some concerns. Three pregnant women who used theophylline and beta-agonist inhalers delivered children with severe congenital heart defects. Studies in chick embryos have shown that high doses of theophylline can cause congenital heart defects. These recent findings suggest that theophylline should be avoided in pregnancy.

Obviously, the ideal drug therapy during pregnancy is no therapy, especially during the first three months of pregnancy when the likelihood of fetal malformation is greatest. However, no matter what is done, remember that three to five percent of all pregnant women will deliver an infant with a birth defect and two-thirds of the time the cause of the birth defect is unknown. Several prospective studies are underway to determine the safety of asthma drugs during pregnancy. Many of these studies will be the first to look at pregnancy outcomes on a prospective basis. GlaxoSmithKline has developed a registry program to evaluate the effects of several drugs during pregnancy. Drugs used for common conditions like migraine headaches, antiviral therapy and anti-epileptic medication will be evaluated. This laudable effort may help to pinpoint those drugs that cause birth defects. The American College of Allergy, Asthma & Immunology has established a registry for pregnant asthmatics to gather more information to enable physicians to choose safe and effective asthma medications during pregnancy.

What about allergy testing and allergy injections during pregnancy? Allergy tests should be postponed until pregnancy is completed. There is a small risk that allergy testing might trigger an allergic reaction which in turn could provoke premature labor. Allergy injections or immunotherapy is safe during pregnancy in experienced hands. One study of 121 pregnancies in 90 women receiving immunotherapy found no increase in perinatal complications in treated patients versus a non-treated control group. It is recommended that allergen immunotherapy be continued during pregnancy in patients who have reached a maintenance dose. I recommend a dose reduction to minimize the risk of a systemic reaction. No competent allergist or asthma specialist would recommend starting allergy injections during pregnancy.

In 1993, the National Asthma Education and Prevention Program established the Working Group on Asthma and Pregnancy. Twelve physicians from various specialties recommended the following integrated asthma and obstetric management program:

- Periodic lung function tests to detect early warning signs of relapsing asthma. This can be accomplished by home monitoring with peak flow meters and in-office assessment with spirometry. The group emphasized the need for fetal monitoring, including ultrasound and daily kick counts to evaluate fetal activity.

- Avoidance of asthma triggers is extremely important during pregnancy, as appropriate environmental controls reduce the need for asthma medications and acute care visits for asthma.

- Ongoing allergy injections can be continued in pregnancy, but allergy injections should not be started during pregnancy.

- Stepwise drug therapy with a careful step-up and step-down approach as discussed in the section on asthma guidelines.

## The Eight-Step AAFA Asthma Plan

The Asthma and Allergy Foundation of America (AAFA) published The Eight-Step Asthma Plan in 2000 that concisely summarizes the proper approach to asthma in pregnancy.

**Step 1:** Form a strong team between your primary care provider, asthma specialist and your obstetrician. Be sure all health-care providers know about your asthma and your pregnancy.

**Step 2:** Keep taking your asthma medications. Avoid all other medications. Be sure to discuss all medications with your team of doctors or nurses. Know which medications to avoid during pregnancy.

**Step 3:** Continue your regular allergy shots. Do not start allergy shots or increase doses during pregnancy.

**Step 4:** Get a flu shot and try to avoid people, especially young children, who have repeated respiratory infections. Frequent hand washing may ward off unwanted viral infections.

**Step 5:** Aim for good control of your asthma every day. Keep a journal of your peak flow readings and use of asthma medications.

**Step 6:** Monitor, monitor, monitor! When asthma is unstable, use your peak flow meters daily. Your doctors should also check your breathing capacity on a regular basis with a spirometer, as peak flow readings may not always portray a true picture of your lung functions. Ultrasound and fetal heart rate monitoring will follow your baby's progress.

**Step 7:** Avoid asthma triggers, irritants and allergens.

**Step 8:** Do not smoke and avoid people who do. If you do smoke, make every effort to stop. Remember those infants exposed to passive smoke or born to smoking mothers have lower birth weights and are three times more likely to die from Sudden Infant Death Syndrome.

Leaders from several agencies, including the FDA, NIH and the pharmaceutical industry have held workshops to review the issues of asthma in pregnancy. They summarized the medical literature and asked the question, "How does the course of asthma change during pregnancy?" The one message that came through loud and clear is that mothers with moderate to severe asthma need to be followed at regular intervals during their pregnancy by both their obstetrician and an asthma specialist. Patients with moderate to severe asthma should undergo fetal ultrasound and fetal heart rate monitoring at appropriate intervals. It is also important that asthma medications be available in the labor and delivery suite. Both the obstetrician and the anesthesiologist should be prepared to treat an asthma relapse.

In summary, the main goals of asthma management during pregnancy should include prevention of asthma episodes that interfere with sleep or normal activity, maintenance of optimal lung function and avoidance of adverse drug effects, thereby enabling the normal birth of a healthy infant. Educational efforts should emphasize appropriate inhaler technique, recognition of symptoms and signs of relapsing asthma, and teaching patients when to seek medical care. Optimal patient education should maximize patient compliance. Allowing the patient to express her concerns can reduce stress associated with asthma. One must reassure the pregnant mother that outcomes in properly managed asthma are not significantly different from outcomes in non-asthmatic women.

## Breastfeeding and Asthma

The concerns of the asthmatic mother do not end with delivery if she decides to breastfeed her baby. Mothers with allergic asthma should be encouraged to breastfeed, as breastfed infants are less likely to develop eczema, food allergy or asthma in infancy and early childhood. Even though 10 percent of any drug she takes ends up in her breast milk and is ingested by her baby, there is usually little or no risk to the feeding infant.

One drug that may be troublesome in breastfed infants is oral theophylline. Small amounts of theophylline transferred by breast milk may cause the infant to become irritable or jittery. When such irritability persists, the mother should stop taking theophylline. Inhaled beta-agonist and cortisone drugs have been a boon to nursing mothers, as only trace amounts of these inhaled drugs end up in the mother's breast milk. Nursing mothers who require oral cortisone (prednisone) on a daily or alternate-day basis to control severe asthma should not breastfeed.

Does breastfeeding prevent the development of eczema, food allergies or asthma? There are conflicting responses to this important question. Controlled trials of breastfeeding can be criticized for a variety of reasons, including inadequate duration of breastfeeding, lack of environmental controls or maternal diet, small sample size and early introduction of solid foods. The theoretical benefits of breast milk derive from the transfer of maternal antibody that protects the infant from bacterial and viral illnesses. More importantly, breastfed infants avoid the ingestion of sensitizing foods like eggs or cow's milk. A *British Medical Journal* report urged pregnant women with a family history of asthma or allergic disorders like hay fever and eczema to avoid eating peanut products during pregnancy or while breastfeeding. Ingestion of such foods during pregnancy or while breastfeeding may sensitize the fetus or newborn to peanut allergen. I recommend that infants who have eczema, egg or milk allergy, asthma or a strong family history of allergy avoid peanut and tree nut products until their third birthday.

Older data suggests that breastfeeding forestalls but does not prevent the onset of asthma or allergic diseases later on in childhood. Newer studies suggest breastfeeding may be permanently protective. Doctor Wendy Oddy believes breastfeeding for four months may prevent childhood asthma. Oddy followed 2,187 Australian children from birth to age six and found that infants who were breastfed for more than four months were less likely to have asthma at age six. Oddy speculated that breastfeeding might modify the immune system and divert it down the non-allergy-asthma Th1 pathway. A long-term study of children in Tucson, Arizona, found that breastfeeding protected against asthma, but only in those infants who had no other allergic problems. Thus, until additional studies are completed, the questions revolving around the protective effects of breastfeeding remain unresolved. In my opinion the scale tips in the direction of protection from asthma and other allergic diseases. Thus, when given the opportunity, I strongly advise all pregnant mothers to breastfeed, especially if they have a strong family history of asthma or other allergic diseases.

# **Adult**
## Asthma

# 23

hile most victims of asthma develop the disease in early childhood, many people start to wheeze in adulthood for the first time in their lives. This form of asthma is called adult-onset asthma. When I first encounter a new patient with adult-onset asthma, I closely question them about their health in childhood. At first, many deny having any asthma during childhood, but on closer questioning they often recall being allergic or "bronchial" during their childhood. To me this suggests that they had undiagnosed childhood asthma that went into remission for several years. Another important variable to look at in adult-onset asthma is the history of exposure to environmental tobacco smoke. Adults with bronchitis or chronic lung disease due to exposure to environmental tobacco smoke are often mislabeled as having asthma.

## *Adult-onset Asthma*

Adult-onset asthma is quite different from childhood asthma. There is often no association with family history, hay fever, eczema or food allergies. The typical case of adult-onset asthma in a non-smoker often begins with a simple respiratory infection that evolves into a bronchitis-like illness that never clears up. Coughing and wheezing may persist for weeks, months and sometimes years before the diagnosis of asthma is entertained. This type of "post-infectious asthma" is the least understood of all forms of asthma.

When I first started practice, I thought that adults with adult-onset asthma got better with age. After following hundreds of these patients for nearly 30 years, I know that this is not the case. Only one in every five patients with adult-onset asthma experiences a significant remission. Adult-onset asthma is usually more severe and less reversible than childhood-onset asthma, especially in women who start wheezing after age 50. Many patients with adult-onset asthma experience a severe decline in lung function. In some cases this occurs soon after the onset of asthma and levels off over time. Smoking asthmatics have the most severe decline in lung function. Most studies on the prognosis or long-term outlook of asthma have focused on children and young adults. There is little solid data looking at the prognosis of adult-onset asthma. One reason that the clinical course of adult-onset is so unclear is that it is often confused with chronic bronchitis or emphysema.

Doctor Charles Reed reviewed the records of 242 Mayo Clinic asthmatics over age 65. Reed found that the majority of elderly patients with asthma had severe airway obstruction and many of these patients had had asthma for only a short period of time. In contrast, patients with a history of childhood asthma had better lung function and less severe disease. Adult patients with positive skin tests and an allergic component to their asthma had milder asthma than those patients with negative skin tests (so-called intrinsic asthma). What accounts for the difference in the level of severity of asthma in this older age group? Obviously, elderly asthmatics who smoke or have previously smoked have more severe asthma. Another answer may be that adult-onset asthma is more likely to cause airway remodeling, where the bronchial tubes are permanently damaged and scarred. This select group of severe adult-onset asthmatics often requires aggressive and persistent use of all four classes of asthma drugs. Many will require an oral cortisone drug to bring their asthma under control when their lung functions do not improve. More studies are needed to unravel the mysteries of adult-onset asthma.

One new and very disturbing finding in adults with asthma is that asthma sufferers may be more prone to heart disease. Kaiser-Permanente investigators in California studied the medical records of 1,062 non-smoking asthmatics. They found that active asthmatics were 32 percent more likely to have heart disease. The reasons for the higher risk of heart disease in these patients is unclear. It is possible that the inflammation in the asthmatic lung might also occur in the coronary arteries.

## Asthma in the Elderly

Throughout most of the twentieth century asthma was considered to be a disease of children and young adults. Several surveys have shown that many older adults who were diagnosed with chronic lung disease have reversible disease, which means that they have asthma. The number of individuals over age 65 is rapidly increasing worldwide. Senior citizens, who now account for one in every eight Americans, represent the fastest-growing segment of developed societies. Health surveys find that the rate of asthma is rising in this population. Nearly two million American senior citizens have asthma and another million probably have undiagnosed asthma. Elderly individuals who develop asthma are more likely to suffer from nasal polyps, sinus problems and gastroesophageal reflux disease (GERD). Like many other diseases, asthma in the elderly is often overlooked. This is ironic, as the prevalence of asthma in the United States is higher among the elderly than in all other age groups except children under age eighteen. Older women are more likely to develop late-onset adult asthma, suggesting that postmenopausal hormonal changes associated with aging may play a role in adult-onset asthma.

The signs and symptoms of asthma do not differ in older patients. Associated allergic diseases such as hay fever and eczema are less common. Asthma is widely under-diagnosed in the elderly. Physicians often label a coughing and wheezing senior citizen as having chronic bronchitis or emphysema. Undiagnosed asthma may explain why the death rate for asthma in the elderly is 10 times that of younger asthmatics. Doctor Paul Enright uncovered a large number of senior citizens with undiagnosed asthma in an ongoing Cardiovascular Health Study at the University of Arizona. Four in every 10 of these patients were not using any asthma medication whatsoever. Enright's study points out the need to improve the rate of asthma diagnosis in the elderly, and dispels the myth that asthma is a disease that rarely starts later on in life.

There are several reasons why asthma is under-diagnosed in the elderly. Physiologic changes associated with aging that can mask asthma include low lung functions, decreased mucus production and an ineffective cough mechanism. Many senior citizens feel that coughing, wheezing or shortness of breath is just part of getting old. Coexisting depression may disguise an underlying chronic disease like asthma. Another consideration is that many elderly asthmatics are "poor perceivers" of asthma. This means they do not feel any shortness of breath or chest discomfort until their lung functions are way below normal. These poor perceivers have an increased risk of fatal or near-fatal asthma due to the fact that they cannot detect mild airway obstruction. They seek treatment only when airflow obstruction is far advanced. This concept was supported by a study of survivors of near-fatal asthma, who were found to have an impaired ability to detect bronchoconstriction. Following lung function with peak flow meters becomes all that more important when treating poor perceivers with asthma. Laboratory studies in the elderly should include full lung function tests, a total eosinophil count and an allergic antibody or serum IgE test.

Should elderly asthmatics undergo allergy skin testing? I used to believe that skin testing was not always indicated in elderly asthmatics as previous studies found that only 20 percent of elderly patients with asthma had positive skin tests to aeroallergens. This picture is changing—even the elderly are becoming more allergic. Doctor Richard Huss of Johns Hopkins recently looked at 80 elderly patients with persistent asthma and found that nearly 75 percent tested positive to at least one aeroallergen. Cat was the most prevalent positive skin test, and Bermuda grass was the second most common. More than half of these patients were exposed to significant levels of dust mites and 30 percent were exposed to cockroach allergen. Nearly two-thirds had moderate to severe asthma. Yet, only two-thirds were taking inhaled cortisone drugs. Huss's study stresses the importance of diagnostic allergy skin testing in elderly asthmatics. In my recent experience a surprising number of elderly patients have unrecognized dust mite, mold or animal allergy. Thus, in my opinion, allergy skin testing is definitely indicated in all elderly patients with asthma.

## Asthma Management in the Elderly

Elderly asthmatics experience significant relief and improvement in symptoms and lung functions with proper asthma treatment. Due to coexisting diseases and complicated drug programs, asthma management in this age group becomes more complex. Asthma therapy in the elderly should focus on the individual's mental and physical capacity. Many patients will require a polypharmacy, or multiple drug, approach that includes the short-acting and long-acting beta-agonists, inhaled cortisone medications, the leukotriene modifiers or theophylline. A few elderly asthmatics will require oral cortisone drugs. Medication errors and misunderstanding of the use of medications are common in the elderly. The high costs of asthma medications and lack of insurance coverage may force elderly asthmatics to cut back on their medications or resort to less effective and more dangerous over-the-counter (OTC) medications.

Drug interactions are more of a problem in this age group, as many of these patients take additional medications for other chronic diseases like high blood pressure or heart disease. The use of metered dose inhalers is a challenge for this group, as studies have shown that only one in three elderly asthmatics correctly use their inhalers. Certain devices that can help the elderly patient to follow an asthma treatment plan include color-coded medications, daily charts, calendars and pillboxes. It is imperative that these patients receive close supervision and instruction in the use of inhalers and spacing devices. Nebulizers are a great help in administering medications when patients have trouble using metered dose inhalers. It is best to instruct senior citizens on a one-on-one basis and provide a written asthma action plan at each visit. I try to find a family member, neighbor or friend to periodically check on compliance with medication programs if an elderly patient lives alone. In some instances it is necessary to request a home visit from the local Visiting Nurse Association or an asthma educator.

## Drug Interactions

Decreased kidney and liver function associated with aging can lead to difficulty in metabolizing asthma drugs. Many elderly asthmatics require lower doses of asthma medications to reduce side effects or drug interactions that may occur with normal doses of asthma drugs.

Common side effects and drug interactions encountered in elderly asthmatics are listed below.

- High doses of inhaled beta-agonists may lower serum potassium levels, especially in patients who are taking prednisone or fluid pills. Low potassium symptoms like muscle cramps are best treated by taking extra potassium in the form of bananas, orange juice or potassium pills.

- Elderly asthmatics are more prone to easy bruising with oral or inhaled cortisone drugs. Oral cortisone drugs may also increase blood pressure.

- It is best to use the closed-mouth technique when using anticholinergic inhalers drugs like Atrovent and Combivent as these drugs may aggravate glaucoma if accidentally sprayed into the eye.

- Senior citizens are more likely to experience adverse reactions to antihistamines, including dry mouth, dizziness, bladder or prostate problems, and sedation. These reactions are minimized with the new non-sedating antihistamines.

- The use of beta blocking drugs for glaucoma, high blood pressure, and heart disease can aggravate asthma.

- Theophylline drugs lower the pressure between the esophagus and stomach, thereby aggravating gastro-esophageal reflux disease (GERD).

Elderly asthmatics should be encouraged to exercise. In my experience, one of the best forms of exercise in this age group is swimming. Many of my elderly patients have unbelievable improvement in their lung functions after joining an aerobic or active swimming program. Calcium and vitamin D help combat osteoporosis. As the need for emergency or elective surgery is more likely in elderly patients, careful preoperative evaluation is necessary. Health-care providers must be sure that both the surgeon and anesthesiologist are aware of the patient's asthma and asthma drug program. All elderly asthmatics should receive an annual flu shot and the pneumonia vaccine, Pneumovax.

# New
## Asthma
# **Guidelines**

# **24**

## *The NHLBI Reports*

**S**everal sets of guidelines for the diagnosis and treatment of asthma have been published worldwide and in the United States. What provoked a need for asthma guidelines? The alarming increase in asthma hospitalizations and mortality seen in the 1980s and 1990s is one reason. Economics is another. The United States's asthma-related, health-care expenses approached $18 billion in 2000. The last and most important reason for the dissemination of asthma guidelines is the dramatic changes in asthma therapy in past 10 years. While asthma specialists were aware of advances in asthma therapy, many primary health-care providers were not. The 1991 set of National Heart Lung and Blood Institute (NHLBI) guidelines were designed to set a "gold standard" for primary care physicians and health providers who treat asthma. This NHLBI report, an outgrowth of the National Asthma Educational and Prevention Program (NAEPP), reflected current state-of-the-art recommendations for the diagnosis and treatment of asthma.

While this report was mainly directed at primary care doctors, it benefited all health-care providers who deal with asthma, including respiratory therapists, health educators, nurse practitioners, school nurses, social workers and psychologists. The recommendations of the 1991 report were based on classifying asthma into three categories based on severity: 1) mild episodic asthma, 2) chronic moderate asthma and 3) chronic severe asthma. While such a classification seems somewhat simplistic, it serves as a blueprint that allows the health-care provider to assess the level of severity of asthma and follow a step-wise treatment plan.

Rapid changes in asthma care in the 1990s prompted the publication of a second set of guidelines in 1997. This report, entitled *NHLBI Expert Panel Report Number 2; Guidelines for the Diagnosis and Management of Asthma*, summarized the recommendations of the NAEPP program. This report stressed that under-treatment and inappropriate therapy were still the major reasons for asthma hospitalizations and asthma mortality. These guidelines, written by asthma experts who spent two years reviewing more than 5,000 scientific papers on asthma, stress the importance of early and aggressive treatment of asthma symptoms, provision of a written asthma management and action plan with patient involvement, and patient education at each visit with the health-care provider. The report is based on the premise that airway inflammation plays a critical role in asthma, and emphasizes environmental controls and patient education. The major recommendations from Expert Panel Report 2 are as follows:

- Diagnose asthma and initiate a patient partnership.
- Reduce inflammation, asthma symptoms and relapses.
- Monitor and manage asthma over time.

## The 1997 NHLBI Report

The 1997 report divides asthma into four groups on the basis of symptoms and peak flow readings.

**Mild intermittent asthma:** less than three episodes per week, less than three nocturnal asthma attacks per month and normal peak flow readings between episodes

**Mild persistent asthma:** symptoms more than twice a week, but not every day, nighttime asthma more than twice a month and variability in peak flow rates

**Moderate persistent asthma:** daily asthma requiring rescue beta-agonist drugs, nighttime asthma more than once a week and up to a 30-percent decrease in peak flow readings

**Severe persistent asthma:** continual asthma which limits activities, frequent nighttime asthma and peak flows less than 60 percent of normal readings

The 1997 report breaks asthma medications into two categories—the "relievers" and the "controllers." The relievers are the broncho-dilator drugs used to relieve acute asthma. The controllers are the anti-inflammatory medications used to control or prevent asthma over the long term. These guidelines, summarized in Figure 24.1, recommend that all patients except those with mild intermittent asthma, receive a long-term controlling medication to reduce the inflammation in the bronchial tubes.

**Treatment of Asthma Based on Severity.**

**Figure 24.1**

| | Daily Long-Term Control | Quick Relief |
|---|---|---|
| **Mild Intermittent**<br>• Symptoms 1–2 times/week<br>• Nocturnal symptoms ≤2 times/month<br>• Exacerbations brief<br>• PFTs: ≥80% predicted | None | Short-acting bronchodilator |
| **Mild Persistent**<br>• Symptoms >2 times/week<br>• Nocturnal symptoms >2 times/month<br>• PFTs: ≥80% predicted | Anti-inflammatory agent (low-dose inhaled corticosteroid or cromolyn or nedocromil) (Alternatives: sustained-release theophylline or leukotriene modifier* for patients ≥6 years old) | Short-acting bronchodilator |
| **Moderate Persistent**<br>• Daily symptoms<br>• Nocturnal symptoms >1 time/week<br>• Exacerbations ≥2 times/week; may last days<br>• PFTs: >60% and <80% predicted | Anti-inflammatory agent (low/medium-dose inhaled corticosteroid) plus long-acting bronchodilator (inhaled beta$_2$-agonist, sustained-release theophylline, or oral long-acting beta$_2$-agonist); if needed, add medium-/high-dose inhaled corticosteroid and long-acting bronchodilator | Short-acting bronchodilator |
| **Severe Persistent**<br>• Continual symptoms<br>• Frequent nocturnal symptoms<br>• Frequent exacerbations<br>• PFTs: ≤60% predicted | Anti-inflammatory agent (high-dose inhaled corticosteroid) and long-acting bronchodilator (inhaled beta$_2$-agonist, sustained-release theophylline, or oral long-acting beta$_2$-agonist) and corticosteroid tablets or syrup | Short-acting bronchodilator |

PFTs = pulmonary function tests.
*The role of leukotriene modifiers in the management of asthma has yet to be fully defined.

323

## *Step-Up Versus Step-Down Therapy*

The 1991 Expert Panel Report stated that the preferred approach to asthma management was to start with less intensive therapy and then step up the therapy as opposed to starting high and stepping down. This contrasts with the 1997 report that recommended a starting-high and then stepping-down method. Personally, I often find these guidelines to be somewhat restrictive. I prefer a middle-of-the-road approach. Some patients need to start high and then step down, while others benefit from starting low and then stepping up. The newly diagnosed patient with mild persistent asthma does not usually need to start with a higher dose of an inhaled anti-inflammatory drug, as they can be easily controlled with low or moderate doses. On the other hand, patients presenting with more moderate to severe asthma will require the more aggressive step-down approach. I will often start these patients on a short course of oral cortisone and higher doses of long-term-controlling medications in an effort to normalize lung functions. Patients with poor asthma control (nighttime wheezing, need for more rescue medications or urgent care visits) require step-up therapy. Step-up therapy may include doubling the dose of an inhaled cortisone drug, starting a short-term pulse of prednisone or adding other long-term-controlling medications like the beta-agonists and the leukotriene modifiers.

While the NHLBI Guidelines precisely outline the use of asthma medicines when the patient is coughing and wheezing, they do not tell the asthma caregiver how to fine-tune asthma medications. Once patients have stabilized, I will fine-tune or step down medications to the lowest possible dose that controls asthma. In general the last medication added can be the first to be reduced or eliminated. In other words—"last in-first out." At certain times of the year, particularly in the change of seasons, patients may require asthma medications on a daily basis, whereas at other times of the year—often mid-summer or mid-winter—some patients can revert to an as-needed schedule. These decisions are more difficult for patients with moderate asthma, whose needs can vary from day to day, week to week, season to season and year to year.

My personal approach to patients with persistent asthma who have varying needs for medications is as follows: If they are taking their asthma medications on a regular basis, say two times a day, I tell them to taper to once a day when they have been symptom-free or have normal peak flow readings for two to three months. If they are symptom-free for another month or so, they may be able to stop their medications completely and revert to an as-needed schedule.

If asthma recurs or peak flow readings fall while tapering medicines, patients (or parents) are instructed to revert to the previous medication schedule that controlled asthma symptoms or kept their peak flow readings at normal levels. When they get a chest cold or a respiratory infection, they should resume or increase their medications. In essence, I try to instruct the patients (or parents) to be their own asthma doctor. Patients and families are taught to contact their primary physician or my office in the early stages of an asthma relapse that may require antibiotics or prednisone. Not every patient or family can be handled in this manner, as self-management requires a certain level of patient motivation, judgment, asthma education and intelligence. No one should attempt to follow these directions without the advice and consent of their personal physician or asthma doctor. Sicker patients who require daily or alternate-day cortisone need to be monitored closely, preferably by an asthma specialist.

Unfortunately, some tightly controlled managed care programs prevent asthma specialists from rendering the type of care that requires several specialty visits a year. Fortunately, most of the primary care doctors I deal with will approve these extra visits when so requested. A recent study in the *British Medical Journal* (August 4, 2001) implies that doctors may be prescribing too much inhaled cortisone drugs to their asthma patients. This study looked at eight asthma studies in 2,324 asthma patients and found that 80 percent of the benefit achieved at higher doses of an inhaled cortisone drug could be obtained at much lower doses. In other words, a low dose may work just as well as a higher dose in most patients. This finding makes it even more imperative to constantly adjust patients to the lowest possible dose of inhaled cortisone that controls their asthma.

## New Pediatric Guidelines

The approach to managing asthma in children under the age of five is really no different than older children and adults. Nevertheless, separate guidelines, entitled *Pediatric Asthma: Promoting Best Practice*, for pediatric asthma were published in late 1999. These are the first set of asthma guidelines devoted entirely to the pediatric patient. This worthwhile document, developed by the Pediatric Asthma Committee of the American Academy of Allergy, Asthma, & Immunology (AAAAI), chaired by Drs. Gary Rachelefsky and Gail Shapiro, was compiled by health-care professionals in general medicine, family practice, pediatrics, allergy, pulmonary medicine, nursing, school health care and health education. The goal of this publication was to ensure that health-care providers who manage pediatric asthma learn about, understand and implement clinical and best-practice information for diagnosing and managing children with asthma. These well-referenced, user-friendly guidelines can be obtained from AAAAI or accessed from the AAAAI Web site at http://www.aaaai.org

## Treat Early and Often?

One of the dilemmas faced by doctors treating newly diagnosed asthma in young children is deciding when to start an inhaled cortisone drug. Published guidelines for young children urged the use of non-cortisone medications such as cromolyn or Intal. While this approach usually works well in children with milder asthma, it does not always control patients with moderate or severe persistent asthma. Patients have to take Intal three to four times a day, and it often takes weeks or months for Intal to take effect. This approach may not be the best way to treat early-onset childhood asthma. In the past few years, asthma specialists have learned that most of the deterioration in lung function that occurs in young asthmatic children occurs by age seven. Thus, one must ask a very important question. Would the early use of inhaled cortisone drugs in young children optimize lung function and prevent permanent lung damage? Let me explain why my answer to this question is yes.

Doctor Terri Haahtela from Helsinki, Finland, studied 103 newly diagnosed children with asthma over a two-year period. These children were assigned to two treatment groups. One group received the inhaled cortisone drug, budesonide (Pulmicort), twice a day. The other group only took an inhaled beta-agonist, terbutaline (Brethine), on an as-needed basis. After two years, children on budesonide (Pulmicort) had better peak flow rates, symptom scores and fewer asthma relapses. This study concluded that early use of inhaled cortisone resulted in greater improvement than the as-needed use of a rescue bronchodilator. A Swedish study followed two groups of asthmatic children for seven years. One group received an inhaled cortisone drug right after they were diagnosed with asthma. The other group did not use inhaled cortisone for nearly five years after they were first diagnosed with asthma. The group that used the inhaled cortisone drug early on had much better lung function than those patients whose treatment was delayed. More importantly, the delayed group never caught up to the early treatment group even after three years of treatment with an inhaled cortisone drug. These studies strongly suggest that the early use of an inhaled cortisone drug in young asthmatic children may prevent permanent lung damage later on in life.

There is no doubt that children with persistent asthma have chronic inflammation in their bronchial tubes. Likewise, there is no question that treatment with inhaled cortisone reduces or even reverses this inflammation. Thus, early intervention with inhaled cortisone drugs may be the treatment of choice in these young children with persistent asthma. Since inhaled cortisone drugs have only been available for a little more than two decades, there are no long-term studies that tell us if early use of inhaled cortisone in a four-year-old child will prevent permanent lung disease when this child reaches age 50 or 60. Some proponents of the leukotriene modifiers suggest that these drugs can take the place of the inhaled cortisone drugs in mild persistent asthma. Evolving studies will eventually answer this important question. At the present time I prefer to use an inhaled cortisone drug in all forms of persistent asthma.

How important is it to diagnose persistent asthma early in the course of the disease? Unfortunately, it is very difficult to pick out those infants and children who are at risk to develop irreversible lung damage or remodeling. One study showed that children and adults who received asthma medications and were instructed in environmental controls early on had a better chance of being symptom-free 25 years later. This study looked at 181 patients diagnosed and treated at the same asthma clinic from 1962 to 1970. These patients were then tested 25 years later. Forty percent were symptom-free, and 25 percent had normal lung functions. This survey showed that the shorter the time between diagnosis and expert asthma treatment, the less likely the person would have a reactive airway 25 years later. Milder disease at the time of diagnosis also improved the chances of being asthma-free. I believe early diagnosis and aggressive treatment may vastly improve one's chances of being wheeze-free later on in life. Let me further explain why there may be a window of opportunity in early childhood asthma where treatment with an inhaled cortisone drug may lead to a permanent asthma remission in adolescence or adulthood.

In my early years of practice in the 1970s, the pre-inhaled cortisone drug era, I treated scores of children and young adults with severe asthma. As inhaled cortisone drugs were not yet available, many of these patients only did well when they took oral prednisone on a daily or alternate-day basis. When I received a phone call from one of these patients or their parents during the evening or on a weekend, I knew that I was in for a long night. Many of these patients had labile asthma that could quickly evolve into severe, life-threatening asthma, which would require immediate hospitalization and treatment in an intensive care unit. Despite the dramatic increase in the incidence of asthma and the size of my practice, I do not encounter this type of patient as often as I did in the pre-inhaled cortisone era. At the time of this writing, none of my children or young adult patients with persistent asthma require alternate-day prednisone! In my opinion the main reason for this change in asthma severity is the availability and early use of inhaled cortisone drugs in childhood.

I have one other observation that supports this concept. I see patients of all ages with asthma. Over the past 10 years I have been impressed with a drop-off in the number of young adults in their twenties and thirties who have severe asthma. Most young asthmatic adults have mild impairment in their lung functions and show no evidence of permanent lung damage, as opposed to my older adult patients who often have poor lung functions. In other words, while like most other asthma specialists, I am seeing more young and middle-aged adults with asthma, they are not as severely impaired as older, non-smoking asthmatics in their fifties and sixties. I believe the decline in severe asthma in young adults is due to the fact they took inhaled cortisone drugs in their childhood, whereas these inhaled cortisone drugs were not available to the older generation of asthmatics earlier in the course of their disease.

## Duration of Treatment

Most patients respond to an inhaled cortisone drug within days or weeks. In moderate to severe asthma three to nine months of treatment may be required to show major improvement. Some patients require more than one year of treatment before reaching a full response. Abrupt withdrawal of a cortisone inhaler may evoke a recurrence of symptoms, usually within a month. It would appear that the need for regular inhaled cortisone therapy, once started, is likely to continue indefinitely except for those patients in whom a causative allergen or irritant can be identified in the home or workplace and then successfully avoided. One question repeatedly posed by patients or their caretakers after they have been placed on inhaled cortisone drug is, "How long will I or my child have to take this drug?" A Netherlands study looked at the effects of stopping inhaled cortisone in a group of children who had been using these drugs for nearly three years. They found that when the inhaled cortisone drug was stopped, most children rapidly relapsed to the level of asthma they had before the drug was started. Thus, the message is that inhaled cortisone drugs do not cure asthma, and long-term treatment may be necessary in patients with moderate to severe asthma.

## Lung Function Tests

One final important point needs to be made regarding the asthma guidelines. Both the adult and pediatric guidelines emphatically state that spirometry or lung function testing is the *"gold standard of asthma diagnosis and management."* Spirometry is recommended at the initial visit, after starting treatment and at least once a year after that to properly evaluate the effectiveness of asthma therapy. I wish to emphasize this critical point. In my experience, most primary health-care providers are not using spirometers in their office or clinic. Due to cost constraints, many health-care providers rely on the less expensive peak flow meters. In my opinion, relying on peak flow meters alone to assess the status of moderate to severe asthma can lead to serious errors in asthma management. I have seen scores of patients with unstable asthma who blow normal readings on their peak flow meter but have lung function or spirometry tests that are markedly abnormal. Every health-care provider who treats moderate or severe persistent asthma must monitor their patients' lung functions with a spirometer.

## Acute Asthma

Prior to 1990, most patients with acute asthma attacks were sent to emergency rooms where oxygen and X-ray facilities were available, and where blood theophylline levels, and arterial blood gasses could be done to assess the severity of the acute asthma attack. Now many patients come to their physician's office or clinic for treatment of acute asthma. There are valid reasons for this emerging trend. First, chest X-rays and blood gas studies are not needed in most cases of acute asthma. Second, acute asthma care is undoubtedly more cost-effective in a clinic or office setting. The majority of patients with acute asthma are not that seriously ill, even though many patients have been wheezing for several days or weeks before they contact their health-care provider. While modern-day emergency room physicians have the expertise and experience to competently resolve an acute asthma episode, they may not have the time to implement the asthma education programs that prevent future asthma relapses. When first evaluating an acute asthma attack in the doctor's office or clinic, it is important to assess the severity of the attack. Danger signals during an acute episode include the following:

- Severe coughing and wheezing
- Using neck and rib muscles to breathe
- Chest tightness
- Inability to talk
- Cyanosis (discoloration of lips and fingernails)

The quickest way to objectively assess the severity of an attack is to measure lung function or peak flow rates. Patients with severe wheezing, cyanosis (discoloration of lips and fingernails), an inability to talk or a previous history of life-threatening asthma should always be referred to a fully equipped emergency room. Severe asthma setbacks can be minimized or prevented when asthmatic patients and their families learn the 10 early warning signs of deteriorating asthma.

1. Excessive absence from school or work

2. Cough and wheezing unresponsive to medications

3. Wheezing with minimal exertion

4. Need for inhaler every two or three hours

5. Constant wheezing during sleep

6. Persistent high fever

7. Severe neck or chest pain

8. Persistent vomiting

9. Difficulty speaking because of wheezing

10. Cyanosis (discoloration of lips and fingernails)

The presence of one or more of these 10 early warning signs is a clear-cut sign that "out-of-control asthma" requires immediate medical attention from a primary care doctor, emergency room or asthma specialist. Additional risk factors that mandate immediate care in relapsing asthma are as follows:

- A prior history of near-fatal asthma

- A recent asthma hospitalization

- Repeated emergency room visits

- Chronic use of prednisone

- Recent withdrawal from prednisone

- A past history of fainting or seizures

- Serious psychosocial problems

## *Acute Asthma Treatment*

When an acutely ill patient is initially seen in the office or clinic, the doctor should quickly evaluate the severity of the asthma episode by noting the patient's overall appearance, listening to the chest and performing a breathing test. The doctor will order an inhalation treatment with a beta-agonist drug. Fortunately, the time-honored practice of administering repeated injections of epinephrine has given way to the more judicious modern-day nebulization or inhalation therapy with short-acting, beta-agonists like albuterol or levalbuterol (Xopenex). Patients no longer have to endure the pallor, tremors, rapid heart rates and vomiting often associated with epinephrine injections. I usually find it necessary to administer a prednisone pulse in acute asthma. I give the first day's dose in the office to avoid any delay in starting prednisone. Patients and families need be constantly reminded that proper use of their peak flow meter at home may enable them to detect an asthma relapse in its early stages and prevent a sick call or emergency room visit. Several home management techniques shown to be ineffective in acute asthma include drinking large volumes of liquid, breathing moist air or mist from a hot shower, breathing into a bag and taking over-the-counter antihistamine or cold remedies.

There are three possible responses to the treatment of acute asthma treatment with a beta-agonist—good, fair and poor. A good response is typified by mild coughing and wheezing, no use of neck or rib muscles, no symptoms at rest and the ability to climb one flight of stairs. Lung function or peak flow rates are usually 70 percent or better of baseline. A fair or incomplete response after one hour of treatment is characterized by persistent coughing and wheezing. The patient is usually alert with no cyanosis, and minimal use of neck and rib muscles to breathe. This patient may have some symptoms at rest and cannot exercise vigorously. Lung function and peak flow rates are usually between 60 and 70 percent of baseline. At this point physicians should start a pulse of prednisone. A poor response to inhaled beta-agonist means just that; severe coughing and wheezing persist, patients need to use their rib and neck muscles to breathe, they cannot speak without gasping and they have cyanosis of their lips and nails. Lung function and peak flow rates are usually less than 50 percent of baseline. These are the asthmatics that can and do die from asthma, especially when they delay seeking emergency care. Those patients who do not respond to routine office treatment should be referred to an emergency room where they may be given more inhalation treatments along with an intravenous cortisone drug. If emergency room care does not break the asthma attack, the patient will be admitted to the hospital for additional treatment. The six telltale signs that signal the need for an asthma hospitalization are the following:

- Fast heart rate and rapid respiration
- Using the neck and rib muscles to breathe
- Severe wheezing or inability to speak
- Persistent sweating
- Cyanosis of lips and fingernails
- A disturbed or confused mental state

While children and young adults are more prone to acute asthma episodes, they are also more likely to respond promptly to treatment and avoid hospitalization. Adult asthmatics coming to an emergency room with acute asthma are a different story. They can be very difficult to treat, as adults are more likely to have put off calling their doctor and seeking care. Delays in seeking care make it harder for emergency room physicians to reverse the asthma relapse. As emergency room docs are fond of saying, "The time to treat your acute asthma relapse and prevent you from being hospitalized was yesterday." When patients require a hospital stay, doctors use the term "status asthmaticus" to describe their medical condition. Once hospitalized, the patient in status is given oxygen, inhalation therapy and intravenous cortisone drugs. Most hospitalized asthmatics improve within 24 to 48 hours.

## Acute Respiratory Failure

A small percentage of patients who do not respond to in-hospital treatment develop a life-threatening condition called status asthmaticus or acute respiratory failure. In respiratory failure, the bronchial tubes are almost totally blocked. The lungs are deprived of life-sustaining oxygen and cannot eliminate the body's toxic waste gas, carbon dioxide. Picture it as a form of very slow suffocation. Machines must now take over the control of breathing. These patients are connected to a breathing machine called a ventilator. A tube is inserted into the trachea or windpipe and the respiratory muscles are deliberately paralyzed. Dials on the machine are then adjusted to deliver the proper amounts of oxygen and remove carbon dioxide. This procedure, called assisted ventilation, may continue for several days. Once the ventilated patient improves, the machine is gradually turned down, and the patient is slowly weaned from the ventilator. Thanks to the development of intensive care units devoted to respiratory care and the ready availability of critical-care doctors, assisted ventilation now has a very low complication and mortality rate. An inpatient asthma death is a very rare event in well-staffed hospitals.

Most asthma deaths now occur suddenly and unexpectedly outside of the hospital. It is my impression, and that of my pulmonary colleagues, that the overall incidence of acute respiratory failure is decreasing. Our practice used to see several asthmatic patients a year who ended up on a ventilator. Now, far fewer patients require this type of intensive treatment. More aggressive use of inhaled cortisone drugs and prompt intervention with prednisone in the early stages of relapsing asthma may be the main reasons for the decline in status asthmaticus.

## Asthma Action Plan

Our practice will often write out an asthma action plan for high-risk asthma patients (Figure 24.2). This written plan is available to the patient, family, primary physicians, school nurses, emergency rooms and any health personnel who may be involved in the care of the patient. The purpose of such a plan is to make everyone involved with the patient aware of the severity of the patient's asthma and convey the need for immediate and appropriate care should the patient suffer an asthma relapse. While it may not be necessary to carry this plan with you at all times, it should be used when traveling or visiting medical facilities unfamiliar with your asthma treatment program.

# Asthma Action Plan

**Figure 24.2**

**ADULT SELF-MANAGEMENT**
**INSTRUCTIONS for ASTHMA ACTION PLAN**

DATE: _____

**When to Monitor Peak Flow Numbers**
- ❑  In the morning soon after waking up
- ❑  Before supper
- ❑  Before bed
- ❑  Before and 5-15 minutes after inhaled treatments
- ❑  With increased respiratory symptoms
- ❑  _____

**Important Peak Flow Numbers**
Baseline _____
_____ % baseline _____
_____ % baseline _____

---

If your peak flow number drops below _____ or you notice:
- • Increased use of inhaled treatments to manage asthma
- • Awakening at night with asthma symptoms
- • Increased asthma symptoms upon awakening •  _____

**Follow these treatment steps:**
- ❑  Increase inhaled steroids
  Take _____ puffs of _____ _____ times a day
- ❑  Begin/increase treatment with oral steroids
  Take _____ mg of _____
  In the ❑ morning and/or ❑ before supper
- ❑  _____

---

If your peak flow number drops below _____ or you continue to get worse after increasing treatment according to the directions above, follow these treatment steps:
- ❑  Begin/increase treatment with oral steroids
  Take _____ mg of _____
  In the ❑ morning and/or ❑ before supper
- ❑  Contact your healthcare provider

---

Contact your health care provider *if:*
- ❑  Asthma symptoms worsen while you are taking oral steroids or,
- ❑  Inhaled bronchodilator treatments are not lasting 4 hours or,
- ❑  Your peak flow number falls below _____
- ❑  If you cannot contact your healthcare provider, go directly to the Emergency Room

---

**Directions for Resuming Normal Treatment:**
- ❑  Continue increased treatment until symptoms and peak flow number have returned to normal, then continue increased inhaled steroids or _____ mg of oral steroids for the same number of days it took to return to normal.  If your peak flow number has not returned to normal in 5 days contact your healthcare provider
- ❑  Call your healthcare provider for specific instructions

If you have questions please call:
- ❑  _____  ❑ Other _____ After hours
- ❑  Your home physician

Physician Signature _____  Date _____

Patient/Family Signature _____  Staff Signature _____

Figure 2. Asthma action plan. Data from the National Asthma Education and Prevention Program, Expert Panel Report 2.[23]

# Near-fatal and
# **Fatal Asthma**

# **25**

sthma doctors know that Oliver Wendell Holmes was dead wrong when he stated, *"Asthma is a slight ailment that promotes longevity."* Sir William Osler also erred when he wrote *"Asthmatics pant on into old age."* The extremely low asthma death rate in this era was undoubtedly the result of inaccurate statistics and poor record keeping. In 1968, investigators in England and Wales reported a sudden increase in the asthma death rate in Great Britain in the 1960s. A similar pattern was seen in Australia and New Zealand, but not in the United States or Canada. Initially, this dramatic rise in asthma mortality was attributed to overuse of metered dose inhalers in young adults. In 1981, a second epidemic of asthma deaths was observed in young New Zealanders. Confirmation of these findings spawned additional surveys that concluded that inadequate care and adverse social factors were the main reasons for the rise in asthma mortality in New Zealand.

## *The Asthma Death Alarm*

In 1984, Doctor Michael Sly reported an alarming increase in asthma mortality in the United States that started in 1979. Regional studies confirmed Doctor Sly's astute findings. An 82-percent increase in asthma mortality was reported in Washington state and Oregon. California investigators found a threefold increase in asthma deaths from 1976 to 1983. The increase in asthma deaths in California was highest in blacks, females and patients over age 55. In 1988, I reviewed asthma mortality data in Massachusetts and found a threefold increase in asthma deaths in Massachusetts from 1977 through 1986. Unlike other studies in England, New Zealand, France and Germany, there was no increase in asthma mortality in children and adults under age 65. The rise in asthma deaths in Massachusetts was concentrated in elderly females. I extended this research into the 1990s and found a twofold increase in the asthma death rate in Massachusetts between 1986 and 1994 that was most apparent in adults between 35 and 49 years of age. There was only a slight rise in asthma deaths in 15- to 35-year-olds. No increase was noted in children under age 14. Massachusetts inner-city black females were more at risk than any other group.

The lack of a physical examination or accurate medical records during fatal asthma makes it difficult to determine the triggers of these fatal episodes. In an effort to identify fatal asthma triggers, researchers have studied patients who have survived life-threatening or near-fatal asthma episodes. The terms near-fatal asthma or sudden asphyxic asthma describe such survivors. Claude Perret and his colleagues from University Hospital in Laussane, Switzerland, analyzed the characteristics of 34 patients with sudden asphyxic or near-fatal asthma who required intubation or mechanical ventilation with a respirator. Approximately one-third of Perret's patients developed severe asthma "out of a clear blue sky." After analyzing the age, sex and allergen exposures in these patients, Perret concluded that near-fatal asthma was more likely to be triggered by allergens or emotions and was more common in young men.

Another near-fatal asthma study in Argentina looked at 10 patients who required mechanical ventilation within 20 minutes of their arrival at the hospital. Nine of these 10 patients experienced sudden deterioration of their asthma. The objective of this study was to determine if an abnormal heartbeat (cardiac arrhythmia) or administration of oxygen was responsible for the sudden deterioration of asthma. The authors found that oxygen administration did not lead to respiratory arrest, and only one of the 10 patients had an abnormal heart rate. This study concluded that the near-fatal asthma was a result of severe oxygen depravation rather than abnormal heart rate, suggesting that under-treatment rather than over-treatment was contributing to near-fatal and fatal asthma.

In 1991, Doctor Mark O'Hollaren from the Mayo Clinic reported that exposure to a mold allergen was a precipitating factor in near-fatal asthma. O'Hollaren reviewed 11 patients (two of whom eventually died) who had 18 episodes of near-fatal asthma. Most patients developed acute respiratory failure within one to two hours after the onset of asthma symptoms. Four patients had seizures, although none had a prior history of seizure disorder. Ten patients had positive skin tests to the *Alternaria* mold, and all episodes of near-fatal asthma occurred during the peak of the *Alternaria* season. This was the first study to provide evidence, albeit circumstantial, that exposure to aeroallergens like an outdoor mold might be a significant risk factor for a sudden near-fatal or fatal asthma episode. Doctor Richard Ruffin of South Australia conducted a follow-up study of 45 patients with near-fatal asthma. These Australians were carefully followed at monthly intervals for one year. Near-fatal asthma was twice as common in females. There was no seasonal pattern, and more than one-third of near-fatal episodes occurred at home. The important message of this Australian study was that none of these patients died in the ensuing year, clearly pointing out the need for close assessment and frequent follow-up visits for patients who have experienced a near-fatal asthma episode.

Doctor Roy Patterson of Northwestern University recently classified 10 near-fatal asthma patients according to their psychological profiles, and specifically studied the issue of non-compliance. Patterson's patients exhibited multiple personality disorders and significant psychiatric problems, all of which resulted in a bottom line of non-compliance. The message of Doctor Patterson's report was clear. Non-compliance issues should be thoroughly addressed by health-care providers in all cases of near-fatal asthma.

Before continuing on with this rather morbid discussion of asthma deaths, I want to emphasize that even though asthma deaths are on the rise, they are very rare when one considers that millions of children and adults have asthma. Approximately 200 American children die from asthma each year, yet nearly six million children have asthma. This makes the odds of dying from childhood asthma about 30,000 to 1. The odds of dying from adult asthma are quite a bit higher, about 2000 to 1. The reason I am discussing asthma deaths in detail is not to frighten the reader, but to point out that many, if not most, asthma deaths are totally preventable. I believe the most common cause of an asthma death in children and adults is a failure by the patient or family to recognize the severity of a serious asthma attack. Doctors at the Aberdeen Royal Infirmary in Scotland found that most asthmatics that died had a very poor understanding of their asthma. Patients and their families failed to recognize the danger signs of deteriorating asthma, and delayed seeking care until they were critically ill. Studies at the Royal Hospital for Sick Children in Bristol, England, found that most of the children who died from asthma did so in the middle of the night before they reached the hospital. Tragically, the parents of these children failed to recognize the severity of the nocturnal attack, and many did not want to bother their family doctor in the middle of the night. Unlike other asthma death studies, the Bristol report did not find that asthma deaths were sudden and totally unexpected. In most cases, there was ample time to treat and save the child. The high risk of nocturnal asthma has been identified in subsequent studies. Seventy percent of all near-fatal and fatal asthma attacks occur between midnight and 8:00 A.M.

## Risk Factors for Near-fatal and Fatal Asthma

In 1985, Doctors Robert Strunk and David Mrazek, from Denver's National Jewish Hospital, reviewed the medical records of 21 patients who died after they were discharged from this world-renowned asthma center and compared them to a similar number of survivors. The profiles of the survivors were quite different from those who died from asthma. The patients who died were more likely to have severe psychological problems not found in the surviving group. As a result of their study, Strunk and Mrazek developed the following profile of the high-risk patient with asthma:

- A history of seizures associated with asthma
- A recent decrease in prednisone doses
- Wheezing at the time of hospital discharge
- A disregard of wheezing and other symptoms
- Poor self-care while in the hospital

- Conflicts with staff and parents
- Use of asthma to manipulate people
- Emotional disturbance and depression
- Severe family disruption

Thanks to Doctors Strunk and Mrazek, asthma specialists now have a specific profile of the high-risk patient, who is often an outwardly hostile, angry, rebellious or depressed patient who comes from a disrupted family. Even though it is easier to identify such patients, providing the necessary medical and psychological care needed for survival is a major challenge.

## Changing Patterns

Prior to 1970, relatively few reports depicted sudden and unexpected asthma deaths occurring outside of the hospital. Most publications on asthma mortality in this era described younger children and older adults with slowly deteriorating disease that culminated in an asthma death in a hospitalized setting. Predisposing factors to this type of asthma included severe "malignant asthma," poor medical care and adverse psychosocial factors. Improvements in emergency room and intensive respiratory care, combined with the availability of advanced pharmacological agents over the past two decades, have virtually eliminated this type of "slow onset-late arriving" asthma demise. However, despite advances in asthma care since the late 1970s, scores of publications have documented a worldwide increase in asthma morbidity and mortality. Now, the clinical features of patients who experience near-fatal or fatal asthma and the typical sites of asthma death have dramatically changed.

National and international reports describe a growing number of patients with varying levels of disease, who no longer experience slowly deteriorating asthma and die in a hospital. Patients now nearly die or die suddenly and unexpectedly at home, en route to the hospital or in public places. While several studies have documented rising asthma mortality rates in the United States, especially in American inner cities, there is a paucity of data from the United States describing the clinical characteristics of patients experiencing near-fatal or fatal asthma. Most studies on near-fatal or fatal asthma

341

come from less populated countries such as Canada, Great Britain, Australia and New Zealand, where the population is more homogenous. Such countries have more centralized data banks and case registries that simplify the collection and analysis of the characteristics of patients experiencing near-fatal or fatal asthma.

In an attempt to identify patient profiles and triggers of near-fatal and fatal asthma, I conducted a survey of asthma specialists to gather case reports and analyze the characteristics of patients experiencing near-fatal and fatal asthma. A questionnaire was distributed to 400 asthma specialists, most of whom practiced in New England. Near-fatal asthma was defined as asthma requiring out-of-hospital CPR, on-site or in-hospital intubation (putting in a breathing tube), and mechanical ventilation (using a respirator). Characteristics assessed in the survey included age, sex, race, duration of asthma, severity of asthma, lability or brittleness of asthma (history of wide swings in peak flow rates or lung function tests) and existence of other allergic diseases like allergic rhinitis, eczema, and food or drug allergy. Additional data collected included date, place and time of onset of the near-fatal or fatal episode. Respondents reported prior need for emergency room visits, hospitalizations or assisted ventilation. The survey inquired about potential clinical triggers, such as respiratory infections; oral, inhaled or injected allergens; prior medication programs; additional medical problems and use of tobacco products. Lastly, patient compliance, peak flow meter use and adverse psychosocial factors were assessed.

This survey of 400 asthma specialists gathered 25 reports of near-fatal and 20 cases of fatal asthma. The average age of those experiencing fatal asthma (22 years) was younger than that of the survivors of a near-fatal event (30 years). Equal sex distribution occurred in patients with near-fatal asthma, while deceased females outnumbered males by a four to one margin. This is a finding in agreement with an Australian study, which noted that most asthma deaths occurred in young women. Whites outnumbered non-whites in both near-fatal and fatal attacks, probably due to the fact that most respondents practiced in suburban areas. The majority of patients experiencing near-fatal and fatal asthma had other allergic diseases. Most patients in both groups had brittle or unstable asthma. Recent studies suggest that unstable asthma, particularly in allergic patients, may be due to a specific asthma gene that renders these patients more at risk for sudden near-fatal or fatal asthma attacks. Prior emergency visits were a common feature, although six patients who died had never been hospitalized. Five patients in each group had previously required assisted ventilation, and two patients with a near-fatal event who required assisted ventilation eventually succumbed to asthma. This supports previous observations that a history of a prior need for mechanical ventilation or an ICU asthma admission is a strong predictor for fatal asthma.

## Survey Summary

My survey supports the disturbing observation that younger allergic patients are experiencing life-threatening asthma suddenly and unexpectedly outside the hospital, as only two near-fatal episodes and one fatal event took place in a hospital setting. Most patients in the survey nearly died or died suddenly and unexpectedly at home, en route to the hospital, in physicians' offices, or in public places such as county fairs, automobiles and schools. Clinical triggers for near-fatal and fatal asthma included respiratory infections and ingested, inhaled or injected allergens. Two patients succumbed to peanut or tree nut ingestion. Four patients experienced near-fatal or fatal asthma after exercising in cold winter weather. Two patients who died after running in colder weather might have over-relied on their home nebulizer and delayed seeking appropriate emergency room care. One patient died at home while setting up a home nebulizer for an inhalation treatment. The tragic sequence of over-relying on home nebulizers has previously been cited as a risk factor in both near-fatal and fatal asthma. The risk factor for near-fatal and fatal asthma posed by exercising in colder weather has been infrequently noted. All patients in both groups were using a short-acting, inhaled beta-agonist drug, and 20 percent of near-fatal and fatal victims were reportedly using a long-acting, beta-agonist. Beta-agonist abuse was cited as a contributing factor in four patients with near-fatal asthma and nine with fatal asthma. Unlike other studies, where under-utilization of inhaled cortisone drugs is commonly noted in life-threatening asthma, the majority of patients in both groups were reportedly using an inhaled cortisone drug. Most patients had unstable asthma, characterized by wide swings in their lung function tests. This observation is in agreement with other reports that noted that patients with severe bronchial hyper-reactivity and blunted perception of the severity of their attack were more prone to life-threatening attacks of asthma.

While approximately 50 percent of the patients in this survey were thought to have poor compliance and severe disease affected by adverse psychosocial problems, good to excellent compliance was noted in half of those patients experiencing near-fatal asthma and fatal episodes. Three patients died on long holiday weekends, where a delay in seeking care may have been a factor. This observation of an increase in near-fatal and fatal episodes on weekends, especially on Sundays, has previously been reported. In one study, 40 percent of asthma deaths took place between Friday night and Monday morning.

The worldwide increase in cases of near-fatal and fatal asthma has many causes. While earlier reports cited adverse psychosocial patterns, poor care and denial as important risk factors, the role played by inhaled aeroallergens and irritants in near-fatal and fatal asthma is receiving increased attention. Reported triggers for near-fatal and fatal asthma include aeroallergens, emotions, molds, house dust mites, cockroaches, nebulized distilled water and sulfur fumes. One report described a 76-year-old woman with chronic asthma who, several minutes before her sudden death, was exposed to a sulfite-containing de-rusting agent called Super Iron-Out. Shortly after the de-rusting agent was placed in her dishwasher in an effort to open a clogged drain, this unfortunate woman opened the dishwasher door and inhaled the emerging hot, steamy vapors. She immediately gasped, wheezed and died within minutes. Subsequent analysis of this de-rusting agent showed that it emits high concentrations of sulfur dioxide, a well-described asthma trigger.

In summary, while many patients in my survey had moderate to severe asthma tainted by adverse psychosocial factors and might be justifiably labeled "doomed to die," nearly half of the collected cases occurred suddenly and unexpectedly in young, allergic and compliant patients who did not have a severe high-risk asthma profile. Tragically, several patients in this survey might not have died had they not exercised in colder weather, over-relied on their home nebulizer, inadvertently ingested nuts or peanuts or delayed seeking medical care on holiday weekends. In order to better identify and appropriately treat patients prone to preventable near-fatal and fatal asthma episodes, additional studies are warranted. My regional survey supports the need to establish a national case registry to collect data and analyze the clinical characteristics of patients experiencing near-fatal and fatal asthma. Data generated from a registry would help to further define the risk factors and lead to the development of preventive programs for patients at risk for near-fatal and fatal asthma.

## New Trends in Asthma Mortality

The Global Initiative for Asthma has set a worldwide goal for a 50-percent reduction in the number of asthma deaths by the year 2005. Studies published in 2001 suggest this is an obtainable objective. In Australia, the country with the highest rate of asthma in the world along with New Zealand, the prevalence of asthma continues to rise, yet there has been no increase in asthma hospitalizations or asthma mortality, suggesting that new asthmatics are receiving better treatment and are more easily controlled. Mortality rates have leveled off in the United States in 1997 and 1998 versus 1994 to 1996. Two reports from Sweden found decreased hospitalizations with the increased use of inhaled cortisone drugs. A review by Doctors Samy Suisa and Pierre Ernst from Royal Victoria Hospital in Montreal, Canada, found that the use of inhaled cortisone drugs, even in low doses, prevented the major portion of asthma hospitalizations and asthma deaths. In my own experience, I am now seeing fewer patients who could be labeled as having severe life-threatening asthma.

# Psychological Factors in Asthma

# 26

In 1903, Sir William Osler wrote: *"All writers agree that there is, in a majority of cases of bronchial asthma, a strong neurotic element. Many regard it as a neurosis."* Unfortunately, Osler's concept of asthma persisted throughout most of the twentieth century. Alexander and French extensively studied the role of psychological factors in asthma in the 1930s at the Chicago Institute of Psychoanalysis. Asthma was included in this study, along with ulcerative colitis, stomach ulcers and other chronic ailments. Alexander and French wrote that asthma was related to the loss of love and care by the maternal figure, and represented a repressed cry for one's mother. Prior to 1980, most medical texts stated that psychological influences played a major role in asthma. The fundamental hypothesis was that asthma was a symbolic representation of an unconscious conflict, and wheezing was the expression of a suppressed cry for a lost relationship.

The role played by psychological factors in asthma is still the subject of debate. Today there is no doubt that asthma is a true immunological driven disease. Yet, asthma specialists agree that psychological factors can be important in many patients with more moderate to severe asthma. Severe asthma leads to stress and emotional strain, which then sets up a vicious cycle of worsening asthma. Asthma sufferers should be aware that a wide range of emotions, including crying or even laughing, may trigger asthma. After the introduction of more effective asthma therapies in the 1980s, interest in the psychological aspects of asthma waned. However, the emerging asthma epidemic has rekindled awareness of this topic.

Many patients with moderate to severe asthma deny their symptoms and knowingly expose themselves to asthma triggers. Doctor Robert Strunk has found that obese asthmatic children are more likely to have severe psychological problems. He has outlined a psychological profile for high-risk asthma. High-risk patients have severe psychological dysfunction, chronic depression and problems interacting with their medical providers and peers. In families where extreme dysfunction exists, intense psychological counseling is indicated. Those families who require intervention include patients with a risk for near-fatal asthma, marital problems, alcoholism, denial or manipulative traits and obvious signs of depression. The most important form of psychological therapy in these situations is family therapy. The aim of family therapy and asthma self-help programs is to fully educate the family and patient in asthma mechanisms, triggers, warning signs and drug management. Appropriate themes to address during family therapy include poor communication patterns, fear of death, denial of disease and non-compliance on the part of the patient or family.

## The Average Family

What are the effects of asthma on the average family with an asthmatic child? The National Jewish Hospital in Denver, Colorado, surveyed several hundred patients and families affected by asthma. These families averaged 10 office visits per year. Afflicted children averaged eight to fifteen lost school days per year. Half of the parents reported that asthma caused depression in their children, and four of ten parents felt that their child was overly concerned about becoming ill. One-third experienced guilt feelings after an asthma attack. Strained relationships were common between family members and directly correlated with the severity of asthma.

## Stress in Asthma

Stress stimulates the nervous system and triggers asthma through multiple mechanisms. Children exposed to inner-city violence in Boston are more than three times as likely to be diagnosed with asthma. Mothers of asthmatic children have more marital problems and higher divorce rates. Stress may increase our susceptibility to viral infections and bronchial reactivity. In cases where stress plays a major role in asthma, relaxation and biofeedback techniques may be helpful. Hypnotic suggestion may also benefit asthma. Other approaches that have been studied include behavior modification, verbal desensitization and keeping a daily journal. Formal psycho-therapy is rarely indicated in asthma, however, unless there is an independent psychiatric problem. Psychoactive drugs are some-times required to treat associated anxiety, panic attacks or depression. When psychotropic drugs are utilized, it may be necessary to adjust doses of asthma drugs, as beta-agonists and theophylline may accentuate anxiety and the cortisone drugs can induce mood changes.

## Non-adherence or Non-compliance

Doctor Robert Strunk notes that emotional issues worsen asthma when they interfere with compliance and the proper use of medications. The medical buzzword for failing to follow instructions is called non-compliance or non-adherence. Doctor Bruce Bender, Professor of Psychiatry at National Jewish Hospital, defines adherence or compliance as the extent to which a patient follows a reasonable treatment plan that has been prescribed by a qualified caregiver. Fifty to 90 percent of all patients given a simple course of oral penicillin for a strep throat infection fail to complete their therapy. Similarly, more than half of all patients with asthma do not take their asthma medicines as prescribed. In 10 pediatric adherence studies, medication compliance averaged 48 percent. In one asthma study only 70 percent of new asthma prescriptions written by general practitioners were actually filled by the pharmacy. Nearly one-third of asthmatic patients do not use their beta-agonists as prescribed. They ignore their peak flow meters and do not carry their EpiPens as recommended. Non-adherence leads to more emergency room visits and hospitalizations and has been closely linked to asthma deaths. For whatever reason, the sickest patients are often the most non-adherent.

Non-adherence behavior accounts for $8 billion a year in asthma health costs. Non-adherence is a very common problem in adolescents with asthma, as peer pressure leads to a total disregard of asthma medications. Inhaler overuse is the biggest threat in this age group. Non-adherence is directly related to lower intelligence.

Poorly informed school personnel unknowingly contribute to non-adherence when they make it difficult for the student to take asthma medications at school or prior to gym classes or sports activities. Surprisingly, non-adherence is less of a problem in elderly adults; however, non-compliance in this age group is usually due to a failing memory and a confusing medication schedule. Patient distrust of their caregiver is another reason for non-adherence. It is human nature not to take a drug if you are feeling well. Insuring adherence is a two-way street in which both the doctor or caregiver and the patient must participate. Adherence is the strongest predictor of improvement in asthma and quality of life. How can doctors improve adherence?

- Whenever possible, simplify the treatment program.
- Establish a relationship of trust with the patient.
- Maintain a schedule of frequent follow-up office visits or telephone contact.
- Monitor refills of rescue inhalers, especially in young adults.
- Allay concerns about asthma drugs generated by the media and friends. Discuss potential side effects of drugs.
- Address depression, a common cause of non-adherence.
- Help the patient or family acquire the knowledge needed to make informed choices. Provide patient education and written treatment plans.

The patient or family also needs to take an active role in managing their asthma. They should

- Keep a written list of medications.
- Learn the names of their asthma medicines.
- Keep a diary of asthma symptoms and medication use.
- Keep accurate pill counts.
- Review instructions on proper inhaler usage.
- Read educational material on asthma.
- Enroll in asthma self-help programs.

## *Anxiety and Depression*

Depression may play a major role in asthma. Depressed mothers living in inner cities are more likely to bring their asthmatic child to the emergency room. A Dutch study in 98 adults with severe asthma found that patients with psychiatric problems were five times more likely to visit their doctor, use the emergency room or be admitted to the hospital. The two most common psychological reactions to asthma are anxiety and depression. The unpredictable nature of asthma may cause a sense of losing control over bodily functions. This leads to a feeling of vulnerability, fear and anxiety. Because breathing is so central to survival, the loss of respiratory function is threatening. Anxiety may also be worsened by reactions of friends and family members. Depression is a reaction to the helplessness and loss of self-esteem caused by asthma. The major signs of severe depression are sleep disturbance, loss of interest in usual activities, loss of appetite, crying spells and difficulty concentrating. When the level of the depression is moderate, antidepressant drugs may help. Relaxation techniques, deep breathing, understanding the effects of anxiety on breathing and learning to differentiate the effects of asthma on breathing are all important steps to combat depression. Severe depression requires a consultation with a psychologist or psychiatrist.

## *Malignant Asthma*

Do psychological factors play a role in childhood asthma? My feeling is that in most cases psychological factors do not play an important role in childhood asthma. Stress and tension, like cold air or exercise, are just one more asthma trigger. However, asthma is an incapacitating illness for a small group of children, who develop what has been labeled "malignant asthma." This term signifies severe, life-threatening asthma, that has led to denial, anger, guilt and a host of other profound problems for the patient and the entire family. Doctor Clifton Furukawa, of Seattle, Washington, has aptly portrayed the family with multiple psychosocial problems due to malignant asthma. Furukawa found that severe asthma in one member of the family leads to a great deal of overprotection by all family members. The entire family structure becomes very rigid. No one in the family is able to deal with or resolve problems. The sick asthmatic child becomes a substitute solution for all conflicts, and may actually assume the role of a holy or God-like person. Strange as it may seem, this family is most at peace when the child is in the midst of an asthma relapse. These families eventually self-destruct. School absenteeism increases. Family trips and vacation plans are cancelled. Income is lost when both parents work. All outside social contact stops, as the parents are unable to transfer responsibility to caretakers or babysitters. These families require intense and continuous psychological support to avoid total destruction. In some instances, the only salvation for such a family is to admit the asthmatic child to a residential asthma care center. Removing the child from the home on a temporary basis allows the family to return to a more normal lifestyle and rebuild the collapsed family structure. Fortunately, cases of this sort are very rare, as malignant asthma affects less than one percent of all children with asthma.

## Difficult Patients

It is important for health-care providers to understand the basic traits of the character disorders in order to better handle the difficult patients. Character disorders present an important area for understanding human interactions between patients and health-care providers. The most difficult patient is one who has a character disorder along with asthma. Asthma becomes a major focus for family, friends and the treating physician. This pattern of behavior may begin in childhood. The four types of difficult asthmatic patients described by Grove in the text *Asthma*, edited by Barnes, Grunstein, Leff, and Woolcock (Lippencourt, Williams and Wilkins 1999), are the dependent clingers, the entitled demanders, the manipulative help-rejecters, and the self-destructive deniers.

## Dependent Clingers

The dependent clingers are helpless, dependent patients (or parents) who rely on health-care providers every step of the way. They constantly bombard their provider or local emergency room with phone calls, office visits and multiple questions. Constant complaints by the patient or parent lead to frequent changes in medication programs. This patient or family is not really in a treatment partnership with the doctor. Behind the dance of dependence, the patient or parent is really orchestrating his or her own show. They maintain control because it is too threatening to depend and rely on the doctor's advice. The physician often senses the false dependency because nothing seems to work. Treatment plans are undermined, and the provider begins to feel an increasing sense of frustration.

## Entitled Demanders

Entitled demanders use intimidation and anger, and place unending demands on their health-care provider. This provokes both anger and guilt on the part of the health-care providers, since they are trained to help people. They become confused and disturbed when they develop hostile feelings toward the patient or family. Several explanations for this type of behavior are that the patient feels fear, helplessness or anger in regarding his or her asthma. The patient or family turns these vulnerable feelings into an attacking, demanding stance with the doctor. Such patients or families avoid the feelings of being flawed by making strong demands from the provider.

## Manipulative Help-rejecters

Groves describes manipulative help-rejecters as patients who feel a sense of victory when they defeat the attempts of the provider to help them. Again it is stressed that all these behavior patterns are due to the patient's suffering and maladaptive means of relating to others. The patient or family who continually undermines the treatment plan is fearful of complying with alternative programs. There may be issues around surrender or submission to others as well as anger and anxiety.

## Self-destructive Deniers

Self-destructive deniers have severe compliance issues. They flirt with danger by not taking medications and exposing themselves to dangerous asthma. Some of these patients have a personality complex in which they feel they are bad and deserve to be punished. They have often been treated poorly by their parents and confuse mistreatment with being loved. They feel if they hurt themselves they may receive love. Others deny their illness because of severe narcissistic issues. If they follow treatment, they are admitting they are sick, which is intolerable to them.

From the descriptions above, many behavior patterns can underlie the characteristics of difficult-to-manage patients or families. The major issue centers on the dependency that arises when a sick patient must form a relationship with a doctor or health-care provider. For most patients, establishing relationships with care providers poses no problem. They are able to form an alliance, depend on the provider and follow advice without the fear of losing total control of their lives. Furthermore, most patients have a stable sense of identity and self-esteem. This allows them to absorb the stress and anxiety associated with the illness so that they are able to deal with the real issues involved with having asthma and its treatment. The difficult-to-manage patient has problems dealing with dependency and relationship issues and the threat to his or her self-concept without resorting to maladaptive coping mechanisms.

What is the best way to approach these difficult-to-manage patients or families? In some instances it can be helpful to consult a psychiatrist who treats personality disorders. Patients will often feel that the asthma doctor is trying to get rid of them by sending them to a psychiatrist. Patients suffering from borderline and narcissistic disorders are especially sensitive to this reaction. For these reasons, the best model is for the psychiatrist to be part of the treatment team. This is best integrated in an asthma center, where a psychiatrist or psychologist is a member of the treatment team. The patient or family should be reassured that psychological intervention is just another aspect of the asthma treatment program. The patient should be reassured that psychological consultation will not remove the primary care provider or the asthma specialist from the picture.

# Asthma
# Education

# 27

The development of newer, more effective asthma drugs in the late 1970s and 1980s was followed by an explosion of asthma education and self-help programs in the 1990s. The increasing awareness of the asthma-allergy epidemic spawned public education efforts by national specialty societies and gave birth to national organizations like The Asthma and Allergy Foundation of America, The National Asthma and Allergy Network, and The Food Allergy and Anaphylaxis Network. The third facet of these asthma educational efforts was the publication of scores of books, magazines and newsletters for asthma sufferers and their families. When I wrote *The Asthma Self-Help Book* in 1989, there were only a handful of asthma education programs worthy of discussion. Just one decade later there are far too many programs to cover in one chapter.

The mission of any educational health program is to fully involve the patient, family, health-care provider, school personnel and allied health personnel in asthma education. Such programs foster improved understanding of asthma, reduce the negative impact asthma has on patients and their families, and lower asthma morbidity and mortality. Their overall goal is to teach patients and their families to recognize asthma symptoms, reduce exposure to asthma triggers, and properly use asthma medications. Educational programs stress the need to allow patients with asthma and their families to learn how to handle asthma in a responsible manner. Hundreds of controlled trials evaluating structured asthma education and management programs show that most programs are successful in achieving one or more of these goals. Given the wide variation in learning skills, the ability to retain information and interest in participating in education programs, it is unlikely that any single educational format is optimally suited for all patients with asthma. Asthma educational programs must be tailored to the individual needs of the patient or family. Three of the more important points in asthma education that my nurses and I emphasize when we see a new patient with asthma involve the correct use of inhalers, spacers and peak flow meters.

## *Proper Inhaler Use*

A pocket inhaler delivers a measured amount of drug and produces excellent results when patients follow instructions and prescribed dosing intervals. Unfortunately, many asthmatics either overuse their inhalers or do not follow instructions. Some patients have never been properly taught how to use an inhaler. The most common patient errors are improper activation of the inhaler, not waiting between inhalations, forgetting to shake the inhaler and not keeping the inhaler clean. The basic steps for proper inhaler use are outlined in Figure 27.1.

- Shake the inhaler thoroughly.
- Breathe out slowly and steadily.
- Hold your breath 6 to 10 seconds.
- Hold the inhaler two inches from your mouth.
- Tilt your head up and activate the inhaler.
- Breathe in very slowly and as deeply as possible.
- Breathe out slowly and steadily.
- Wait one minute between sprays.

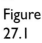

Figure
27.1

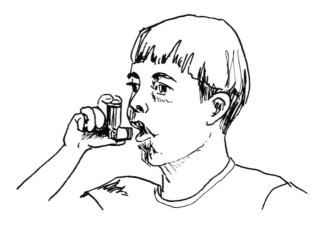

## Dry Powder Inhalers

Non-pressurized or dry powder inhalers (DPIs) are becoming more widely available. Many patients find them easier to use. As these devices are breath-activated, patients do not need to coordinate breathing in with the discharge of the aerosol. DPIs reduce the incidence of the voice huskiness or throat irritation caused by the propellants present in the MDI. The DPIs have some disadvantages. In contrast to the MDI, they require a strong inspiration to maximize drug delivery. They may be less effective in severe asthma or unsuitable for children younger than four years of age. A DPI is an acceptable alternative to the MDI, provided the patient can generate enough of a deep breath to inhale the powder. Many DPIs come with a dose-counting device that lets you know when the inhaler is running low.

## Need for Caution

Three recent reports highlight the need for caution when using an MDI. One case describes a 25-year-old male who awoke with an acute asthma attack in the middle of the night and reached for his bedside MDI. In the process of doing so, he did not remove the inhaler cap and subsequently inhaled the cap of the MDI, which resulted in obstruction of his upper airway. Fortunately, he was able to remove the cap from his upper airway on his own. The only adverse reaction he experienced was pain and hoarseness that persisted for two months. The second report involved a 46-year-old man who developed acute respiratory distress after using his MDI. He kept his uncapped MDI together with some loose change in his pants pocket. After he developed choking and coughing, a chest X-ray showed a coin in his bronchial tube that was subsequently removed by passing a tube down his windpipe. The third case involved a 19-year-old woman who had acute throat pain and difficulty breathing after using her metered-dose inhaler. This patient was in the habit of storing her tetracycline capsules in the mouthpiece. Shortly after using her inhaler, she began coughing and successfully expectorated the tetracycline capsule fragment. These cases should alert asthma sufferers and health-care providers of the potential hazards of MDIs. At least five other instances of inhalation of foreign objects have been reported with the use of these devices. In all these cases, foreign objects in the mouthpiece were propelled into the airway during delivery of the aerosolized medication. Patients should check the inhaler mouthpiece before use and cap the device after using.

## Asthma Spacers

One of the more subtle advances in asthma therapy has been the development of inhaler devices, known as spacers or holding chambers that make it easier to use the MDIs. These inhaler aids allow young children, uncoordinated patients and elderly asthmatics with arthritis to use their inhalers more effectively (Figure 27.2). Spacers allow more aerosol spray to penetrate deeper into the lungs of patients who cannot coordinate the release of the spray with taking a deep breath. The big advantage of the spacing devices is that large particles of the medications are deposited on the sides of the tube, leaving only the smaller particles that are more easily inhaled into the lung. Fewer large particles end up being deposited in the mouth or the back of the throat. Using inhalers with spacers is the most versatile and cost-effective way to deliver an aerosol. Provided it is used properly, a large-volume spacer may double the amount of the drug that is delivered to the lung in comparison with

Figure
27.2

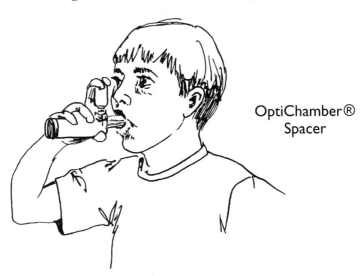

OptiChamber®
Spacer

what a well-trained patient can achieve using an MDI. The addition of a spacer to the MDI limits the amount of medication deposited in the mouth and throat, and also reduces the systemic absorption of the inhaled drug.

## Home Nebulizers

Patients with mild or moderate asthma usually do quite well with a DPI, or an MDI with a spacer. Some patients with more severe asthma need home compressors to administer aerosol medications at home (Figure 27.3). Devices like the DeVilbis Nebulizer, Pulmo-Aide, or the portable DuraNeb 2000 are actually mini-versions of the equipment used in the hospital by respiratory therapists. Medication added to a nebulizer is inhaled via a facemask or a mouthpiece. New versions of nebulizers are very portable, and can be powered by small batteries or automobile cigarette lighters. The best candidates for nebulizers are infants and young children and elderly asthmatics who have difficulty with hand-held metered dose inhalers and cannot grasp the concepts of the MDIs even when spacers are used. The availability of unit dose packs for cromolyn (Intal), albuterol and inhaled cortisone drugs have improved the nebulizer's overall

Figure
27.3

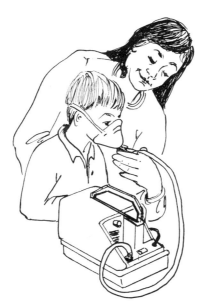

Nebulizer

effectiveness and ease of use. Some of my patients and families who prefer to use the DPIs or MDIs and spacers for routine daily medications only use nebulized drugs in acute attacks that do not respond to the hand-held inhalers. Nebulizers have no inherent advantage over the hand-held inhalers in terms of local deposition of particles, dose or clinical response.

## Peak Flow Meters

Lung function or breathing tests are essential yardsticks in the asthma diagnosis and management. Breathing tests can be compared to monitoring blood pressure in people with hypertension and blood sugar levels in diabetics. What is the peak expiratory flow rate, commonly called the peak flow? The peak flow is the amount of air one can exhale during a forced expiration after taking as full a breath as possible. Your peak flow rate can be measured by a relatively inexpensive portable device called a peak flow meter, that measures the amount of air in liters (a liter is about a quart) you exhale per minute (Figure 27.4).

■
Figure
27.4

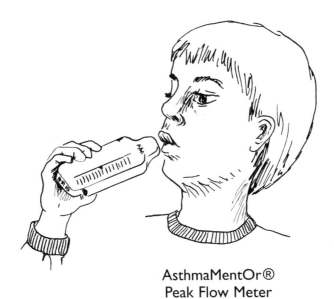

AsthmaMentOr®
Peak Flow Meter

Poor perception of asthma severity is a known factor in patients exhibiting asthma relapses. The peak flow meter is a much more accurate instrument than the doctor's stethoscope in assessing the severity of an asthma relapse. The peak flow meter lets you know how well you are breathing. Peak flow meters come in various forms. There are approximately a dozen or so peak flow meters on the market. The typical device consists of a plastic or metal tube with a mouthpiece at one end. When you blow into the tube, a pointer moves along a scale and records how much and how fast you can blow air out of your lungs. When asthma is active, it is harder to exhale air, and the peak flow meter measures how much obstruction you have in your airways. The peak flow meter has many uses. It can assess the severity of acute or chronic asthma in the health-care provider's office or the emergency room. It is used before and after exercise to determine the presence or absence of exercise-induced asthma. It enables the patient or family to monitor asthma at home and guide the need to step up or step down asthma medications.

School personnel can use the peak flow meter to assess the student who experiences acute asthma in the gymnasium, playing field or classroom. Lastly, it can detect what type of occupational exposures may be triggering asthma in the workplace. The peak flow meter is not a perfect instrument. It is effort-dependent—or in other words, it depends on the patient's ability and willingness to exhale as hard and as fast as possible. Also, it only measures function of the larger airways. Asthma affecting the smaller airways may go undetected by the peak flow meter. Patient and family education is of the utmost importance for the peak flow meter to be an effective instrument. Education should include how and when to use the peak flow meter, how to record peak flow rates, how to interpret the readings and when to communicate with health-care providers.

Most adults and older children, occasionally even a three- or four-year-old, can be taught to generate a peak expiratory flow rate. As the peak flow rate is effort dependent, patients need to be coached to put forth their best effort. Peak flows can be recorded in a notebook, table or graph. The NHLBI Guidelines recommend that peak flow decisions be based on the patient's "personal best," rather than using a percentage of a normal predicted value. Many patients exhibit a wide variation between their morning and evening peak flow rate. A 20-percent swing in peak flow readings is a normal variation on a day-to-day basis. Those patients whose peak flow rate drops in the morning are called "morning dippers." One's personal best peak flow rate often occurs in late afternoon or evening after maximum asthma therapy. Sometimes a course of oral cortisone may be needed to establish one's personal best. I usually advise a new asthma patient to record their peak flow rate two to three times a day for two to three weeks after they have been placed on daily asthma medications. Once asthma stabilizes, the peak flow rates can be charted when warning signs occur or during an asthma relapse.

Doctors Guillermo Mendoza and Thomas Plaut strongly recommend using the Asthma Management Zone System, that uses a traffic light color code to develop an asthma action plan. Three zones based on the individual's personal best or predicted value are established. The green zone represents 80 percent or better of one's personal best—this signals a go or all clear signal that asthma is stable and routine treatment should continue. The yellow zone ranges from 50 to 80 percent of one's personal best, and indicates the need to proceed with caution. An acute relapse may be imminent, and you need to take action to get your asthma under control. A peak flow below 50 percent of personal best signals a red or dangerous medical alert. Bronchodilator drugs should be administered and health-care providers should be notified if peak flow measurements do not immediately return to the yellow or green zone.

Some health-care providers advocate the use of peak flow meters for all asthmatics. Others feel the widespread use of peak flow meters is unnecessary, as it results in too intense a focus on asthma by the family or patient. Doctor Donald Cockroft, Professor of Respiratory Medicine at University Hospital in Saskatchewan, Canada, is not overly enthusiastic about using peak flow meters in the adult population. Cockroft feels that only five percent of his adult patients have the type of asthma where home peak flow measurements are helpful, and that peak flow meters are more beneficial in the management of children with persistent asthma. On the other hand, Doctor Thomas Plaut feels that any patient who requires daily asthma treatment needs a peak flow meter. The NHLBI Guidelines strongly state that all patients with asthma should utilize peak flow meters. I believe that the peak flow meter should be part of any asthma education program, but simply providing a peak flow meter as a means of measuring airway obstruction may not achieve the desired effect.

Utilization of peak flow meters ultimately depends on patient compliance. Retrospective studies on diabetics asked to measure their blood sugar at home have shown a high rate of non-compliance even among well-educated diabetics and their families. Similar problems with compliance occur with the use of the peak flow meter. Nearly half of the patients I see during an asthma relapse have not used a peak flow meter prior to coming to the emergency room or my office. I prescribe peak flow meters to every patient with persistent asthma that requires daily asthma medications. I do not "zone" all of my patients into green, yellow and red zones. I prefer to use this approach in patients with more moderate to severe unstable asthma. I also utilize peak flow meters to determine the presence or absence of occupational and exercise-induced asthma. Furthermore, the peak flow meter allows the on-call doctor to make a more objective analysis of asthma relapses by phone during the evening or on weekends. I do not think peak flow meters should be routinely utilized in patients with mild asthma, as such use could potentially cause social hang-ups or emotional dysfunction similar to those seen in patients with hypertension who monitor their own blood pressure on a daily basis.

In summary, the peak flow meter is a vital component of the management of persistent asthma, and one that should be used in combination with education programs that stress appropriate use of medications, recognizing the early warning signs of relapsing asthma and implementing appropriate environmental controls. The peak flow meter should not replace spirometery or lung-function testing in a clinic or medical office as a way to assess patients with moderate to severe asthma. Several studies have shown that the peak flow meter reading may be normal when the more accurate method of following asthma, the FEV1 or one second vital capacity, is profoundly depressed.

## *AsthmaPACK.III*

Respironics has created AsthmaPACK.III, a clever personal asthma care kit, which provides an AsthmaMentOr Peak Flow Meter, the OptiChamber Valved Holding Chamber or spacer and instructional video and booklet in English and Spanish. The AsthmaMentOr's Peak Flow Meter built in AutoZone automatically calculates color-coded peak flow zones based on your best peak flow rates. The OptiChamber Valved Holding Chamber allows smaller particles of inhaled medications to reach the lower lung airways.

This all-inclusive kit incorporates the key elements and devices needed to properly use medications, monitor symptoms and better understand asthma. This kit and products are available from Respironics-Health Scan Asthma & Allergy Products, 41 Canfield Road, Cedar Grove, NJ 07009-1292. 1-800-962-1266, Fax 973-239-0831.

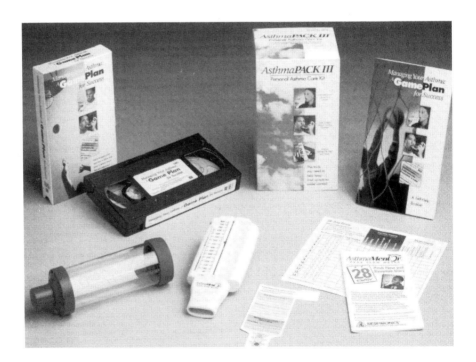

# Appendix

---

## *Asthma Education Programs*

### Childhood Programs

Most asthma education programs developed for children share several common elements. They provide families with a series of learning opportunities—typically four to eight sessions lasting an hour—so that families can fully explore all aspects of managing childhood asthma. Programs provide the opportunity for families to learn new information, acquire and practice new skills, and review their experience in applying these skills in the home situation. Most of these programs review basic asthma mechanisms, asthma symptoms, environmental controls and proper use of asthma medications. These programs encourage families to develop an active partnership with their care providers. Some of the more successful childhood asthma educational programs are discussed below.

### Teaching Myself About Asthma

Developed by Health Education Associates, the Teaching Myself About Asthma program is offered in schools to groups of children six to twelve years of age. This program encourages at-home participation by parents. The program is delivered in weekly sessions by a team of teachers, school psychologists and nurses. Parents occasionally participate in meetings with children at school to learn more about the curriculum and to discuss asthma-management issues with a physician associated with the program. Children also work at home alone or with parents on assignments contained in the program workbook.

## Asthma Care Training (ACT) for Kids

ACT is a program designed by a team at the University of California at Los Angeles. Made available through the Asthma and Allergy Foundation of America, ACT is offered in both English and Spanish in outpatient medical settings for children eight to twelve years of age. The program has five sessions. Parents and children meet in separate groups for 45 minutes and then come together for 15 minutes of shared learning. Children who complete the ACT program have fewer emergency visits, fewer hospital days and improved self-management skills.

## Air Power-Air Wise

Air Power, developed by the American Institutes of Research and sponsored by the National Heart, Lung, and Blood Institute (NHLBI), uses a group format with four one-hour sessions for parents and children nine to thirteen years of age. Air Wise is an individualized version of Air Power, designed for children with difficult-to-manage asthma. The asthma educator meets with child and parent to assess the child's specific needs. Air Wise is designed for use in a clinic or other medical or community setting. Children in the Air Power program had significantly greater self-management skills than controls at follow-up. Children who completed the Air Wise Program had fewer emergency treatments and hospitalizations.

## Open Airways

Open Airways is a group program designed for low-income, inner-city children and their parents. English and Spanish materials are designed for readers with low literacy skills. The program has seven 60-minute sessions, and uses an educational approach where group members share problems and develop solutions. The aim is to ensure that barriers to asthma treatment are identified. This program can be used in both a medical care and community setting.

Open Airways for Schools is an adaptation of the Open Airways program, sponsored by the American Lung Association. This program focuses directly on children with asthma eight to eleven years of age. Six educational sessions are held at school. Parents do not take part in the sessions, but are involved through interactive homework assignments at home. Children who participated in this program had improved self-management behavior, better school performance and fewer symptom days when compared to controls.

## Living With Asthma

The Living With Asthma program, developed at the National Asthma Center, consists of eight one-hour sessions held separately, but simultaneously, with parents and children eight to thirteen years of age. The program uses a group format with written diaries and checklists for responding to problems and developing asthma management skills. It requires a higher literacy level than other programs. Living With Asthma was developed for a rural population, but it can be used in both a medical care and community setting. A post-research analysis found reductions in the frequency of asthma attacks and improved school attendance among children who completed the program.

## You Can Control Asthma

The You Can Control Asthma program combines individual and group components. It uses slides and videotapes that teach the recognition of asthma triggers, early warning signs of attacks and the value of early treatment. In addition, nurses and the physicians discuss the key points of the management plan with patients during their regular medical encounter. Using a pre-post research design without controls, children increased their knowledge of self-management skills and the sense of personal control over asthma.

## Superstuff

Superstuff is another program of the American Lung Association, uniquely designed for in-home use by families who cannot afford the time off from work to attend classes during the day or evening. Superstuff contains a folder of games, books, puzzles and posters that are very helpful for elementary school children. Superstuff stresses knowing the early warning signs of asthma and the proper techniques of abdominal breathing. Superstuff materials can be obtained from your local chapter of the American Lung Association.

## Childhood Asthma: Learning to Manage (CALM)

CALM is an asthma-management program approved by the Medical Scientific Council of the Asthma and Allergy Foundation of America. CALM uses peak flow monitoring and educational materials to provide a unique resource for children with asthma. CALM emphasizes the use of the home peak flow meter to measure lung function. As many patients frequently over- or underestimate their lung function, daily peak flow readings allow asthma care to be based on objective data. This allows the care provider to determine if the program is controlling asthma at home. CALM offers an in-depth view on asthma medications, asthma triggers, warning signs and responding to asthma attacks. Unlike other programs, it does not require group sessions or a trained instructor. Patients and families can use the materials at their own pace. The uniqueness of this program is that it recognizes the needs and learning abilities of children at different ages. Separate booklets are provided for children and their parents for pre-readers (one to seven years), pre-adolescents (eight to twelve years) and teenagers (thirteen to nineteen years). For further information contact: the Asthma and Allergy Foundation of America or the CALM Coordinator, IOX Assessment Associates, 11411 West Jefferson Boulevard, Culver City, California, 90230. (213-391-6245)

## The Neighborhood Asthma Coalition (NAC) Program

NAC is a community organization approach to promoting basic understanding of asthma and improved care within low-income African-American neighborhoods in St. Louis, Missouri. NAC involves a partnership between university-based asthma specialists and community organizations. This program concentrates on promoting awareness of asthma, preventive measures and appropriate use of health-care services in a large, urban minority population through community organization. Like the Open Airways program, the NAC program was based on the difficulties in finding or paying for good medical care and poor appreciation of the seriousness of the disease by the patients and their families.

## Adult Programs

While most asthma education programs are directed at children, many adult education programs have been developed. Most adult education models consist of single sessions to review educational materials like video and audiotapes or printed booklets. Another type of adult program involves efforts to improve asthma management through special asthma clinics or asthma centers where more intensive medical management is coupled with asthma education. A review of adult programs suggests that brief patient education programs may lead to gains in asthma knowledge. Unfortunately, many programs have not demonstrated a long-lasting effect on patient self-management behavior or health outcomes.

To date, the most comprehensive study on asthma education in adults was reported by Wilson and colleagues. These investigators randomized 323 adults with asthma into four groups who received either 1) small group education, 2) individualized, structured teaching, 3) information only or 4) usual care. Data included self-reports, physician judgments and audits of medical records. Patients were followed for two years. At the end of one year, improvement was noted in the education groups with respect to asthma symptoms, use of environmental control and increased skill in metered-dose inhaler techniques. While physician assessment of asthma suggested that educated groups had improved, health-care utilization did not differ among groups at the end of one year. However, at the two-year follow-up, individual instruction was associated with a greater reduction in acute visits for asthma.

The mode of delivering patient education may influence outcomes. Some patients respond to group offerings, while others do best with one-on-one instruction. A Great Britain study compared patients educated in groups to those educated one-on-one. Both modes of delivery produced gains, with neither group being better than the other. However, the amount of staff time required to administer the program was different. Group education required four-and-a-half hours of staff time, compared to 14 hours for individual sessions. As the knowledge gains between those educated in groups were equal to those educated individually, the cost-benefit analysis clearly favored group education. However, other researchers reported major difficulties in recruiting and maintaining participation in group education programs. Even though group education may be more cost-effective, participation rates are higher when patients are individually scheduled. A final concern is the lack of any attempt to build educational programs that address adult learning. Many researchers note that adults differ from children in terms of educational needs and response to educational programs.

# *Asthma and Allergy Organizations*

## The Asthma and Allergy Foundation of America

The Asthma and Allergy Foundation of America, or AAFA, is a national, nonprofit, patient organization dedicated to improving the quality of life for people with asthma and their caregivers. AAFA provides practical information, community-based services, educational programs, support and referrals through a national network of chapters and educational support groups. AAFA is the only asthma and allergy patient advocacy organization that sponsors research toward identifying better treatments and a cure for asthma and allergic diseases.

AAFA's programs are designed to improve the quality of life and care for people with asthma and allergies in communities across the country. These programs and resources include the following:

- *Asthma Management and Education for Allied Health Professionals*
- *Asthma and Allergy Essentials for Child Care Providers*
- *Power Breathing* (for 10- to 18-year-olds)
- *You Can Control Asthma* (for 4- to 12-year-olds)
- *You Can Control Asthma (ACT) for Kids* (for 6- to 12-year-olds)
- *Meeting in a Box* (adults, parents, school personnel)
- *The Student Asthma Action Card*
- *AAFA's Child Care Asthma/Allergy Action Card*
- Online continuing education courses for health-care professionals

AAFA's advocacy and outreach efforts have played an integral role in establishing national guidelines for the diagnosis and management of asthma and allergies; setting national standards to improve quality care for patients; obtaining federal funding for asthma prevention programs, for state health departments; and strengthening laws that protect patient rights. In 1984, AAFA established, by presidential proclamation, that the month of May be Asthma and Allergy Awareness Month that is observed by communities, organizations and federal agencies.

To obtain more information on AAFA, its programs, ask a question of a board-certified allergist, chat and exchange tips with others afflicted with asthma and allergies, or locate an AAFA chapter in your area, contact AAFA at 1233 20th St. NW, Suite 402, Washington, DC 20036; 1-800-7-ASTHMA, 202-466-7643; or visit their Web site at www.aafa.org

## Allergy and Asthma Network Mothers of Asthmatics

In 1985, Nancy Sander, a mother of a child with asthma, founded the Allergy and Asthma Network Mothers of Asthmatics known as AANMA. AANMA is committed to eliminate suffering and death due to asthma and allergies through education, advocacy and community outreach and research programs. AANMA offers original books, videos and pamphlets that are carefully reviewed by medical experts. It provides discounts for allergy and asthma products like peak flow meters or nebulizers. AANMA depends on membership support for its programs and publications. A donation of any amount brings you a year of award-winning publications, up-to-the-minute news and research developments.

### AANMA Publications and Programs

- *Allergy & Asthma Health,* an award-winning quarterly magazine with hands-on advice, medical news and a *"Just for Kids"* section. Well-written and nicely illustrated, this magazine covers all aspects of allergic disorders and asthma.
- The MA Report, published eight times a year, provides readers with news, tips, events and research findings.
- *Asthma, Allergies and School: Parents, Students and Teachers Together.* This is a customized tool kit that deals with the issues of allergies and asthma in the school.
- The *"Mickey Campaign"* launched by AANMA in 2000, the result of the tragic death of an eight-year-old boy named Mickey. After Mickey's mother learned that his death could have been prevented, she became involved with AANMA and published the *Mickey Booklet,* which tells parents how to avoid a tragic outcome.
- *Breatherville USA* is a unique feature of their educational Web site. It is a charming town containing 14 buildings, which offer solid educational advice on various topics including asthma, childcare, food allergies and environmental controls.
- *The Peak Flow Meter Book* and *What Everyone Needs to Know About Peak Flow Meters*—state-of-the-art guide books for peak flow meter use.

Contact AANMA at 2751 Prosperity Ave., Suite 150, Fairfax, Virginia, 800-878-4403. To view or download their resources visit their Web site at www.aanma.org

## The American Academy of Allergy, Asthma & Immunology

The American Academy of Allergy, Asthma & Immunology, or AAAAI, is a membership organization of 4,000 practicing physicians, academicians and researchers from the United States and 42 foreign countries. AAAAI fosters new advances and education in the field of asthma, allergy and immunology and promotes research and professional competence in the field of medicine. AAAAI's Web site (www.aaaai.org) offers pollen counts, a listing of asthma camps and a physician referral guide.

*Asthma and Allergy Advocate* is an informative newsletter published by the American Academy of Allergy, Asthma & Immunology that offers practical information and health tips for asthma and allergy sufferers. To obtain it, call (414) 272-6071 or write the AAAAI at 611 East Wells St., Milwaukee, WI 53202.

## The American College of Allergy, Asthma & Immunology

The American College of Allergy, Asthma & Immunology, or ACAAI, is an organization of 3,000 doctors dedicated to educating physicians and improving patient care by addressing the needs of practicing physicians and specialists in the field of asthma and allergy. ACAAI encourages research and maintains the skills of its members by sponsoring educational programs and scientific publications. For additional information, contact ACAAI at 85 Algonquin Road, Suite 550, Arlington Heights, IL 60005; 847-427-1200 or visit their Web site at www.allergy.mcg.edu

## The American Lung Association

The American Lung Association, or ALA, has produced a broad range of informative literature for sufferers of all types of lung diseases, including asthma. ALA sponsors public information programs, anti-smoking programs and camps for children with asthma. The Web site also provides the latest news about asthma, tips for patients and parents, and information about your local lung association. You can also sign up for their e-mail digests: *Breath/Easy Asthma Digest*, a monthly summary of asthma news, and *Weekly Breather*, a weekly summary of lung-health news.

*The Asthma Handbook*, published by the ALA, is a self-teaching booklet written expressly for adults and older teens with asthma. It covers basic asthma topics including asthma triggers, medications, asthma prevention and control. The ALA also publishes *The Asthma Alert*, a file folder for school personnel to aid them in recognizing asthma and dealing with youngsters stricken by an asthma attack at school. To contact the ALA, call or write the national office, 1740 Broadway, New York, NY 10010-4374; 212-315-8700, or consult your local phonebook to find the ALA chapter nearest you. For more information, you can visit the ALA Web site at www.lungusa.org. ALA has opened a new service called Ask Us at their Web site. They will answers questions on all lung diseases via e-mail within 24 hours.

## The National Institute of Allergy and Infectious Diseases

The National Institute of Allergy and Infectious Diseases (NIAID) is a division of The National Institute of Health (NIH), which conducts broad-based research training programs dealing with the causes, prevention, control and treatment of all allergic diseases. NIAID publishes several informative pamphlets for people with asthma. These materials can be obtained by contacting NIAID at 9000 Rockville Pike, Bethesda, MD 20205; 301-496-5717, or visiting their Web site at www.nhlbi.nih.gov/nhlbi/nhlbi.htm

### Global Allergy Information Network (GAIN)

The Global Allergy Information Network (GAIN) was launched by the World Allergy Organization in September 2000 during their annual Congress in Sidney, Australia. GAIN aims to be the premier Internet Web site specializing in allergic disorders. Its intended audience includes both professional and lay people. A key feature of the Web site is a series of links to lay organization Web sites around the world. Each month a new topic in allergy and asthma will be reviewed. Visit GAIN's Web site at www.worldallergy.org and register for the GAIN e-newsletter, which will alert you when new features and topics are added to the Web site.

## Asthma Education Program

The Asthma Education Program, sponsored by the National Heart, Lung, and Blood Institute, has developed a reading and resource list for patients and families with asthma. They have published *Check Your*

*Asthma IQ; Managing Asthma, A Guide for Schools;* and several other pamphlets on asthma. Their publication list can be obtained by writing to them at P.O. Box 30105, Bethesda, MD 20824-0105, 301-951-3260 or visiting their Web site at www.nhlbi.nih.gov/index.htm

## Asthma and Allergy Publications

*Asthma Magazine* is an outstanding asthma publication edited by Rachel Butler who did a great job in editing this book. *Asthma Magazine* strives to promote public education and create a partnership between the patient, physician and other health-care professionals through education and awareness. Published five times a year by Mosby. To order *Asthma Magazine,* call 800-654-2452 or e-mail them at hhspcs@harcort.com

*Allergies and Asthma for Dummies* by William Berger, M.D. (IDG Worldwide Inc., 2000) is an interesting, motivating, and amusing book written by my good friend Doctor Bill Berger. This easy-to-read text covers asthma, hay fever, food reactions and more. It is a valuable addition to one's allergy-asthma library.

*Taking Charge of Asthma: A Lifetime Strategy* by Betty Wray M.D. (John Wiley and Sons, Inc., 1998) outlines strategic ways to prevent asthma and control your environment. Doctor Wray accurately defines the latest medical and alternative therapies in asthma and reviews the foods that may trigger asthma.

*Asthma Guide for People of All Ages* by Thomas Plaut, M.D. A guide for controlling your asthma includes information on medication, tracking of symptoms and how to handle a variety of asthma symptoms. Doctor Plaut has also written *One Minute Asthma,* a concise pamphlet highlighting the principles of asthma therapy and *Children With Asthma: A Manual for Parents,* an informative book for the parents of asthmatic children that contains many interesting anecdotes written by patients and their parents. These publications are available from Pedi Press, Inc., 125 Redgate Lane, Amherst, MA 01002.

*A Parent's Guide to Asthma* by Nancy Sander (Plume 1994). The founder of Mothers of Asthmatics has written an informative book for parents that covers all aspects of asthma from a parent's viewpoint. The book reviews asthma basics, asthma triggers and the use of peak flow meters. Any parent who wants to learn more about asthma should obtain this well-written book from their local bookstore or AANMA.

*Patient's Guide to Asthma* by Fred Leffert, M.D., is a brief but informative 15-page booklet for individuals not interested in reading a full-length book on asthma. This publication is free and can be obtained from GlaxoSmithKline, at 5 Moore Drive, Research Triangle Park, NC 27709.

*Cooking for the Allergic Child* by Judy Moyer is an informative cookbook with over 300 recipes, nutritional facts and a fine resource section. Order through your bookstore or send $15.95 to Allergy Control Products, 89 Danbury Road, Ridgefield, CT 06877.

*Understanding Asthma* (University Press of Mississippi, Jackson, Mississippi) was written by my friend and scholarly colleague Phil Lieberman, M.D. This book provides a comprehensive review of how asthma affects the lungs. The section on immunology is well written and illustrated. Lieberman gives thoughtful insight into current research and future asthma therapies.

*Guide to Your Children's Allergies and Asthma* edited by Michael Welch, M.D. Published by Villard Books, New York, NY 10171. This is the latest in a series of parenting books published by the American Academy of Pediatrics. A good resource book for parents who want up-to-date information on their child's allergies or asthma. The user-friendly format includes real-life case studies.

*Allergies: The Complete Guide to Diagnosis, Treatment, and Daily Management.* A Plume Book published by Penguin Group. This revised edition of an earlier publication by Stuart H. Young, M.D., Bruce Dobozin, M.D., and Margaret Miner is a comprehensive review of all allergic diseases including asthma. The book provides self-education and clarifies misconceptions in the field of allergic disorders.

*My House is Killing Me! The Home Guide for Families with Allergies and Asthma.* Written by home inspector and science teacher, Jeffrey May, and published in 2001 by Johns Hopkins

University Press. This very readable and informative book takes the reader through the home on a room by room basis. May details how to identify and remove asthma and allergy triggers. Available at bookstores or at www.jhupbooks.com

*Essential Guide to Asthma* published by the American Medical Association provides the keys to understanding asthma with reliable scientific information on the diagnosis and treatment of this puzzling disease. Contains a detailed section of frequently asked questions, resources lists and a glossary of medical terms. Published by Pocket Books, New York, NY.

*Lung Line Letter.* A newsletter called LUNG LINE is available from the National Jewish Medical & Research Center as an additional service from their educational hotline. Call toll-free 1-800-222-LUNG for additional details.

*Asthma and Allergy Alert* is a newsletter for allergy and asthma sufferers and their families that will begin publication in late 2002. This newsletter will be published by Lighthouse Press and edited by me. This bimonthly publication is intended to keep readers abreast of any and all new important developments in the field of asthma and allergic disorders. To order in advance, call 1-800-245-0512, or write Lighthouse Press, P.O. Box 602, Marblehead, MA 01945.

## Asthma Treatment Centers

In the late 1920s, Doctor Murray Peshkin admitted a group of severely ill asthmatic children to New York's Mount Sinai Hospital. Much to Doctor Peshkin's surprise, many children improved dramatically without specific treatment. It was obvious that an unstable home environment and family stress played a major role in asthma, and when children were removed from the parental home, they were able to overcome their asthma. Doctor Peshkin appropriately coined the term "parentectomy." This innovative program, which eventually moved to the more favorable climate of Denver, Colorado, led to the establishment of the world's leading asthma-allergy research center, now known as National Jewish Hospital. This center and others like it became residential treatment facilities for the care of children with severe asthma. Children were admitted to such centers for several weeks or months. Due to changes in the economics of medical care, virtually all of these programs have either closed or have converted to short-term treatment facilities.

At National Jewish Hospital, the outdated approach that required a hospital stay of several weeks or months has been replaced by a new program called *Time Out for Asthma.* This program for children and adults with difficult-to-manage asthma averages 10 days in length. *Time Out for Asthma* combines a multi-specialty approach along with an intense psychological and social evaluation. The first step is to bring the asthma under control by closely regulating medications to the lowest possible dose that maximizes breathing functions. Patients are taught how to use their medications and monitor their daily lung functions with peak flow meters. The overall goal of the program is to allow the patient to improve his or her quality of life through a better understanding of asthma. After completing this intense program, patients return home and are followed by a Care Manager Nurse, who provides ongoing follow-up and telephone support to the patient, family and local medical care providers for one year after the patient returns home. A 12-month study of 44 patients who completed this program revealed dramatic results. Unscheduled doctor visits decreased by nearly 90 percent, emergency visits decreased 88 percent, hospitalizations were lowered by 67 percent, and missed school or work days were lowered by 80 percent. For additional information, call 1-800-NJC-9555 or visit their Web site, www.nationaljewish.org

## Asthma Summer Camps

Another very successful educational approach for asthmatic children is the asthma summer camp. Many camps for asthmatic children have been established throughout the United States. Most are modeled after the Camp Bronco Junction in Redhouse, West Virginia, which was founded by Doctor Merle Scherr, the pioneer of asthma summer camps. The American Lung Association sponsors most of these asthma camps. At last count there were 80 camps, serving 4,500 kids each summer. Programs vary from day camps to two-week overnight camps. Most camps have well-structured programs that stress self-help and basic asthma education. All approved camps have good medical supervision. While it may cost $350 to $400 per week for an overnight camp, the ALA or the camp sponsor will often pick up the tab for families who cannot afford the camp fee.

Doctor William S. Silver, medical director of Camp Champ in Colorado, recently surveyed the children and families involved in his asthma camp and found that 100 percent of the children and their families felt they had a positive experience. Doctor Silver advises parents to check out any camp by making sure that there is a physician and trained support staff on hand. At Camp Champ there is always a doctor, nurse and respiratory therapist available. Contact your local chapter of the American Lung Association or the Asthma and Allergy Foundation of America to locate the nearest asthma summer camp in your area.

## Employee Education Programs

Employers are now demanding improved quality of care and cost efficiencies through disease-management programs. The demands of employers are due in large part to the development of managed care programs. Purchasers of health care are urging their insurers to implement asthma-management programs. When you consider that asthma costs American employers $4 billion a year, it is no surprise that many corporations have implemented asthma-education programs. Such programs are aimed at reducing emergency room visits, asthma hospitalizations and work absenteeism. Most of these employer programs that were started in the early 1990s have shown a dramatic reduction in the costs of asthma care and improved quality of life for the participants.

## Web Sites for Asthma Education

Health-care providers or interested consumers who want to learn about the most up-to-date diagnostic and treatment protocols for asthma can now access almost all the medical literature on asthma. One new Web site, called the Asthma Management Model System or AMMS, was designed by the NHLBI's National Asthma Education and Prevention Program (NAEPP). This wide-ranging system will search major scientific databases from MEDLINE, CRISP and CORDIS, as well as documents from the CDC and the FDA. This

AMMS Web site can be accessed via the NHLBI home page at www.nhlbi.nih.gov

### National Allergy Bureau

The National Allergy Bureau, or NAB, is the leading source for pollen and spore count information in the United States. The AAAAI and ACAAI have joined forces to promote this valuable network. It serves as a public service to Americans who are concerned about allergens in their environment. NAB keeps patients informed about aeroallergens in their environment and enables them to make proper decisions regarding medication use and environmental controls. For more information regarding NAB, contact the AAAAI at 414-272-6071 or visit their Web site at www.aaaai.org/nab.

## Asthma and Allergy Supply Companies

The companies listed below all provide a wide range of allergy and asthma products including allergen barriers, cleaning supplies, air cleaners, respiratory products and educational materials required to institute proper environmental controls in your home. Very few, if any, retail stores offer the quality of material and pricing available through these mail order houses. Most, if not all of these companies, have attractive brochures and Web sites that display their prices and products.

**Asthma and Allergy Relief.** 3095 Tilghman Street, Allentown, PA 18104; 610-770-6849; Fax 610-770-6879. Environmental control products-mattress encasings, HEPA Air Purifiers and Asthma Products

**Allergy Asthma Technology LTD.** 8224 Leigh Avenue, Morton Grove, IL. Offers quality products for asthma and allergy care and environmental controls. Colorful and complete brochure. 800-621-55454; Fax 847-966-3068; www.allergyasthmatech.com

**Allergy Control Products** 96 Danbury Road, Ridgefield, CT 06877. 800-422-3878; Fax 203-431-8963. An 18-year-old company with a proven line of allergy avoidance products designed to reduce allergen exposure in the home. www.allergycontrol.com

**Allergy Direct** 2020 SW Fourth Avenue, Suite 750, Portland, OR 97201; 877-283-2323; www.allergyydirect.com. Offers a wide selection of name-brand, physician-approved products and educational materials.

**Allergy Etc.** A one-stop source for allergy and environmental products. Their full line of products is listed in their award-winning Web site. 800-804-6022; www.allergyetc.com

**Allergy Free.** 6835 Flanders Drive #500, San Diego, CA 95746; 916-789-4165; Fax 916-789-4159. Manufactures Aller-Pure Gold electrostatic filters. They also provide a complete line of allergen avoidance products.

**National Allergy Supply.** 1620 Satellite Blvd., Suite D, P.O. Box 1658, Duluth, GA 30096; well-established company that offers full line of allergen avoidance products. Offers new membrane-free encasements for bedding materials. 800-522-1448; www.nationalallergy.com

**Allergy Solutions, Inc.** 7 Crozerville Road, Aston, PA 19014; 404-840-0363; Fax 484-840-0366. A complete source of environmental control, allergen avoidance and asthma management products.

**Mission Allergy.** 28 Hawleyville Road, Hawleyville, CT 06440; 203-364-1570; Fax 203-426-5607. Manufactures high-quality microfiber pillow and mattress encasings. Offers Self-Help Guide for accurate information on allergen avoidance.

# Glossary

**Adrenalin.** The trade name for epinephrine, the natural product of our adrenal gland that doctors use to treat acute allergic reactions.

**Aeroallergens.** Term used to describe airborne allergens.

**Aerosols.** Drugs sprayed or inhaled into the nose or lung.

**Albuterol.** An asthma drug that relieves bronchospasm.

**Allergen.** Any substance or antigen like pollen, foods or drugs which is capable of causing an allergic reaction.

**Alveoli.** The tiny air sacs in the lung where oxygen enters and carbon dioxide leaves the body.

**Anaphylaxis.** The medical term for a severe or life-threatening allergic reaction.

**Antibody.** A protein produced by the immune system after an exposure to an antigen or allergen.

**Anticholinergic.** Term used to describe drugs that counteract the cholinergic side of the nervous system.

**Antigen.** See allergen.

**Antihistamines.** A class of drugs which counteract histamine

**Aspirin disease.** The medical term used to describe the co-existence of nasal polyps, asthma and aspirin allergy. Also called Samter's Syndrome

**Autonomic Nervous System.** The part of the nervous system which regulates control of blood pressure, pulse rate and bronchial muscle tone.

381

**Beta-agonist.** The name given to the adrenaline-like bronchodilating drugs.

**Beta receptor.** The receptor in the nervous system which regulates the tone of the bronchial tubes.

**Bronchial tubes.** The tubes or airways that conduct air in and out of the lung.

**Bronchodilator.** A drug that dilates or relaxes the bronchial tubes.

**Bronchioles.** The smaller bronchial tubes which lead to the alveoli.

**Bronchiolitis.** An infection of the smaller bronchial tubes in infants caused by the RSV virus.

**Compliance.** The term used when a patient correctly follows medical instructions. Failure to follow instructions as directed is called non-compliance.

**COPD.** Abbreviation for chronic obstructive pulmonary diseases such as chronic bronchitis and emphysema.

**Cortisone.** Group of drugs or steroids derived from the adrenal gland used to control asthma and many other medical conditions.

**Carbon dioxide.** The waste gas of the body which is eliminated from our lungs when we exhale.

**Cystic fibrosis.** A severe lung disease of children which sometimes can be confused with asthma.

**Eosinophil.** The white blood cell which signals the presence of asthma or an ongoing allergic reaction.

**Eczema.** A skin disease associated with allergies and asthma.

**Epinephrine.** A drug used to treat acute allergy attacks or anaphylaxis, also called adrenaline.

**ETS.** Abbreviation for environmental tobacco smoke.

**FDA.** Abbreviation for the Food and Drug Administration.

**Fungi.** Plants that lack stems whose spores are capable of causing an allergic reaction.

**GERD.** Abbreviation for gastroesophageal reflux disease.

**HEPA Filter.** An effective air purifier. HEPA stands for high energy particulate air purifier.

**Hygiene hypothesis.** Theory that proposes that the asthma epidemic is due to being raised in too clean an environment.

**Immune system.** The body system made up of our bone marrow, thymus gland and lymph nodes which protects or gives you immunity against disease. An overactive system leads to the development of allergic conditions (asthma and hay fever) or allergic reactions to food and drugs.

**Immunoglobulins.** The antibodies produced by the immune system in response to exposure to allergens or any infectious agents like bacteria and viruses.

**Immunoglobulin E.** Also called IgE. This is the specific immuno-globulin or allergic antibody produced by the immune system which triggers allergic reactions.

**Immunotherapy.** Refers to the administration of antigens or allergens in the form of allergy shots. Also known as desensitization or hyposensitization.

**Leukotrienes.** Chemicals that can cause bronchospasm—that can be blocked by leukotriene-modifiers.

**Lymphocytes.** White blood cells program the immune system. The two most important groups of lymphocytes are the T-cells and B-cells.

**Mast cell.** A cell present throughout our body, especially in areas exposed to the outside environment. This cell contains dozens of potent chemicals which cause swelling and inflammation when they are released into the surrounding tissues.

**Mediators.** The chemicals released by the T-cells and mast cells.

**Metabolize.** To use up or eliminate from the body.

**Micron.** A unit of length equal to one-millionth of a meter.

**Mold.** See Fungi.

**Non-adherence.** See Compliance.

**OTC.** Abbreviation for non-prescription or over-the-counter drugs.

**Particulate matter.** Air particles arising from fossil fuel combustion, wood stoves and industrial smoke stacks.

**Placebo.** An inactive substance like salt water used in drug studies.

**Pollen.** Plant parts released by trees, grasses and weeds that can trigger allergic reactions.

**Prednisone.** The oral cortisone or steroid drug that doctors use to reduce inflammation in asthma.

**Prick test.** A skin test in which a drop of allergen is placed on the skin and then pricked with a needle.

**PRN.** Medical abbreviation for "take as needed."

**Pulmonologist.** A medical doctor who specializes in either pulmonary or lung diseases.

**RAST test.** A blood test that detects the presence of allergic antibodies in the bloodstream.

**Remodeling.** The term used to describe permanent lung damage in asthma.

**RSV.** The respiratory syncytial virus or RSV virus which causes bronchiolitis in young infants.

**Scratch test.** Skin test in which the skin is lightly scratched and a drop of the allergen is placed on the scratched area.

**Sensitization.** An allergic reaction due to repeated exposures to an allergen.

**Serum IgE test.** A blood test which measures how much IgE antibody you have in your system.

**Sweat test.** A test done to rule out cystic fibrosis.

**Sympathetic nervous system.** Part of the autonomic nervous system that controls blood pressure, heart rate and bronchial muscle tone.

**Trachea.** The airway connecting the mouth to the bronchial tubes.

# Index

## A

AAFA asthma plan in pregnancy, 310–312
Accolate, 196, 198
Acid reflux and asthma, 97
Acupuncture, 215, 221
Acute
    asthma, 330–331, 332–333
    respiratory failure, 333–334
Adolescent-onset asthma, 290–291
Adrenal glands
    function of, 176
    suppression of, 186–187
Adrenaline, as asthma treatment, 159, 160, 161–162
Adult-onset asthma, 315–316
Advair, 3, 164, 178
Aeroallergens, 27, 61, 62, 71, 99–100, 102–103, 123–124
    animals, 107–112
    cockroaches, 103, 104–105, 231–232
    dust mites, 100–103
    in fatal and near-fatal attacks, 339
    molds, 103, 106–107
    pollens, 112–114, 238–239
AeroBid, 178
Aerosols, 162, 163
Aesculapius, 48
African Americans, asthma in, 11, 34
Agricola, Georgius, 55–56
Air conditioners, 242–243
Air pollution

alerts, guidelines for, 122–123
asthma and, 118
controlling, 128–129, 240–242
diesel exhaust, 121
health effects of, 118
indoor, 120, 123–128
outdoor, 37, 117–123, 129–130
Air purifiers, 240–242
Air travel, risks of, 244–246
Airway remodeling. *See* Remodeling
Albuterol, 163, 279, 308, 332
Alcohol-induced asthma, 148–149
Allegra, 201
Allergic
    rhinitis, 13, 89–92, 102–104. *See also* Hay fever
    salute, 91, 152–153
    shiners, 91
Allergies
    animal, 36, 107–112, 235–238
    blood tests, 79–80, 224
    cockroach, 103, 104–105, 231–232
    controversial therapies, 223–225
    definition, 69
    ethnicity and, 34
    food, 131–151
    frequency of, 10–11, 13
    genetic patterns, 21, 34–35
    IgE antibodies and, 25, 26, 29
    latex, 114–115
    pollen, 112–114, 238–239
    risk factors, 33–34, 129–130

Atropa belladonna, 216
Atropine, 171
Atrovent. *See* Ipratropium bromide
Avicenna, 52, 131
Azathioprine, 205
Azelastine, 201–202
Azmacort. *See* triamcinolone

**B**
Bacteria exposure, 44–45
Barcelona asthma, 122
Barium swallow, 98
B-cells, 23, 28
BCG vaccine, 43–44
Beclomethasone, 177, 178
Beclovent. *See* Beclomethasone
Benadryl, 138, 139, 201
Bennich, J., 70
Beta-agonist drugs, 18, 160, 161–163
    albuterol, 163
    debate over, 165–168
    fenoterol, 166, 167
    formoterol, 3, 163, 164
    levalbuterol, 165
    metaproterenol, 162
    salmeterol, 3, 163, 164
    side effects, 163–164, 320
    theophylline, 18, 97, 160, 161, 168
Birth
    date and asthma, 37–38
    order and asthma, 43
Blackley, Charles, 62
Blood tests, 75–76, 79–80, 134. *See also*
        Laboratory tests, Tests
Bostok, John, 61
Boys, asthma in, 76, 290, 291
Breastfeeding and asthma, 312–313
Breathing
    technique therapy, 215
    tests, 76–77
Bronchial
    hyperreactivity, 19, 103
    tubes, 15, 16–17
Bronchiolitis, viral, 80, 154
Bronchitis, chronic, 81
Bronchodilators, 3, 5, 18, 159, 160,

161–171. *See also*
        Beta-agonist drugs
Bronchoprovocation testing, 70
Bronkaid Mist, 163
Budesonide, 3, 178, 179, 189, 308, 327

**C**
Cardano, Gerolamo, 54–55
Caretakers, role in managing asthma,
        293
Cat allergy, 108–112, 228, 237–238
    in children, 287
Cataracts, side effect of cortisone
        drugs, 193
Categories of asthma, 84
Cell-mediated immunity, 24–25
Celsus, Aulus, 49–50
Chest X-ray studies, 80, 81
Children. *See also* School asthma
        management programs
    allergies in, 13, 287
    anesthesia, effect of, 292
    antibiotics in, 44–46
    asthma in, 9, 10, 12, 13, 285–302
    conditions that mimic asthma in,
        80–81
    croup in, 292
    diagnostic procedures, 78, 80,
        288–289
    dust mite sensitivity in, 103
    eczema in, 92
    environmental tobacco smoke (ETS)
        and, 124
    exercise-induced anaphylaxis in,
        141–142
    food allergies in, 133, 134–135,
        139–140, 287
    growth patterns and cortisone
        therapy, 187–190
    IgE levels in, 75–76
    immunotherapy in, 4, 252, 255–256
    inhaled cortisone and, 19, 188–189
    lactobacillus in, 44–45
    long-term prognosis, 291–292
    respiratory syncytial virus (RSV) in,
        80, 152, 153–154

risk factors, 11, 34–40, 41, 43, 92–93,
103–105, 124–125, 287, 292
school absenteeism, 7, 12
sinus infections in, 94
skin testing of, 288–289
symptoms in, 8, 287–289
treatment of, 19–20, 175, 178, 180,
196, 326
vaccines in, 44
viral infections in, 152–155
wheezing in, 153, 285–286, 287
Chinese restaurant syndrome, 147–148
Chlamydia pneumoniae, 156
Chiropractic manipulation, 222–223
Chondroitin sulfate, 216
Chronic bronchitis, 81
Churg-Strauss Syndrome, 198
Cimetadine, 97
interaction with theophylline, 169
Claritin, 201
Clarithromycin, 156
Clinical ecologists, 225–226
Coal stoves, 127–128
Coca, A.F. and R. A. Cooke, 70
Cockroach allergy, 36, 103, 104–105,
231–232
College students, guidelines for, 302
Combivent, 171, 320
Common cold, and asthma, 151,
152–153
Controller drugs, 18, 159, 161, 173–183,
323
Control
of animal allergens, 235–238, 242
of cockroach allergen, 231–232
of dust mite exposure, 228–231, 242,
245
of indoor humidity levels, 239–240
of indoor pollution, 128–129
of mold allergens, 232–234, 245
of pollen exposure, 238–239
Cooke, R. A., 70
Cortisone drugs, 160, 161, 176–177,
179–180
and leukotriene modifiers, 196–197
effect on adrenal glands, 187

inhaled, 3, 5, 18, 177–178, 308, 325
oral, in motherhood, 309, 312
pediatric treatment with, 326–329
side effects, 176, 185–194, 202, 320
Couch potato theory, 38–40
Cough-variant asthma, 259–260
Cromolyn, 214
action of, 174
-like drugs, 18, 160, 161
sodium, 173–175, 279, 308, 326
spinhaler, 174
use with children, 175–176
Croup, risk factor for children, 292
Cullen, William 58–59
Cystic fibrosis, 81
Cytotoxic testing, 224

**D**
Dale, Henry, 67
Dehumidifiers, 243
Dendritic cells, 27
Dependent clinger patients, 352–353
Depression and asthma, 348, 351
Diagnosis
breathing tests, 76–77
lab tests, 75–76, 79–80
medical history in, 73–74
physical examination, 74–75
skin tests, 77–78
X-ray studies, 80
Diesel exhaust fumes, 121
Dietary therapy, 220
DNA, 20, 21
Dog allergy, 107–108, 235–237, 287–288
Drug interactions
in the elderly, 319–320
with aspirin, 264
Drug therapies
antibiotics, 202, 203
antifungals, 206–207
antihistimines, 201–202
anti-inflammatory, 18, 159, 161,
173–183, 323
bronchodilating, 3, 5, 18, 159, 160,
161–171
controlling, 18, 159, 161, 173–183, 323

Scuba diving and asthma, 282–284
Self-destructive denier patients,
     353–354
Serevent. *See* Salmeterol
Severe persistent asthma, 322
Sick building syndrome, 125–126
Side effects
     of antihistamines, 201–202
     of beta-agonist drugs, 163–164, 320
     of cortisone, 176, 185–194
     of herbs, 217–218
     of leukotriene modifiers, 197–198
     of theophylline drugs, 169–170, 320
Sighing syndrome, 82
Singulair, 196, 197, 279
Sinus disease
     and asthma, 94–95–96
     diagnosis of, 80, 95
     prevalence of, 93
     symptoms, 94
     treatment of, 95–96
Skin testing, 69, 77–78, 134–135
     of children, 288–289
     risks of, 253–254
Smoke, tobacco
     asthma and, 124–125
     by-products of, 120
     chronic bronchitis and, 81
     emphysema and, 81
     nitrogen dioxide and, 120
Sneeze, wheeze, itch (SWI) reaction,
     26–27
Social effects of asthma, 7–8, 12–13, 293
Spacers, 358–359
Specialist care, 75, 79, 83–88
Spinhaler, 174
Spirometry. *See* Pulmonary function
     studies
Sports and asthma, 270–271, 273–278,
     280–284
Sputum smear, 75
SRS-A, 71, 195
Stachybotrys mold, 234
Status asthmaticus, 333
Step-up therapy, versus step-down,
     324–325

Stethoscope
     invention of, 61
     use in physical exam, 75
Stoves
     gas, 120
     wood and coal, 120, 127–128
Stramonium, 51, 65, 66, 160, 171
Stress in asthma, 348–349
Substance P, 155
Sulfite reactions, 146–147
Sulfur dioxide, 120
Supply companies, asthma and allergy,
     379–380
Surgery
     childhood asthma and, 292
     cortisone therapy and, 187
     gastroesophageal reflux disease
          and, 97
     sinus disease and, 95
Sweat test, and cystic fibrosis, 75, 81
Symbicort, 3
Sympathetic nervous system, 161–162
Symptoms, asthma, 16–18, 73, 83,
     317–318, 322–323, 330–331
Systemic reactions to immunotherapy,
     253–254

**T**
Tacrolimus, 93
Tagamet. *See* cimetadine
TAO therapy, 202
T-cells, 24, 29
     Interaction with RSV, 155
Teacher's role in asthma management,
     296, 297
Tedral, 168
Terbutaline, 308, 327
Tests
     blood, 75–76, 79–80, 134
     breathing, 76–77
     laboratory, 74–75, 77–78, 318
     skin, 77–78, 134–135
Th cells, 29, 30–31
Thachrah, Charles Turner, 63
Theophylline drugs, 6, 18, 97, 160, 161,
     168–169, 214

**Order Form**
# *Asthma—An Emerging Epidemic*

**Order through your local bookstore or directly from Lighthouse Press**

I wish to order _____ copies of *Asthma—An Emerging Epidemic* for $24.95 each plus $3.95 shipping and handling for one book. Add $1.95 for each additional book.

Payment must accompany orders. Allow 3 weeks for delivery.

My check or money order for $_____ is enclosed.

*Make your check payable to Lighthouse Press and return to:*
Lighthouse Press
P.O. Box 602, Marblehead, MA 01945

Please charge my credit card
____ Visa     ____ MasterCard     ____ American Express

Name _____

Organization _____

Address _____

City/State/Country/Zip _____

Phone_____ E-mail_____

Signature_____

Credit Card #_____ Expiration Date_____

*To order via e-mail contact Lighthouse Press:*
LHTpress@aol.com

*For additional information or large discount orders:*
Tel: (800) 225-9886 • (978) 740-0648
Fax: (978) 745-6208 • (781) 631 2225

*Visit our Web sites:*
www.lighthousepress.org *or* www.asthmaepidemic.org